Palliative Care: A Practical Approach

Palliative Care: A Practical Approach

Editor: Lily Bowen

FOSTER ACADEMICS

www.fosteracademics.com

www.fosteracademics.com

FOSTER ACADEMICS

Cataloging-in-Publication Data

Palliative care : a practical approach / edited by Lily Bowen.
p. cm.
Includes bibliographical references and index.
ISBN 978-1-63242-854-7
1. Palliative treatment. 2. Care of the sick. 3. Medical care. I. Bowen, Lily.
R726.8 .P353 2019
616.029--dc21

Foster Academics,
118-35 Queens Blvd., Suite 400,
Forest Hills, NY 11375, USA

ISBN 978-1-63242-854-7 (Hardback)

Printed and bound in China.

Contents

Preface IX

Chapter 1 **Bereaved parents' experiences of research participation** 1
Ashleigh E. Butler, Helen Hall and Beverley Copnell

Chapter 2 **Using co-design to develop an intervention to improve communication about the heart failure trajectory and end-of-life care** 10
Lisa Hjelmfors, Anna Strömberg, Maria Friedrichsen, Anna Sandgren, Jan Mårtensson and Tiny Jaarsma

Chapter 3 **Comparing unplanned and potentially planned home deaths: a population-based** 20
Camilla Kjellstadli, Bettina Sandgathe Husebø, Hogne Sandvik, Elisabeth Flo and Steinar Hunskaar

Chapter 4 **Use of hospital palliative care according to the place of death and disease one year before death in 2013** 31
Claire Poulalhon, Laureen Rotelli-Bihet, Sébastien Moine, Anne Fagot-Campagna, Régis Aubry and Philippe Tuppin

Chapter 5 **The degree of social difficulties experienced by cancer patients and their spouses** 41
Takashi Takeuchi, Kanako Ichikura, Kanako Amano, Wakana Takeshita and Kazuho Hisamura

Chapter 6 **Adding a second surprise question triggers general practitioners to increase the thoroughness of palliative care planning: results of a pilot RCT with case vignettes** 50
F. Weijers, C. Veldhoven, C. Verhagen, K. Vissers and Y. Engels

Chapter 7 **"It doesn't exist…": negotiating palliative care from a culturally and linguistically diverse patient and caregiver perspective** 59
Emma Kirby, Zarnie Lwin, Katherine Kenny, Alex Broom, Holi Birman and Phillip Good

Chapter 8 **The availability and effectiveness of tools supporting shared decision making in metastatic breast cancer care** 69
Inge Spronk, Jako S. Burgers, François G. Schellevis, Liesbeth M. van Vliet and Joke C. Korevaar

Chapter 9 **Does special education in palliative medicine make a difference in end-of-life decision-making?** 77
Reetta P. Piili, Juho T. Lehto, Tiina Luukkaala, Heikki Hinkka and Pirkko-Liisa I. Kellokumpu-Lehtinen

Chapter 10 **Building Bridges, Paediatric Palliative Care in Belgium: A secondary data analysis of annual paediatric liaison team reports from 2010 to 2014** 88
Marie Friedel, Bénédicte Brichard, Christine Fonteyne, Marleen Renard, Jean-Paul Misson, Els Vandecruys, Corinne Tonon, Françoise Verfaillie, Georgette Hendrijckx, Nathalie Andersson, Ilse Ruysseveldt, Katrien Moens, Jean-Marie Degryse and Isabelle Aujoulat

Chapter 11 **Access to palliative care for homeless people: complex lives, complex care** 99
Anke J E de Veer, Barbara Stringer, Berno van Meijel, Renate Verkaik and Anneke L Francke

Chapter 12 **Experiences and challenges of home care nurses and general practitioners in home-based palliative care** 110
Britt Viola Danielsen, Anne Marit Sand, Jan Henrik Rosland and Oddvar Førland

Chapter 13 **Feasibility, acceptability and adaption of dignity therapy: a mixed methods study achieving 360° feedback** 123
Sandra Stephanie Mai, Swantje Goebel, Elisabeth Jentschke, Birgitt van Oorschot, Karl-Heinz Renner and Martin Weber

Chapter 14 **Palliative care for patients with cancer: do patients receive the care they consider important?** 133
Marianne Heins, Jolien Hofstede, Mieke Rijken, Joke Korevaar, Gé Donker and Anneke Francke

Chapter 15 **Chemotherapy and palliative care near end-of life: examining the appropriateness at a cancer institute for colorectal cancer patients** 140
Ilaria Massa, Oriana Nanni, Flavia Foca, Marco Maltoni, Stefania Derni, Nicola Gentili, Giovanni Luca Frassineti, Andrea Casadei Gardini, Martina Valgiusti, Dino Amadori, Elena Prati, Mattia Altini, Davide Gallegati and Elisabetta Sansoni

Chapter 16 **Exploring the meaning and practice of self-care among palliative care nurses and doctors** 147
Jason Mills, Timothy Wand and Jennifer A. Fraser

Chapter 17 **Negative pain management index scores do not necessarily indicate inadequate pain management** 159
Naoki Sakakibara, Takahiro Higashi, Itsuku Yamashita, Tetsusuke Yoshimoto and Motohiro Matoba

Chapter 18 **A public health approach to palliative care in the response to drug resistant TB: an ethnographic study** 166
Joseph M. Sawyer, Rahul Asgr, Florence N. Todd Fordham and John D. H. Porter

Chapter 19 **Allow natural death versus do-not-resuscitate: titles, information contents, outcomes, and the considerations related to do-not-resuscitate decision** 177
Sheng-Yu Fan, Ying-Wei Wang and I-Mei Lin

Chapter 20 **First year experiences with a palliative out-patients structure for patients with COPD: a qualitative study of health professionals' expectations and experiences** **184**
Dorthe Gaby Bove, Marie Lavesen, Maria Omel Jellington, Kristoffer Bastrup-Madsen Marsaa and Suzanne Forsyth Herling

Chapter 21 **The experience of caring for patients at the end-of-life stage in non-palliative care settings** **194**
Xiao Bin Lai, Frances Kam Yuet Wong and Shirley Siu Yin Ching

Chapter 22 **Intranasal fentanyl for respiratory distress in children and adolescents with life-limiting conditions** **205**
Lucas Pieper, Julia Wager and Boris Zernikow

Chapter 23 **Addressing the needs of terminally-ill patients in Bosnia-Herzegovina: patients' perceptions and expectations** **213**
S. Aebischer Perone, R. Nikolic, R. Lazic, E. Dropic, T. Vogel, B. Lab, S. Lachat, P. Hudelson, C. Matis, S. Pautex and F. Chappuis

Chapter 24 **Attitudes to specialist palliative care and advance care planning in people with COPD: a multi-national survey of palliative and respiratory medicine specialists** **222**
Natasha Smallwood, David Currow, Sara Booth, Anna Spathis, Louis Irving and Jennifer Philip

Chapter 25 **Benchmarking time to initiation of end-of- Life homecare nursing: a population-based cancer cohort study in regions across Canada** **230**
Hsien Seow, Danial Qureshi, Lisa Barbera, Kim McGrail, Beverley Lawson, Fred Burge and Rinku Sutradhar

Permissions

List of Contributors

Index

Preface

This book has been an outcome of determined endeavour from a group of educationists in the field. The primary objective was to involve a broad spectrum of professionals from diverse cultural background involved in the field for developing new researches. The book not only targets students but also scholars pursuing higher research for further enhancement of the theoretical and practical applications of the subject.

Palliative care refers to the medical and nursing care meant for people struggling with life-limiting illnesses. It aims at controlling symptoms, reducing pain and providing relief in physical and mental stress at any stage of illness. It focuses on improving the quality of life for the patient as well as their family. The health professionals commonly involved in a palliative care team include nurses, physicians, occupational therapists, physiotherapists and speech-language pathologists. Edmonton Symptoms Assessment Scale (ESAS) is a common method used to assess the symptoms of the patients receiving palliative care. The book studies, analyzes and upholds the pillars of palliative care and its utmost significance in modern times. It aims to shed light on some of the unexplored aspects of palliative care and the recent researches in the subject. This book includes contributions of experts and researchers, which will provide innovative insights into this field.

It was an honour to edit such a profound book and also a challenging task to compile and examine all the relevant data for accuracy and originality. I wish to acknowledge the efforts of the contributors for submitting such brilliant and diverse chapters in the field and for endlessly working for the completion of the book. Last, but not the least; I thank my family for being a constant source of support in all my research endeavours.

Editor

1

Bereaved parents' experiences of research participation

Ashleigh E. Butler[1,2*], Helen Hall[2] and Beverley Copnell[3]

Abstract

Background: As understandings of the impacts of end-of-life experiences on parents' grief and bereavement increase, so too does the inclusion of bereaved parents into research studies exploring these experiences. However, designing and obtaining approval for these studies can be difficult, as guidance derived from bereaved parents' experiences of the research process are limited within the current literature.

Methods: We aimed to explore bereaved parents' experiences of research participation in a larger grounded theory study exploring experiences of the death of a child in the paediatric intensive care unit. Data were obtained during follow-up phone calls made to 19 bereaved parents, five of whom provided data from their spouse, 1 week after their participation in the study. Participants were asked to reflect on their experiences of research participation, with a focus on recruitment methods, timing of research contact, and the location of their interview. Parents' responses were analysed using descriptive content analysis.

Results: Our findings demonstrate that despite being emotionally difficult, parents' overall experiences of research participation were positive. Parents preferred to be contacted initially via a letter, with an opt in approach viewed most favourably. Most commonly, participants preferred that research contact occurred within 12–24 months after their child's death, with some suggesting contact after 6 months was also appropriate. Parents also preferred research interviews conducted in their own homes, though flexibility and parental choice was crucial.

Conclusions: Findings from this study offer further insight to researchers and research review committees, to help ensure that future studies are conducted in a way that best meets the unique needs of bereaved parents participating in research.

Keywords: Research, Bereavement, Parent, Child, Death, Experience

Background

Over the past few decades, research has begun to highlight the impacts of the end-of-life care experience on parental grief, bereavement, and coping [1–7]. Consequently, in order to gain insights into their experiences of end-of-life care across a variety of locations and healthcare climates, the rates of inclusion of bereaved parents in research studies has also risen. However, despite studies which demonstrate participation in research studies is usually not harmful for bereaved parents [8–13], anecdotal evidence suggests that designing and obtaining approval for such sensitive research projects can be challenging.

Ongoing assumptions that bereaved parents are especially vulnerable and need to be protected from the perceived 'harms' or 'risks' of research may cause research review committees to be more hesitant in approving bereavement research [8–10, 13]. The research review committee's role in assessing bereavement research can be challenging, as there is little empirical evidence to guide them in the 'best' way that these studies should be conducted. To date, the voices and opinions of bereaved parents on how to conduct bereavement research have largely been absent from the literature, with only a very limited number of studies published [8, 9, 11–13]. Many of these studies have attempted to provide guidance on important considerations when including bereaved parents into research studies, such as

* Correspondence: Ashleigh.butler@ucl.ac.uk
[1]The Louis Dundas Centre for Children's Palliative Care, University College London Great Ormond Street Institute of Child Health, London, UK
[2]School of Nursing and Midwifery, Monash University, Melbourne, Australia
Full list of author information is available at the end of the article

preferred contact methods; however such guidance is typically provided as vague, non-specific recommendations. More specific guidance around recruitment methods, contact timeframes, and data collection locations, based on the opinions of bereaved parents themselves, is urgently needed to assist both researchers and research review committees in moving forwards in bereavement research. We aim to address this gap by specifically exploring bereaved parents' opinions of the research process, covering their experiences of being recruited into a bereavement study, the timeframe between their child's death and their participation, and the location of their research interview. By specifically exploring these three key areas of research participation, we hope to provide concrete guidance for both bereavement researchers and research review committees, so that future studies may best meet the needs and preferences of bereaved parents and facilitate their ongoing inclusion into paediatric end-of-life care research.

Methods

Study design

The Bereaved Paediatric Intensive Care Unit (PICU) Parent Study explored bereaved parents' experiences of the death of their child in the PICU, and their subsequent follow-up care [14]. In order to check on the wellbeing of participants, follow-up phone calls were undertaken by the research team 1 week after their interview, with parents asked to reflect on their experiences of research participation.

Setting and participants

Twenty-six bereaved parents from 18 families took part in The Bereaved PICU Parent Study. Parents were recruited using purposive and theoretical sampling from four Australian PICUs by social workers involved in routine bereavement follow-up or via mailed letters 6–48 months after their child's death in 2015–2016. For the primary study they took part in audio-recorded, semi-structured interviews at a time and location of their choice, conducted by the first author, a PICU nurse with prior qualitative research experience who was unknown to the participants. Participants were also advised that they would be called by a member of the research team within 1 week of their interview to ensure their wellbeing and to discuss their experiences of participating in the study.

Research process

Parents' reflections on their participation in bereavement research and the research process were collected during follow-up phone calls, lasting approximately 15–30 min. Parents were contacted 1 week after their interview by A.B, primarily to check on their wellbeing. During these phone calls, we asked six open-ended questions to explore their experiences of the research process, as outlined in Table 1. Parents' responses were recorded verbatim in writing by the interviewer and checked with parents during the phone call.

Data analysis

Data from the follow-up interviews were subjected to descriptive content analysis, informed by the processes described by S Elo, et al. [15]. Content analysis is used to explore common issues and experiences within a set of data from both a qualitative and quantitative perspective [15, 16]. It involves establishing categories which describe the data, and identifying the frequency with which they occur, proving both a qualitative overview of the key concerns for participants and an indication of how commonly they occurred [17].

Data analysis was primarily undertaken by the first author, in consultation with the research team. The 'preparation' phase of content analysis commenced by identifying each individual question within the follow-up interview as the units of analysis, and re-reading the data multiple times to facilitate familiarity. During the 'organising' phase, open coding was undertaken, with common codes within each question grouped into categories. Where possible, these categories were further grouped based on similarities, which allowed key concepts in each question to be described and explored. Frequencies of each code and category were also identified at this stage, and analysed using descriptive statistics.

Ethics

This study was reviewed and approved by four human research ethics committees. Written informed consent was provided by all participants prior to their interview, with verbal consent reconfirmed at the commencement of each follow-up phone call. Participants were encouraged to rely on personal coping strategies during and after their interviews, with breaks from the interview process utilised as required. Social workers associated with the study were also available for follow-up care of participants if ongoing distress was noted during the interviews or follow-up calls. In order to protect

Table 1 Follow-up interview questions

1. How did you feel in the hours and days after your interview?
2. Could you tell me a little bit about why you preferred to do the interview at home/over the phone/at the university?
3. When we first contacted you about this study, it had been xx months/years since [insert child's name] had died. Did you feel this was appropriate, or would there have been a better timeframe for us to contact you?
4. You were initially contacted through a letter from the research team/ a letter from the hospital/your bereavement social worker. How did you find this process?
5. Was there anything about the letter that you received that you liked or didn't like?
6. How did you find participating in this research study overall?

participants' privacy, all data have been de-identified, and pseudonyms are used for all participants and their children.

Results

Twenty-four out of the 26 participants in The Bereaved PICU Parent Study provided data on their experiences of research participation during follow-up phone calls. Direct follow-up was undertaken with 19 parents, five of whom also provided comments from their spouse. Two parents had mentioned they may be unavailable for further contact after their interview, and were subsequently lost to follow-up. Characteristics of all participants and their children are provided in Table 2. During follow-up phone calls, parents were asked how they felt after participating in their interviews, and were asked to reflect on the timing between their child's death and researcher contact, the method of contact and the location of their interview.

The timing of research contact

Initially, we contacted parents 6–18 months after the child's death in the PICU. This time frame was chosen to avoid early intense grief, and to minimise the impacts of memory and recall bias on data collection. However, due to lower than anticipated recruitment within this timeframe, we extended an invitation to all bereaved parents up to 48 months after their child's death.

At participation, most families were 12–24 months into their bereavement (See Table 2). This was also the most commonly preferred timeframe for research contact, both for parents contacted at 12–24 months and for four parents who were contacted later in their bereavement (See Table 3). Parents suggested that this timeframe ensured that they still remembered what happened, how they felt, and what they needed very clearly. Many parents also noted that talking about their experiences would always hurt, but felt that at 12 months, enough time had passed that the interview was not significantly painful for them.

Table 2 Characteristics of participants and their children

Direct follow up	Child's name	Child's age	Cause of death	Illness type	Time since death
Layla	Lucas	Infant	Neurological injury	Chronic	7 months
Daniel	Olivia	Teenager	Metabolic condition	Chronic	8 months
Lucy	William	Toddler	Septic shock	Acute	1 year, 1 month
Alice	James	Toddler	Accident	Acute	1 year, 2 months
Emma	Charlotte	Infant	Sudden Infant Death Syndrome	Acute	1 year, 4 months
Evelyn	Henry	Infant	Congenital heart disease	Chronic	1 year, 6 months
Jasmine	Mason	Infant	Metabolic condition/Liver failure	Acute	1 year, 6 months
Zara	Noah	Teenager	Multi-organ dysfunction	Acute	1 year, 8 months
Abigail	Amelia	Infant	Congenital heart disease	Chronic	1 year, 10 months
Sarah & Connor	Sophie	Infant	Sudden Infant Death Syndrome	Acute	2 years
Isabelle	Ava	Teenager	Cardiac arrest	Acute	2 years, 10 month
Vicki & Nate	Emily	Infant	Sudden Infant Death Syndrome	Acute	2 years, 10 month
Piper & Edward	Ethan	Teenager	Neurological injury	Chronic	3 years
Charlie	Liam	Infant	Liver failure	Acute	3 years
Erin	Ruby	Toddler	Congenital heart disease	Chronic	3 years, 6 months
Eva	Thomas	Teenager	Anaphylaxis	Acute	3 years, 8 months
Comments relayed by spouse					
Hannah	Olivia	Teenager	Metabolic condition	Chronic	8 months
Hudson	William	Toddler	Septic shock	Acute	1 year, 1 month
Joshua	Henry	Infant	Congenital heart disease	Chronic	1 year, 6 months
Ryan	Noah	Teenager	Multi-organ dysfunction	Acute	1 year, 8 months
Zoe	Liam	Infant	Liver failure	Acute	3 years
Lost to follow up					
Jessica	Ella	Infant	Congenital heart disease	Chronic	2 years, 6 months
Imogen	Chloe	Toddler	Multi-organ dysfunction / Septic shock	Acute	4 years

Table 3 Actual and preferred research contact timeframes

Direct follow up	Contacted at:	Contact preference:
Layla	7 months	Prior to 12 months
Daniel & Hannah	8 months	Prior to 12 months
Lucy & Hudson	1 year, 1 month	12–24 months
Alice	1 year, 2 months	12–24 months
Emma	1 year, 4 months	12–24 months
Evelyn & Joshua	1 year, 6 months	12–24 months
Jasmine	1 year, 6 months	12–24 months
Zara & Ryan	1 year, 8 months	Prior to 12 months
Abigail	1 year, 10 months	12–24 months
Sarah & Connor	2 years	Around 12 months
Isabelle	2 years, 10 months	Around 12 months
Vicki & Nate	2 years, 10 months	2–3 years
Piper & Edward	3 years	3–4 years
Charlie & Zoe	3 years	No opinion
Erin	3 years, 6 months	3–4 years
Eva	3 years, 8 months	12–24 months

Though five parents specifically suggested avoiding contact within the first 12 months as "the pain might be too fresh" (Erin), this opinion was not shared by parents who actually took part before the 12-month anniversary of their child's death (Layla, Hannah, and Daniel). These three parents all felt that waiting longer than 12 months may have impacted their ability to remember exactly how they felt and what they needed, and felt that talking about their experiences helped them realise what they currently wanted and needed for support, as none of these parents had received follow-up care from the hospital or other bereavement services. In addition, one couple (Zara and Ryan) who participated at 18 months also mentioned they would have preferred to be contacted before 12 months, as the interview offered them a chance to debrief after their child's death that they had otherwise not received, as no follow-up care was provided for them.

For the 9 parents who took part more than 2 years after their child's death, four parents felt this timeframe was "okay" (Eva) but would have preferred to take part earlier in their bereavement because they felt they would have remembered their experiences more clearly. The remaining parents were happy with the contact time frame, suggesting that it provided sufficient time to work through any issues they had experienced. Erin also suggested that opportunities to discuss her child with family and friends lessened over time, and noted that the interview offered a forum to talk about her child when there was otherwise "no space to talk about [her]" in daily life.

The method of research contact

Due to differences in local site requirements, we used three methods to invite potential participants into the study. At hospital 1, we were able to obtain contact information for eligible families and send an invitation letter directly from the research team. Hospitals 2 and 3 requested that social workers approach eligible families to obtain permission for research letters to be sent from the research team. Invitation letters at Hospital 4 were sent from a hospital based research nurse on behalf of the research team, with an enclosed 'consent to contact' card for interested parents to return. All mailed letters were then followed up with a phone call 2 weeks later. Further detail of our recruitment procedures has been published elsewhere [18].

Overall, 17 out of the 19 parents who provided direct comments felt that letters were an appropriate form of initial contact with bereaved families, regardless of whether the letter came directly from the research team or from another hospital staff member. Only 1 parent suggested a phone call would have been preferred as the initial contact method (Layla), and one parent did not share an opinion. Parents commented that a letter was a sensitive way to invite them into research participation, as it gave them time to consider the research project and make an appropriate decision, rather than being "put on the spot" (Connor). Many parents also felt a 'cold-call', or an unsolicited phone call from a research team member, would be an invasion of privacy and would be too shocking to enable them to consider what was being asked. Three parents from hospital 4 did mention they were confused by the arrival of a letter from the hospital, particularly in the absence of any previous contact, and noted it was helpful to have the name of the researcher and the research study on the back of the envelope. Many parents from hospital 4 also commented favourably on the use of an 'opt-in' card they could fill in and return if they were interested in the study; they suggested that this method of contact left the decision to participate entirely up to them without any pressure from the research team or hospital, and required no effort if they did not want to take part.

Four out of five parents who were initially approached by social workers also provided comments during follow-up phone calls. These parents all felt that contact through social workers was appropriate, but noted that this was only because they already had ongoing personal relationships with the social work team through routine bereavement follow-up. A follow-up letter and phone call from the research team was still desired, as it gave parents time to recall what the social worker had mentioned during the initial phone call, think of questions for the research team, and make a decision.

The location of the interview

Parents in our study were encouraged to choose an interview type (face to face or phone) and location that was comfortable and convenient for them. The vast majority of parents (20 parents from 12 families) preferred face to face interviews in their own homes. Parents commented that discussing their child's death was easier in their own home environment as it provided comfort, reduced feelings of vulnerability, and offered sufficient privacy for emotional expression. In addition, the home environment contained positive memories of the deceased child; for some parents, these memories provided comfort, whilst others felt more able to share their child's life with the interviewer. For these reasons, the family home was often considered a "safe place" (Edward). In contrast, nine parents specifically mentioned that returning to the hospital for interviews would be too difficult, as that was "where it [the child's death] happened" (Edward). In addition, parents commented that returning to the hospital added many logistical challenges to an already difficult task, such as locating and paying for parking, and having to drive home afterwards.

Only one parent (Emma) chose to do a face to face interview in a location other than her home. At her request, Emma's interview was conducted in a private office in one of the university buildings. At the time of her interview, Emma was living in shared accommodation, and did not feel her home offered adequate privacy. However, Emma was also uncomfortable returning to the hospital, and noted she would not have participated in the study if the only alternative location for her interview was at the hospital, reinforcing the need for flexibility in interview locations.

Five parents preferred to participate in phone interviews. All three of the parents who were followed up noted that it would have been "too hard to meet face-to-face" (Eva). These parents commented that they would have either felt uncomfortable expressing their emotions in the presence of a stranger, or felt that they would have been more emotional talking about their experiences face-to-face than over the phone. One mother appreciated that there were options and that she could choose what suited her best, stating that if the only option was a face-to-face interview, she would not have taken part because she felt it would have been too difficult to talk about her experiences in person.

Overall experiences of research participation

Although comments such as 'It was difficult' and 'it was painful to talk about' were common, all 24 of the parents who provided feedback on their research experiences mentioned that they were pleased and thankful to have taken part. They saw having a forum to talk about their child as a benefit; Erin said "It was good to talk. I haven't told the story in a long time", while Layla expressed gratitude to the researchers: "Thank you for listening and taking the time to know his story." Importantly, none of the parents who participated expressed any regret over taking part, nor any concerns about their experience. Instead, many commented that they had "got a lot out of it [the research interview]" (Charlie).

Overall, half of the parents who were followed-up mentioned that they experienced increased fatigue, and increased episodes of crying, numbness, or heightened emotional distress in the 24–48 h after their interviews. However, the parents did not view these emotions negatively; instead, most commented that the interview provided a sense of emotional release that allowed them to "get [things] off your chest" (Charlie) or "take the weight off your shoulders" (Zara). Evelyn said "It really hit home ... but it was a good release" while Alice commented "I cried, but I'm not too upset. Overall, it's a positive experience." Many suggested that despite the difficulties, it was "better to talk about it" (Eva) and remember their experiences, both positive and negative. Three couples suggested that the interview provided a space for them to talk about their experiences together for the first time, whilst another mother appreciated the opportunity to have a conversation entirely focused on her child, suggesting that research participation may be highly valued by bereaved parents. This is supported by the fact that not all parents in our study noted significant emotional distress after their interviews. Twelve parents commented that they felt okay or even 'good' after their participation, suggesting that perceptions of bereaved parents as especially 'vulnerable' to emotional distress might not be accurate.

Finally, many bereaved parents shared their motivations for participation in the research study. For most, the desire to help others and improve the experiences of families in the future was the main influencing factor in their decision to take part. Some parents, like Evelyn, felt like they were "flying blind" in the PICU, with no idea of what would happen during or after the death, and no support available to them. As a result, many wanted to take part in the research study because "if some of the systems can change because of Henry and because of what we put into this research, all the better for it" (Evelyn). For some parents, participation in research also allowed them to keep their child's memory alive, "connect[ing] us with our child" (Charlie) or "acknowledg[ing] her life" (Erin), or create something positive from what had often been an otherwise traumatic experience.

Discussion

Despite a vast number of studies demonstrating that bereaved persons, particularly bereaved parents, find value in participating in research studies and talking about their experiences [8–13, 19], little is known about their experiences of the research process itself. Without this information, it is difficult to design recruitment strategies and identify appropriate locations for data collection that best facilitate the inclusion of bereaved families into research studies. As part of routine follow-up after participation in a bereavement study, we explored parental experiences of the research process, in order to shed light on their preferred recruitment timeframes, contact methods, and locations for data collection.

The majority of bereaved parents in our study felt that the most appropriate timeframe to contact them regarding research participation was 12–24 months after their child's death, with five parents preferring contact from 6 months. In previous studies, researchers have attempted contact somewhere between 6 months to 4 years after death [9, 20–30], but there is little empirical research to support these decisions. Studies of parental grief trajectories indicate that the passage of time is only one factor in a complex process [6, 13, 31–33], and thus there may be no time period that is universally appropriate. Respecting parents' autonomy by giving them the opportunity to participate if they wish to do so may be more important than attempting to find a timeframe that will be least painful [13]. Parents in our study also supported the timeframe of 12–18 months as being optimal for recall. This presents a very narrow window for researchers that, as in our study, may be impractical. Researchers may need to balance parental preferences with pragmatic considerations. Though more research exploring bereaved parents' preferred research contact timeframes is urgently needed, we suggest researchers consider approaching families 6 months- 2 years after a child's death.

It is important to note that none of the parents in our study who expressed a wish for research participation prior to 12 months after their child's death received any follow-up care from the hospital or other bereavement services. It is possible that their views are reflective of a desire for follow up care [34], rather than actual research participation. This presents a potential ethical dilemma for researchers, who could be seen as exploiting parents' vulnerability. Though we recommend that parents still be given an opportunity to participate in research at this stage, heightened caution may be required. In addition, whilst research participation may be therapeutic for families, it cannot replace appropriate bereavement support, which should be provided by the child's hospital or by local bereavement services [34–36]. It is important that researchers do not attempt to assume a counselling role.

During follow-up phone calls, we also asked the bereaved parents to comment on the way they were initially contacted for research participation and whether they would have preferred a different contact method. Consistent with previous studies of bereaved parents [9, 10] and bereaved adults more generally [19], parents in this study typically preferred that initial contact be undertaken via a mailed letter, rather than from an unexpected phone call. This was particularly true for letters that utilised an 'opt-in' approach, which placed parents in control of any further contact with the research team. Bereaved adults have also shown a preference for initial research contact through hospital personnel [19], though our experiences have suggested that this preference largely depends on a positive ongoing or pre-existing relationship with the staff member making contact. As such, we suggest that initial research contact with bereaved parents occur via a mailed letter that includes a reply-paid 'opt-in' card (with the study name on the outside to provide some warning), which both promotes parental autonomy and minimises intrusion and distress as much as possible.

Consideration of the location of research interviews is also particularly important when conducting bereavement research. Many parents in our study expressed a strong aversion to returning to the hospital, citing an association with negative memories and heightened distress. Instead, bereaved parents strongly preferred to be interviewed in their own homes. This location typically provided appropriate privacy and comfort, was noted to be a "safe place" for parents, and minimised parental inconvenience. The preference for interviews in the family home is not unique to our study, and has also been expressed by bereaved parents and siblings in previous studies [9, 10, 12]. However, five parents in our study preferred to do their interviews over the phone and did not find this format caused additional distress, and one parent preferred to be interviewed at the university, demonstrating the importance of providing parents with choices over where their interview takes place. As such, we strongly recommend that flexibility is ingrained into the research protocol, with bereaved family members offered various options for where or how their interview takes place, including in their own homes, to ensure they feel as comfortable as possible.

Within the current literature, it is becoming increasingly apparent that though bereaved parents find research participation emotionally painful, they still describe it as a positive experience and are thankful to have taken part [8–10, 12]. Our findings add weight to this concept, further demonstrating the importance of facilitating the inclusion of bereaved parents into research studies. For most parents, including those in this study, research participation provides a valuable opportunity to talk about their child that can often be missing in their daily lives, helps preserve their bond with their child by keeping their memory alive, and may help them to feel their child's life and death had meaning and would be helpful to other families in the future [8–10, 12, 13, 37]. These findings also offer valuable insights into societal views of childhood death and longer-term parental bereavement. The fact that less-recently bereaved parents value research participation as a place to talk about their child that they do not have in daily life suggests a societal expectation to 'move on' from grief and, in a sense, act as though the deceased child did not exist [37]. However, research demonstrates that bereaved parents never 'get over' their child's death, and want to continue to incorporate their deceased child into their lives and talk about them no matter how much time has passed [38, 39]. Though a detailed discussion on ways to change societal perceptions of 'acceptable' parental bereavement is beyond the scope of this article, it is important for bereavement researchers to publicise these findings to the public as well as the academic community, in order to begin to 'normalise' parental bereavement experiences and needs.

Whilst including parents in bereavement research may provide some therapeutic benefits, it is also important that they are fully aware of all potential risks before deciding to take part. Aside from emotional distress during the interview, over half of the parents in our study reported ongoing heightened emotions and fatigue in the days following their interview. Though post-interview fatigue is briefly mentioned by both K Dyregrov [9] and JL Buckle, et al. [8], it has not been extensively discussed within the literature, nor noted as a consideration for bereavement research planning. Therefore, in addition to the likelihood of ongoing emotional distress, we suggest that the likelihood of increased fatigue in the 24–48 h following research participation be made explicit on participant information sheets. This way, bereaved parents are able to make informed decisions about research participation, and are empowered to schedule interviews so that they do not cause significant disruption to their lives.

Strengths and limitations

Our study was strengthened by the inclusion of both mothers and fathers from four different hospitals, whose children suffered from a variety of acute and chronic illnesses and injuries, and who experienced varied follow-up care, increasing the transferability of our findings. Findings are also reported according to the Consolidated Criteria for Reporting Qualitative Research [40]. However, there are some limitations to our study.

Firstly, the opinions of bereaved parents provided are only from those who had agreed to participate in the study, and who may have been more inclined to view bereavement research favourably. The views of parents who had chosen not to take part are unknown, and as such it is unclear whether some aspect of the recruitment process or contact timeframe influenced their decision not to participate. Where possible, we did attempt to enquire about the reason for their decision not to take part. Though responses were limited, most parents cited a lack of time or the desire to 'move on' as the primary reason for not taking part, rather than any specific concerns about recruitment timing or methods.

The findings were also limited by the fact that not all parents were able to be followed up directly. Two parents were lost to follow up, and five parents had comments relayed by their spouses. It is possible that these parents had negative comments that were not expressed to the research team, or were misrepresented by their spouses. However, the comments provided were consistent with the broader comments offered and offer valuable insights into the parents' experiences.

Finally, participant feedback during follow-up phone calls was solicited by the same researcher who met with the parents and undertook the research interviews. Some parents may not have felt comfortable expressing negative or critical opinions of the research process to someone they had already met, which may have led to a higher incidence of positive feedback. However, similarly to the findings of J Hynson, et al. [10], a significant number of participants also spontaneously expressed positive feedback on the research process during or after their recruitment or interview participation, which suggests that our method of soliciting feedback was not a major limitation to the trustworthiness of the findings. In future studies, it may be beneficial to adopt alternative methods of seeking feedback about the research process, such as a survey or through a non-interviewing member of the research team, to ensure parents feel free to express both positive and negative feedback without fear of offending the interviewer.

Conclusion

Despite ongoing research demonstrating that bereaved parents may find research participation beneficial rather than harmful, it can be difficult to design and gain approval for such emotionally laden studies. In part, this difficulty is caused by a lack of empirical evidence that explores how and when to approach bereaved parents in a way that promotes autonomy and safety whilst minimising harm and distress. Though further research is needed, our findings begin to offer suggestions for appropriate research contact timeframes, contact methods, and interview locations. These suggestions can help researchers design studies which empower bereaved parents, and assist research review committees in evaluating research proposals to facilitate the ongoing inclusion of bereaved parents into studies which are best suited to their needs.

Abbreviation

PICU: Paediatric Intensive Care Unit

Acknowledgements

Nil.

Funding
This work was supported by the Australian College of Critical Care Nurses [Novice Researcher Grant]; and the Australian College of Children and Young People's Nurses [Sister Mary Dorothea Sheehan Scholarship]. A. Butler was supported by an Australian Government Research Training Program Scholarship.

Authors' contributions
All authors made substantial contributions to conception and design, or acquisition of data, or analysis and interpretation of data; were involved in drafting the manuscript or revising it critically for important intellectual content; gave final approval of the version to be published; and have agreed to be accountable for all aspects of the work in ensuring that questions related to the accuracy or integrity of any part of the work are appropriately investigated and resolved.

Competing interests
The authors declare that they have no competing interests.

Author details
[1]The Louis Dundas Centre for Children's Palliative Care, University College London Great Ormond Street Institute of Child Health, London, UK. [2]School of Nursing and Midwifery, Monash University, Melbourne, Australia. [3]School of Nursing and Midwifery, La Trobe University, Melbourne, Australia.

References
1. Butler AE, Hall H, Copnell B. Bereaved parents' experiences of the police in the paediatric intensive care unit. Aust Crit Care. 2018. https://doi.org/10.1016/j.aucc.2018.02.004.
2. Butler AE, Hall H, Willetts G, Copnell B. Parents' experiences of healthcare provider actions when their child dies: an integrative review of the literature. J Spec Pediatr Nurs. 2015. https://doi.org/10.1111/jspn.12097.
3. Contro N, Larson J, Scofield S, Sourkes B, Cohen H. Family perspectives on the quality of pediatric palliative care. Arch Pediatr Adolesc Med. 2002;156:14–9.
4. Gold KJ. Navigating care after a baby dies: a systematic review of parent experiences with health providers. J Perinatol. 2007;27:230.
5. McCarthy MC, Clarke NE, Ting CL, Conroy R, Anderson VA, Heath JA. Prevalence and predictors of parental grief and depression after the death of a child from cancer. J Palliat Med. 2010. https://doi.org/10.1089/jpm.2010.0037.
6. Meert KL, Thurston CS, Thomas R. Parental coping and bereavement outcome after the death of a child in the pediatric intensive care unit. Pediatr Crit Care Med. 2001;2:324–8.
7. van der Geest IM, Darlington AS, Streng IC, Michiels EM, Pieters R. Van den Heuvel-Eibrink MM. Parents' experiences of pediatric palliative care and the impact on long-term parental grief. J Pain Symptom Manag. 2014. https://doi.org/10.1016/j.jpainsymman.2013.07.007.
8. Buckle JL, Dwyer SC, Jackson M. Qualitative bereavement research: incongruity between the perspectives of participants and research ethics boards. Int J Soc Res Methodo. 2010;13:111–25.
9. Dyregrov K. Bereaved parents' experience of research participation. Social Sci Med. 2004;58:391–400.
10. Hynson J, Aroni R, Bauld C, Sawyer S. Research with bereaved parents: a question of how not why. Palliat Med. 2006. https://doi.org/10.1177/0269216306072349.
11. Scott DA, Valery PC, Boyle FM, Bain CJ. Does research into sensitive areas do harm? Experiences of research participation after a child's diagnosis with Ewing's sarcoma. Med J Aust. 2002;177:507–11.
12. Steele AC, Kaal J, Thompson AL, Barrera M, Compas BE, Davies B, Fairclough DL, Foster TL, Gilmer MJ, Hogan N. Bereaved parents and siblings offer advice to healthcare providers and researchers. J Pediatr Hematol Oncol. 2013;35:253.
13. Schafer C, Scarth B. Resilient vulnerabilities: bereaved persons discuss their experience of participating in thanatology research. In: Tolich M, editor. *Qualitative ethics in practice* edn. London: Routledge; 2016. p. 85–95.
14. Butler AE, Hall H, Copnell B. The changing nature of the relationships between parents and healthcare providers when a child dies in the paediatric intensive care unit. J Adv Nurs. 2018. https://doi.org/10.1111/jan.13401.
15. Elo S, Kyngäs H. The qualitative content analysis process. J Adv Nurs. 2008. https://doi.org/10.1111/j.1365-2648.2007.04569.x.
16. Vaismoradi M, Turunen H, Bondas T. Content analysis and thematic analysis: Implications for conducting a qualitative descriptive study. Nurs Health Sci. 2013;15:398–405.
17. Crowe M, Inder M, Porter R. Conducting qualitative research in mental health: thematic and content analyses. Aust N Z J Psychiatry. 2015. https://doi.org/10.1177/0004867415582053.
18. Butler AE, Hall H, Copnell B. Ethical and practical realities of utilising letters for recruitment in bereavement research. Res Nurs Health. 2017. https://doi.org/10.1002/nur.21800.
19. Beck AM, Konnert CA. Ethical issues in the study of bereavement: the opinions of bereaved adults. Death Stud. 2007. https://doi.org/10.1080/07481180701537220.
20. Abib El Halal G, Piva J, Lago P, El Halal M, Cabral F, Nilson C, Garcia P. Parents' perspectives on the deaths of their children in two Brazilian paediatric intensive care units. Int J Palliat Nurs. 2013. https://doi.org/10.12968/ijpn.2013.19.10.495.
21. Brooten D, Youngblut JM, Seagrave L, Caicedo C, Hawthorne D, Hidalgo I, Roche R. Parent's perceptions of health care providers actions around child ICU death: what helped, what did not. Am J Hosp Palliat Med. 2013. https://doi.org/10.1177/1049909112444301.
22. Brosig CL, Pierucci RL, Kupst MJ, Leuthner SR. Infant end-of-life care: the parents' perspective. J Perinatol. 2007. https://doi.org/10.1038/sj.jp.7211755.
23. Keene Reder E, Serwint JR. Until the last breath: exploring the concept of hope for parents and health care professionals during a child's serious illness. Arch Pediatr Adolesc Med. 2009. https://doi.org/10.1001/archpediatrics.2009.87.
24. Lamiani G, Giannini A, Fossati I, Prandi E, Vegni E. Parental experience of end-of life care in the pediatric intensive care unit. Minerva Anestesiol. 2013;79:1334–43.
25. Macdonald ME, Liben S, Carnevale F, Rennick J, Wolf S, Meloche D, Cohen SR. Parental perspectives on hospital staff members' acts of kindness and commemoration after a child's death. Pediatrics. 2005. https://doi.org/10.1542/peds.2004-1980.
26. McGraw S, Truog R, Solomon M, Cohen-Bearak A, Sellers D, Meyer E. "I was able to still be her mom" parenting at end of life in the PICU. Pediatr Crit Care Med. 2012. https://doi.org/10.1097/PCC.0b013e31825b5607.
27. Meert K, Briller S, Myers Schim S, Thurston C, Kabel A. Examining the needs of bereaved parents in the pediatric intensive care unit: a qualitative study. Death Stud. 2009. https://doi.org/10.1080/07481180903070434.
28. Meert K, Thurston C, Briller S. The spiritual needs of parents at the time of their child's death in the pediatric intensive care unit and during bereavement: a qualitative study. Pediatr Crit Care Med. 2005. https://doi.org/10.1097/01.PCC.0000163679.87749.CA.
29. Meyer E, Burns J, Griffith J, Truog R. Parental perspectives on end-of-life care in the pediatric intensive care unit. Critical Care Med. 2002;30:226–31.
30. Robinson M, Thiel M, Backus M, Meyer E. Matters of spirituality at the end of life in the pediatric intensive care unit. Pediatrics. 2006. https://doi.org/10.1542/peds.2005-2298.
31. Alam R, Barrera M, D'Agostino N, Nicholas DB, Schneiderman G. Bereavement experiences of mothers and fathers over time after the death of a child due to Cancer. Death Stud. 2012. https://doi.org/10.1080/07481187.2011.553312.
32. Barrera M, O'connor K, D'Agostino NM, Spencer L, Nicholas D, Jovcevska V, Tallet S, Schneiderman G. Early parental adjustment and bereavement after childhood cancer death. Death Stud. 2009;33:497–520.

33. Meert KL, Shear K, Newth CJL, Harrison R, Berger J, Zimmerman J, Anand KJS, Carcillo J, Donaldson AE, Dean JM, et al. Follow-up study of complicated grief among parents eighteen months after a Child's death in the pediatric intensive care unit. J Palliat Med. 2011. https://doi.org/10.1089/jpm.2010.0291.
34. Butler AE, Hall H, Copnell B. Gradually disengaging: parent–health care provider relationships after a Child's death in the pediatric intensive care unit. J Fam Nurs. 2018. https://doi.org/10.1177/1074840718783470.
35. Donovan LA, Wakefield CE, Russell V, Cohn RJ. Hospital-based bereavement services following the death of a child: a mixed study review. Palliat Med. 2015. https://doi.org/10.1177/0269216314556851.
36. October T, Dryden-Palmer K, Copnell B, Meert KL. Caring for parents after the death of a child. Pediatr Crit Care Med. 2018. https://doi.org/10.1097/pcc.0000000000001466.
37. Klass D. Solace and immortality: bereaved parents' continuing bond with their children. Death Stud. 1993. https://doi.org/10.1080/07481189308252630.
38. Decinque N, Monterosso L, Dadd G, Sidhu R, Macpherson R, Aoun S. Bereavement support for families following the death of a child from cancer: experience of bereaved parents. J Psychosoc Oncol. 2006;24:65–83.
39. Woodgate RL. Living in a world without closure: reality for parents who have experienced the death of a child. J Palliat Care. 2006;22:75.
40. Tong A, Sainsbury P, Craig J. Consolidated criteria for reporting qualitative research (COREQ): a 32-item checklist for interviews and focus groups. Int J Qual Health Care. 2007. https://doi.org/10.1093/intqhc/mzm042.

2

Using co-design to develop an intervention to improve communication about the heart failure trajectory and end-of-life care

Lisa Hjelmfors[1*], Anna Strömberg[2,3], Maria Friedrichsen[1], Anna Sandgren[4], Jan Mårtensson[5] and Tiny Jaarsma[1]

Abstract

Background: The aim of this paper was to describe the development of an intervention that is developed to improve communication about the heart failure (HF) trajectory and end-of-life care. We also present data that provides a first insight in specific areas of feasibility of the intervention.

Methods: Co-design was used and patients, family members and health care professionals were constructive participants in the design process of the intervention. Feasibility of the intervention was tested in two areas; acceptability and limited efficacy.

Results: Two communication tools were designed and evaluated; 1) a Question Prompt List (QPL) for patients and family members and 2) a communication course for professionals which was web -based with one face-to-face training day with simulation. Data on feasibility was collected with questionnaires that were developed for this study, from the 13 participants who completed the course (all nurses). They reported improved knowledge, confidence and skills to discuss the HF trajectory and end-of-life care. The QPL was evaluated to be a useful tool in communication with patients and family members.

Conclusions: In a co-design process, future users identified the need for a QPL and a communication course. These communication tools can be used as a dual intervention to improve communication about the HF trajectory and end-of-life care. The QPL can help patients and families to ask questions about the HF trajectory and end-of-life care. The communication course can prepare the professionals to be knowledgeable, confident and skilled to discuss the questions in the QPL. Before the tools are ready for implementation in clinical practice, further studies testing the feasibility of the intervention are needed, including also patients and their families.

Keywords: Heart failure, Illness trajectory, End-of-life care, Communication, Co-design, User perspective

Background

Heart Failure (HF) is a life threatening illness, often with a poor prognosis [1]. The HF trajectory is unique for each individual person, and it may include recurrent, unpredictable exacerbations, including decreased functional status [2–5]. Death from HF can be sudden, due to an ischemic event or electric instability of the heart, or it can be slow, due to episodes of decompensation or progressive organ failure [6]. Patients with HF also often have several comorbidities that can cause death [7]. Guidelines recommend health care professionals to have an open communication with patients and their families about the HF trajectory, including discussing their preferences for future care, acknowleding the risk of a sudden death, and the possibility of deactivation of implantable defibrillators in the end-of-life [8, 9]. A lack of insight in the HF trajectory, including disease progression and functional decline, can increase anxiety and uncertainty in patients and family members which may affect quality of life and also increase use of health care resources [10]. Additionally, if the HF trajectory is not adequately discussed, issues around end-of-life care tend to be addressed too late, possibly resulting in an unsatisfactory end-of-life care for both patients and families

* Correspondence: lisa.hjelmfors@liu.se
[1]Department of Social and Welfare Studies (ISV), Faculty of Health Sciences, Linköping University, 581 83 Linköping, Sweden
Full list of author information is available at the end of the article

[11]. There seems to be a reluctance to talk about death and dying in clinical HF practice, and conversations focus mostly on disease management and less on preferences and goals of care [12]. Health care professionals are often hesitant to have these conversations as they are afraid of taking away hope and cause anxiety in patients and their families [12, 13].

However, patients with HF and their families would often welcome conversations about the HF trajectory and end-of-life care, but do not always know how to initiate the discussion with health care professionals [12]. Several studies [12, 14–17] have described the needs for improved communication about the HF trajectory and end-of-life care in HF care. However, there is limited knowledge on the most appropriate communication strategies that meet the specific needs of patients with HF, their families and the health care professionals. Interventions to improve communication should be developed in accordance with the future users' needs and preferences to increase their usefulness. During the last decades, methods in which patients, family members and health care professionals are involved in the design of health care services have become more common [18]. Examples of such methods are Experienced-based design, Co-design and experienced-based co-design, in which staff and patients (or other service users) co-design services and/or care pathways, together in partnership [19]. A core methodological approach in these methods is involving the experiences of future users in the design process [19], focusing on both understanding and improving a person's experiences of a product/service as well as the product/service itself [20, 21]. Key benefits of co-design methods in development studies include the possibility to engage and empower patients, family members, and health care professionals to become active participants in the development of services that they will use in the future [19]. The aim of this paper was to describe the development of an intervention that is developed to improve communication about the HF trajectory and end-of-life care. We also present data that provides a first insight in specific areas of feasibility of the intervention.

Methods

Co-design

Patients with HF, family members and health care professionals were invited to be constructive participants in the design process of the intervention. After that, health care professionals participated in a first feasibility testing of the intervention. The intervention was developed and tested in two phases, (phase 1: Development, and phase 2: Testing, Fig. 1), which took place from September 2015 to March 2017 (Fig. 2). In the co-design process, the concepts "Ideas groups" and "Prototyping" were used as described in the Health Service Co-design toolkit [20]. Ideas groups is a tool that can be used to brainstorm ideas for improvement and ways of implementing them in clinical practice. Prototyping can be used to test new products to see if they will work and it is a useful way to engage and stimulate creativity among the stakeholders taking part in ideas groups [20].

Phase 1- developing the intervention

First, stakeholders came together in ideas groups at two different time points to brainstorm improvement ideas and ways to implement them in clinical practice. The goal with the ideas groups was described to the participants as to develop communication tools/support to improve communication between patients, family members and health care professionals about the HF trajectory and end-of-life care. At the first ideas group, the goal was to discuss ideas that could improve communication,

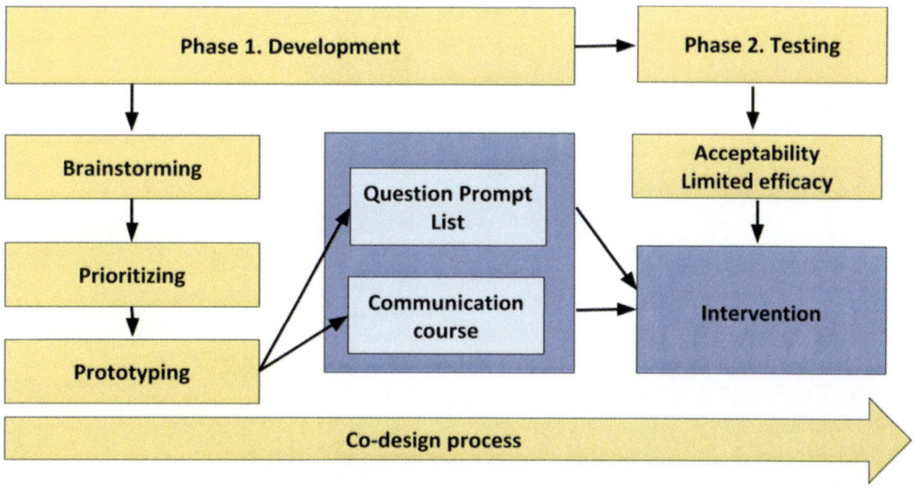

Fig. 1 The co-design process used in the study included phase 1, developing the intervention, and phase 2, testing the acceptability and limited efficacy of the intervention

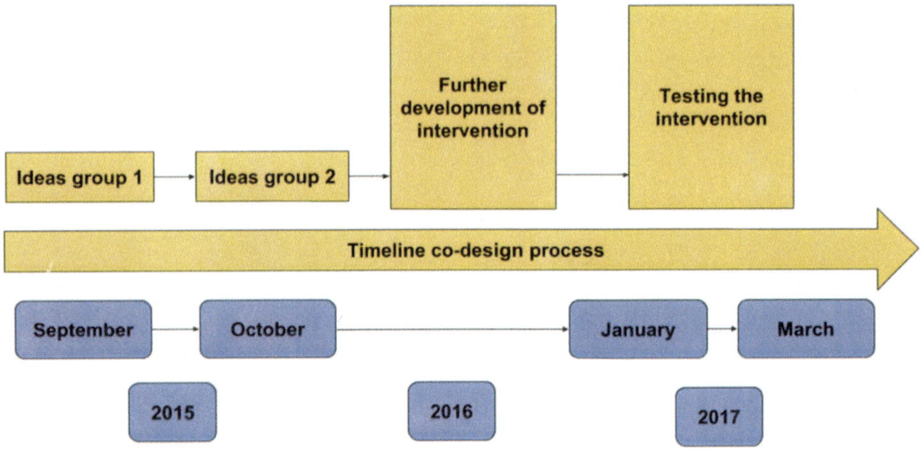

Fig. 2 Timeline of the co-design process including two ideas groups with patients, family members and health care professionals, participating in the development of the intervention. During 2016 the intervention was further developed by the research group and in 2017, acceptability and limited efficacy of the intervention was tested

and at the second ideas group, the goal was to further develop and discuss the ideas that were suggested in the first ideas group. Patients with HF, their family members, and health care professionals, were invited to participate in the ideas groups. A HF nurse in an outpatient HF clinic identified suitable patients and provided their names, ages, and information on their New York Heart Association Functional Classification (NYHA class). The first author sent a study invitation letter to the patients and then called them a few days later to ask if they were interested to participate in the study, with or without a family member. The researchers used their own network of physicians and nurses with expertise in HF care and palliative care, and invited them by email to participate in the study. The patients ($n = 9$) who agreed to participate were in NYHA class I-III and had a mean age of 75 years. The family members ($n = 2$) who agreed to participate in the study had a mean age of 70 years. None of the patients were recently diagnosed, most of them had lived with HF for several years. Some of them had medical devices such as an Implantable Cardioverter Defibrillator (ICD), or Cardiac Resynchronisation Therapy (CRT). The professionals (1 physician and 8 nurses, mean age 50 years) had extensive experience of working in HF care or palliative care. The researchers ($n = 5$) were 4 nurses with experience in co-design, HF care and palliative care, and 1 behavioural scientist with experience in medical education. The researchers led the ideas groups, facilitated and summarized the discussions, took field notes and made audio recordings.

Phase 2- testing the intervention

The intervention was tested in phase 2 of the study. The testing focused on two areas of feasibility; acceptability and limited efficacy of the intervention [22]. Acceptability refers to the participants' satisfaction with, and reactions to the intervention. The limited efficacy testing evaluated the intervention's potential of being successful among the intended users, meaning that the intervention can have an impact on knowledge, skills and confidence of health care professionals in the future [22]. To measure acceptability and limited efficacy in the testing of the intervention, data were collected pre-post intervention, using questionnaires that were developed for this study. The questionnaire that measured the participants' satisfaction with, and reactions to the intervention (acceptability), included open- and closed ended questions and statements using a 4-point Likert scale (1 = strongly agree to 4 = strongly disagree). The questionnaire that measured the participants' knowledge, confidence and skills to discuss the HF trajectory and end-of-life care (limited efficacy), included statements using a 4-point Likert scale (1 = strongly agree to 4 = strongly disagree). A 2-week test-retest reliability of the questionnaire evaluating limited efficacy, was assessed in a group ($N = 13$) of cardiac health care professionals before it being used in the present study. The test-retest reported the kappa values of the 50 items in the questionnaire. Thirty-four items had a good to moderate agreement, 0.41–0.80, and 16 items had a fair agreement 0.20–0.40 [23].

To test the intervention (the Question Prompt List, QPL and the course) an invitation letter was sent out to HF clinics in all regions in Sweden. All cardiac professionals who were interested in the content of the course were eligible to participate. Twenty-one cardiac professionals working in a clinical setting signed up for the course, 3 physicians and 19 nurses. Before the course started and during the first weeks of the course, 6 participants (all nurses) withdrew due to changes in their work situation or due to private matters. Sixteen participants (Table 1) followed web-lectures, completed the 2

Table 1 Course content and teaching methods

Three individual tasks (online)	1) The participants reflect on when they think is the best time to discuss about the HF trajectory with a patient for the first time and give reasons for their choices. 2) The participants familiarize themselves with the QPL and reflect on their own knowledge and ability to converse with the patient and family about the different questions in the QPL. 3) The participants use the QPL in their clinical work with one patient and/or one family member.
Lectures (online)	1) Why do we need to talk about the HF trajectory and end-of-life care? -15 min 2) Discussing the HF trajectory and end-of-life care - Who, what and when? -25 min 3) Patients with heart failure pacemaker or ICD- how to end the treatment – 15 min 4) Patients' experiences of, and preferences for communication about the HF trajectory – 10 min 5) The existential conversation – 15 min 6) End-of-life care communication in HF -20 min 7) Communication with the family members – 10 min
Group discussions (training day)	Participants are divided into small groups with a group leader. The participants reflect on what questions in the QPL they perceived as easy or difficult to discuss. Through group discussions, participants can learn from each other's experiences.
Simulation (training day)	Two actors simulate the role of a patients with HF who want to discuss questions in the QPL and the participants act as health care professionals. The participants take turns to simulate a family member in the conversations and take part in the discussion afterwards.

QPL Question Prompt List, *ICD* Implantable cardioverter defibrillator, *HF* Heart Failure

assignments (Table 2) and attended the training day. None of the 3 physicians completed task 3 (Table 2). The reasons for this is not known.

Data analysis

Data from the ideas groups (field notes and audio recordings) and data from the open-ended questions in the questionnaires were evaluated, discussed and summarized in the research group. As the aim was to identify improvement ideas expressed by the participants, and evaluate the intervention, the data were summarized without an in-depth qualitative analysis. Descriptive statistics were used to describe the participants' background characteristics. Frequencies and proportions were used to describe the outcomes in the questionnaires.

Table 2 Background characteristics of the course participants

N = 16	
Sex (*N*, %)	
Females	16 (100%)
Age (years, mean)	24–57, 39
Occupation (*n*, %)	
Physician	3 (19%)
Nurse	13 (81%)
Workplace	
Hospital	13 (81%)
Public health care centre	2 (13%)
Hospitalized home care	1 (6%)
Specialist education[a]	
Yes	10 (60%)
Time working with HF patients (years, mean)	0–25, 9

HF Heart Failure. [a]Physicians- general or internal medicine, nurses- cardiology or public health

Results

Phase 1- developing the intervention

Brainstorming

Ideas group 1 started with a short presentation by the research group, introducing some background information of life-limiting nature of HF. After that, during a brainstorming session, participants were encouraged to share their experiences of bad or good communication situations in health care. Some patients described a lack of information of their HF from the health care, and emphasised the possibility to get repeated information at different time points. It was considered a problem to remember information as well. The patients also believed that bad communication could depend on the patients themselves, as many might have difficulties to pose questions to the health care professional. Family members described a lack of information on the seriousness of the illness and a wish to receive the same information as the patient. Some kind of a communication tool that could help patients and family members to ask questions would be helpful. Meeting other patients in a group discussion with a nurse as a facilitator of discussion, was suggested as one way to enhance communication.

In the brainstorming, the health care professionals described that it was difficult in clinical practice to know what had already been discussed with patients/family members. Continuity in care was considered important, and a HF nurse could have a crucial role to play in communication, as the nurse is the one that most often meets the patients/family members. Communication training for professionals as a way to improve communication was also suggested.

After hearing and discussing the participants' experiences of communication and various ideas of communication tools/support, the researchers also presented communication interventions that had previously been used in cancer care, to be used as examples to discuss and draw inspiration from [24–26].

In summary, suggested ideas for interventions for the patient and their family members included:

- patient meetings in groups in which patients can support each other
- family conversations in which patients, family members and all health care professionals involved in the care can meet and discuss the future
- a list for patients and family members with questions about the HF trajectory and end-of-life care to be used as a communication tool.

Suggested ideas for interventions for health care professionals included:

- communication training in groups
- individual web-based education in communication
- role play or a film that provides a good example of a conversation
- simulation training of conversations about the HF trajectory and end-of-life care.

An important comment from the participants was that instead of focussing on one group of users (e.g. only make a tool for patients) both an intervention for the patients/family members and an intervention for the professionals could be useful to improve communication.

Prioritizing

The participants voted for the two ideas that came up in the brainstorming that they thought could make the biggest difference in improving communication. The idea of a list with questions about the HF trajectory and end-of-life care for patients and family members, and communication training for health care professionals were the two most popular ideas.

Prototyping

Two months after the first ideas group, the participants met again in an ideas group to further discuss and develop the list of questions and the communication training into prototypes. The participants brainstormed useful questions that could be included in the list and discussed useful wording and language. Following the second ideas group, the prototype of the list was further refined by the researchers, based on the suggestions from the ideas groups and relevant literature. The prototype of the list was sent to the ideas group participants for evaluation. The participants were asked to comment on the layout as well as the content. The majority of the participants found the list to be in concordance with their suggestions.

Further on, the communication training was refined into a communication course prototype by the researchers, based on the suggestions from the ideas groups. Suggested content for the course included, for example, theoretical knowledge about communication, as well as practical training using simulated conversations and role play.

The intervention

When finalizing the prototypes, the research group decided that the two prototypes, the list of questions and the communication training, should be combined into a dual component intervention and be used together. The list of questions will from now on be referred to as the QPL and the communication training will be referred to as the communication course.

The question prompt list

The QPL was designed to stimulate and facilitate patient and family member communication about the HF trajectory and end-of-life care with a health care professional. The QPL is a 7-page A4 booklet, containing 45 questions grouped into the topics: 1) Heart failure and what to expect in the future 2) Help and support at deterioration 3) End-of-life care issues 4) Additional questions for the family members 5) Additional questions for the person with an ICD/CRT/PM. The purpose of the QPL is to function as an aid for patients and family members at clinical appointments, and encourage them to ask questions that are relevant to them about the HF trajectory and end-of-life care. They can also add more questions that are not in the list. The QPL is expected to function as a communication tool to help the patients and families to be more involved in the care.

The communication course

The communication course is web-based with one face-to-face practical training day, designed to be applicable for health care professionals who work in cardiology. Nurses in cardiology and palliative care and a behavioural scientist act as course leaders. Participants take the course at their own convenience. It is based on adult learning principles using self-directed learning [27] and includes several teaching methods (Table 2).

The learning goals of the course are for the participants to expand their knowledge about communication about the HF trajectory and end-of-life care, and to improve on their own knowledge, confidence and skills in communications. The QPL is an important tool in the course and the participants are expected to learn to use the QPL as a communication tool in the course and to gain the needed knowledge, confidence and skills required to discuss the questions in the QPL with patients and family members. Another important part of the course is the practical training with simulated patients (actors) and family members (volunteer course participants), where the participants practice using the QPL in a simulated conversation. Constructive feedback on their performance is provided by course leaders, the simulated patients and family members, as well as the other participants in the course.

Phase 2, testing the intervention

Acceptability: Participants' satisfaction with, and reactions to the course

The participants were asked to evaluate the course, using close-ended (Table 3) and open-ended questions. They described that they took the course simultaneously with their clinical jobs and reported to have spent 10–30 h on the course. The participants expressed that the course had helped them to reflect on their professional role in discussions about the HF trajectory and end-of-life care, which made them more confident in discussions without worrying about providing the "correct" answers to patients and family members. All the participants evaluated the seven lectures to be of importance for their learning and most evaluated the three individual tasks worthwhile to do. They reported that meeting colleagues to discuss and learn from each other as well as practicing having conversations with simulated patients and family members during the training day was valuable. Overall, the participants were satisfied with the content of the course and how it was delivered, but some ($n = 5$) would have preferred to have one additional face-to-face training day as a follow-up. The majority of the participants had no technical problems with the web-site, but 3 participants reported difficulties to view one of the lectures. All participants would recommend the course to a colleague. After completing task 3 (using the QPL in clinical practice), most ($n = 11$) reported that the QPL would be useful in future clinical conversations, but they thought that the QPL could be shortened.

Limited efficacy

In a pre-post-test, questions from the QPL that would mirror the learning goals of the course were included, assessing the participants' self-reported knowledge, confidence and skills for each question. For the majority of the participants, on most of the questions their knowledge, confidence and skills was reported to have

Table 3 Acceptability: Participants' satisfaction with, and reactions to the course ($N = 13$)

Statements	Strongly agree /agree
Lecture 1- "Why do we have to talk about the HF trajectory and end-of-life care with patients and their families?" was a worthwhile lecture	13 (100%)
Lecture 2- "Discussing the HF trajectory and end-of-life care" was a worthwhile lecture	13 (100%)
Lecture 3- "Patients' experiences and preferences of discussing the prognosis" was a worthwhile lecture	13 (100%)
Lecture 4- "Patients with pacemaker and/or ICD- decisions on determination of treatment" was a worthwhile lecture	13 (100%)
Lecture 5- "Enabling existential communication" was a worthwhile lecture	13 (100%)
Lecture 6- "Palliative communication in HF care" was a worthwhile lecture	13 (100%)
Lecture 7- "Communication with family members" was a worthwhile lecture[a]	12 (92%)
Task 1 was worthwhile to do	11 (85%)
Task 2 was worthwhile to do	12 (92%)
Task 3 was worthwhile to do	11 (85%)
The group discussions during the training day was worthwhile	12 (92%)
The Question Prompt List will be a useful tool in my future communications with patients and their families	11 (85%)
The course literature have contributed to my learning	11 (85%)
The provided web -sites on the course site was worthwhile to watch	12 (92%)
It was good that the course was web-based	13 (100%)
The web-site of the course worked well	13 (100%)

[a]One participants could not view this lecture and therefore did not agree with the statement

increased after the course (Figs. 3 and 4). However, the participants reported after the course to have less knowledge, confidence and skills to discuss two of the questions in part 2 of the questionnaire, concerning who the patient/family member can talk to about the things that worry them.

Discussion

To our knowledge, this is the first study to use a co-design method and invite the future users in the development of an intervention aimed to improve communication about the HF trajectory and end-of-life care in HF care, and test the acceptability and limited efficacy of the intervention. In co-design, the 'co' is pivotal, emphasizing a collaborative effort by patients, families, professionals and the researchers facilitating the process [28]. The co-design method made it possible for patients, their families, and health care professionals to share their experiences. Through a partnership with the researchers, the patients and their families contributed to the design and development of the intervention, which ensured that the intervention was based on their needs [20]. In the co-design process, two ideas were suggested and developed into prototypes, a QPL and a communication course that formed the intervention. To evaluate if the intervention could be useful in clinical practice, the two areas of feasibility that were found most important at this stage of the study were tested; acceptability and limited efficacy [22]. The results show that the course was well received by all the nurses who finalized the course. The QPL was tested by nurses in clinical practice with positive results and was reported to be a valuable tool in communication, helping the patients and the family members to ask questions about the HF trajectory and end-of-life care. Similar results have been found in a recent extensive literature review on Question Prompt Lists in cancer care, reporting that most patients find using a QPL useful to frame questions and enhance the consultation [29]. A study from 2001 [30] described the use of a checklist with questions to improve patient education in cardiology and in the evaluation of the long-term efficacy of the checklist, it was concluded that the it could be a useful tool for preparing the patient for the visit to the cardiologist [31]. Our QPL showed similar results, but it is different as it is supposed to be used in discussions between patients, their families and several cardiac professionals, not only by a cardiologist in a doctor-patient communication.

The participants' perceived knowledge, confidence and skills to discuss the HF trajectory and end-of-life care in HF care, increased after the course, with the biggest changes concerning issues around ICD/CRT. This is not surprising as these are areas that are difficult to discuss with patients and family members [32], and health care professionals might have little knowledge about them. The participants reported decreased knowledge, confidence and skills in two questions that concerned who the patient or the patient's family can talk to if they feel a need for help and support. This, however, does not necessarily mean that the participants' knowledge, confidence and skills actually decreased. Rather, during the course, they might have become more aware of the fact that there are more aspects related to certain topics then they originally thought. The participants might have

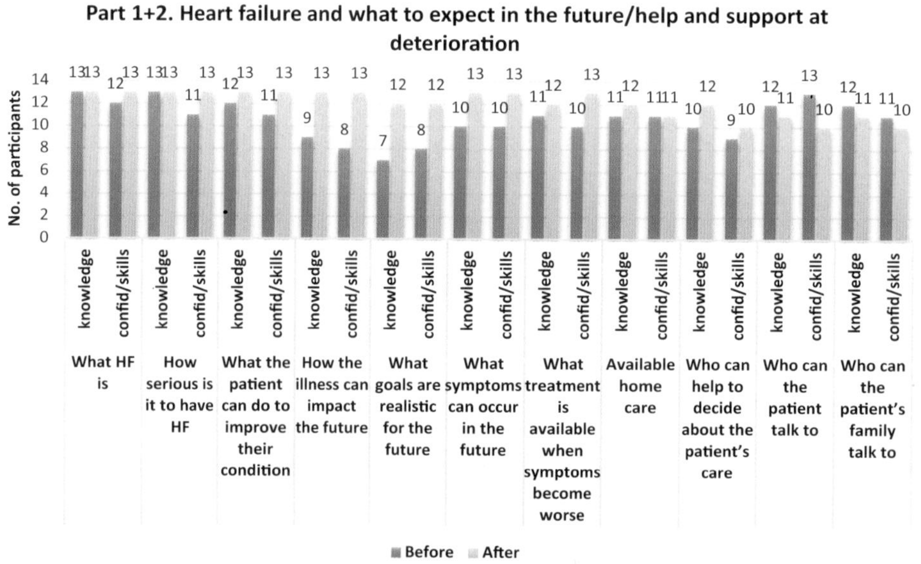

Fig. 3 The number of participants agreeing (strongly agree/agree) to have knowledge/confidence/skills to discuss questions in part 1–2 of the QPL, before and after the course, $N = 13$. Abbreviations: QPL Question Prompt List

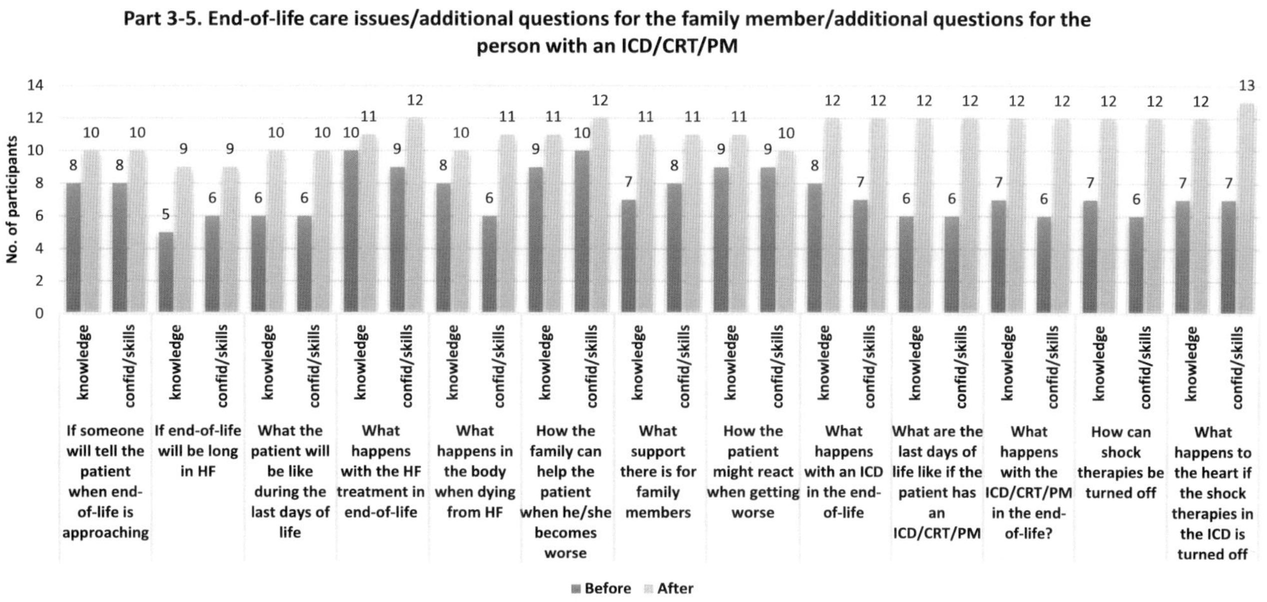

Fig. 4 The number of participants agreeing (strongly agree/agree) to have knowledge/confidence/skills to discuss questions in part 3–5 of the QPL, before and after the course, N = 13. Abbreviations: ICD Implantable Cardioverter Defibrillator, CRT Cardiac Resynchronisation Therapy, PM Pacemaker, QPL Question Prompt List

become aware of their lack of competence, which can be an important first step towards gaining the needed knowledge, confidence and skills to discuss these topics [33]. This is in line with the adult learning principles that aim to facilitate a problem-solving process for the learning individual by identifying a lack of knowledge in order to gain new knowledge [34].

We chose to assess not only the participants' knowledge, but also their confidence and skills to discuss the HF trajectory and end-of-life care, as our previous studies found that even if a person has knowledge to discuss those topics, it does not mean that they have the confidence and skills to actually take on the conversation [13].

To further improve the intervention, other areas need to be tested, such as implementation and demand [22]. These areas of feasibility can be explored in a later phase.

There are some important limitations to consider in this study. First, although the results of the testing are promising, it has to be recognised that due to the limited number of participants and the lack of statistical analyses, more information is needed to draw definite conclusions about the efficacy of the course. Although we are further developing the materials, we find it important to share our results in this stage so readers can be inspired to use or further develop the intervention to improve their care to HF patients. Secondly, input from family members was limited as only two family members participated in the development of the intervention. Thirdly, as we only send an evaluation form to those who completed the final task, we missed specific data on the satisfaction from the three physicians, who did not complete task 3, which limits the possibility to state anything about the physicians' perceptions of the intervention, and also raises the questions if the final task was useful for training physicians. The lack of physicians must also be seen as limitation of the generalizability of the intervention to non-nurse professionals. Preferably, physicians from both general care and cardiology should have participated in all parts of the study in order for it to be more effective and strengthen the validity.

In addition, the data were self-reported and not based on direct observations of the participants' knowledge, confidence and skills, and, due to the small sample size, we could not calculate for any significate changes pre- and post the intervention, but only look at positive trends in the data. It is also important to consider that no men participated in the testing of the intervention and that there might be a potential selection bias if only professionals that were already motivated to learn more about communication about the HF trajectory and end-of-life care, are represented in the sample. Most participants attending the course already had some knowledge, confidence and skills to communicate about the HF trajectory and end-of-life care. At the same time, the majority of the participants also reported having learned more during the course.

To evaluate knowledge, confidence and skills related to the QPL, a questionnaire was developed especially for this study instead of using a general one. However, the results from the questionnaire need to be interpreted with caution, as the questionnaire was only psychometrically tested in a limited extent.

Additionally, it also should be noted that the patients involved in the development of the intervention were not the ones with the most advanced HF; hence this intervention was developed with HF patients at earlier stages of the illness and their ideas for effective interventions may differ from those with more advanced HF.

One important advantage in the co-design process was the diverse sample of participants that participated in both the development and the testing of the intervention. This strengthens our findings and entails that the intervention is based on the needs of future users, which is crucial in order for the it to be useful [35]. Many patients, families and health care professionals are interested in taking part in development studies as they want to see a change and improvement in practice [19]. In this study, some participants contributed more and were more creative than others, but everybody showed an interest in the co-design process and contributed to some extent. The researchers took on a facilitator's role in the design process, bringing knowledge and expertise from their own professional backgrounds, thus guiding and inspiring the design process [21].

Conclusions

We have developed and evaluated an intervention containg a QPL for patients and family members and a communication course for cardiac health care professionals using a co-design approach including those groups representing the future users in the process. This intervention can be a first step towards improving communication about the HF trajectory and end-of-life care in HF care. The intervention has a dual approach to communication, where the QPL can help patients and family members to initiate discussions about the HF trajectory and end-of-life care, whereas the communication course can help professionals to gain the knowledge, confidence and skills required to discuss the questions raised by patients and their families. Before the tools are ready for implementation in clinical practice, further studies testing the feasibility of the intervention are needed, including also patients and their families.

Abbreviations

CRT: Cardiac Resynchronisation Therapy; HF: Heart Failure; ICD: Implantable Cardioverter Defibrillator; NYHA class: New York Heart Association functional classification; PM: Pacemaker; QPL: Question Prompt List

Acknowledgements

We want to thank all the patients, family members and health care professionals who participated in the study. A special thank you to Katarina Karlsson (nurse and simulation expert), Annika Pohl (palliative care physician), Yvonne Hajradinovic (nurse and communication educator), Svante Malm (actor), and Kajsa Eriksson (actor) for valuable contributions to the set-up of the course.

Funding

This work was supported by the Medical Research Council of South east of Sweden [FORSS-645591]; and the Research and scholarship management in Region Östergötland [LIO-656941].

Authors' contributions

All authors qualifies as an author according to the International Committee of Medical Journal Editors (ICMJE) guidelines. All authors (LH, AS1, MF, AS2, JM and TJ) have been part of the design and planning of the study, the analysis of data and interpretation of results, and preparation of manuscript. All authors have given their approval of the final version of the manuscript.

Competing interests

The authors declare that they have no competing interests.

Author details

[1]Department of Social and Welfare Studies (ISV), Faculty of Health Sciences, Linköping University, 581 83 Linköping, Sweden. [2]Department of Medical and Health Sciences, Division of nursing, Faculty of Health Sciences, Linköping University, Linköping, Sweden. [3]Department of Cardiology, Linköping University, Linköping, Sweden. [4]Department of Health and Caring Sciences, Center for Collaborative Palliative Care, Linnaeus University, Växjö, Sweden. [5]Department of Nursing, School of Health Sciences, Jönköping University, Jönköping, Sweden.

References

1. McMurray JJ, Adamopoulos S, Anker SD, Auricchio A, Böhm M, Dickstein K, et al. ESC guidelines for the diagnosis and treatment of acute and chronic heart failure 2012: The Task Force for the Diagnosis and Treatment of Acute and Chronic Heart Failure 2012 of the European Society of Cardiology Developed in collaboration with the Heart Failure Association (HFA) of the ESC. Eur J Heart Fail. 2012;14(8):803–69.
2. Jaarsma T, Beattie JM, Ryder M, Rutten FH, McDonagh T, Mohacsi P, et al. Palliative care in heart failure: a position statement from the palliative care workshop of the heart failure Association of the European Society of cardiology. Eur J Heart Fail. 2009;11(5):433–43.
3. Dickstein K, Cohen-Solal A, Filippatos G, McMurray JJ, Ponikowski P, Poole-Wilson PA, et al. ESC guidelines for the diagnosis and treatment of acute and chronic heart failure 2008: the Task Force for the diagnosis and treatment of acute and chronic heart failure 2008 of the European Society of Cardiology Developed in collaboration with the Heart Failure Association of the ESC (HFA) and endorsed by the European Society of Intensive Care Medicine (ESICM). Eur J Heart Fail. 2008;10(10):933–89.
4. National Institute for Health and Clinical Excellence. Chronic heart failure: management of chronic heart failure in adults in primary and secondary care. National Institute for Health and Clinical Excellence; 2010. Available from https://www.nice.org.uk/guidance/Cg108. Accessed 5 June 2018.
5. Goodlin SJ, Quill TE, Arnold RM. Communication and decision-making about prognosis in heart failure care. J Card Fail. 2008;14(2):106–13.
6. Ørn S, Dickstein K. How do heart failure patients die? Eur Heart J Suppl. 2002;4(suppl_D):D59–65.
7. van Deursen VM, Urso R, Laroche C, Damman K, Dahlström U, Tavazzi L, et al. Co-morbidities in patients with heart failure: an analysis of the European heart failure pilot survey. Eur J Heart Fail. 2014;16(1):103–11.
8. Ponikowski P, Voors AA, Anker SD, Bueno H, Cleland JG, Coats AJ, et al. 2016 ESC Guidelines for the diagnosis and treatment of acute and chronic heart failure: The Task Force for the diagnosis and treatment of acute and chronic heart failure of the European Society of Cardiology (ESC) Developed with

the special contribution of the Heart Failure Association (HFA) of the ESC. Eur Heart J. 2016;37(27):2129–200.
9. Allen LA, Stevenson LW, Grady KL, Goldstein NE, Matlock DD, Arnold RM, et al. Decision making in advanced heart failure: a scientific statement from the American Heart Association. Circulation. 2012;125(15):1928–52.
10. Strömberg A, Jaarsma T. Thoughts about death and perceived health status in elderly patients with heart failure. Eur J Heart Fail. 2008;10(6):608–13.
11. Friesinger GC, Butler J. End-of-life care for elderly patients with heart failure. Clin Geriatr Med. 2000;16(3):663–75.
12. Barclay S, Momen N, Case-Upton S, Kuhn I, Smith E. End-of-life care conversations with heart failure patients: a systematic literature review and narrative synthesis. Br J Gen Pract. 2011;61(582):e49–62.
13. Momen NC, Barclay SI. Addressing 'the elephant on the table': barriers to end of life care conversations in heart failure - a literature review and narrative synthesis. Curr Opin Support Palliat Care. 2011;5(4):312–6.
14. Hjelmfors L, Strömberg A, Friedrichsen M, Mårtensson J, Jaarsma T. Communicating prognosis and end-of-life care to heart failure patients: a survey of heart failure nurses' perspectives. Eur J Cardiovasc Nurs. 2014;13(2):152–61.
15. Hjelmfors L, van der Wal MH, Friedrichsen MJ, Mårtensson J, Strömberg A, Jaarsma T. Patient-nurse communication about prognosis and end-of-life care. J Palliat Med. 2015;18(10):865–71.
16. Goodlin SJ. Palliative care in congestive heart failure. J Am Coll Cardiol. 2009;54(5):386–96.
17. van der Wal MH, Hjelmfors L, Mårtensson J, Friedrichsen M, Strömberg A, Jaarsma T. Variables related to communication about prognosis between nurses and patients at heart failure clinics in Sweden and the Netherlands. J Cardiovasc Nurs. 2017;
18. The Kings Fund. Experience-based co-design toolkit. 2011. Available from https://www.kingsfund.org.uk/projects/ebcd. Accessed 11 Mar 2017.
19. van der Wal MH, Hjelmfors L, Mårtensson J, Friedrichsen M, Strömberg A, Jaarsma T. Variables related to communication about prognosis between nurses and patients at heart failure clinics in Sweden and the Netherlands. Journal of Cardiovascular Nursing. 2018;33(2):E1–6.
20. Boyd H, McKernon S, Old A. Health service co-design: working with patients to improve healthcare services: guide and toolkit: Waitemata District health board; 2010. Available from http://www.healthcodesign.org.nz/tools/TOOLKIT_WEB_DOWNLOAD.pdf. Accessed 6 June 2018.
21. Borgstrom E, Barclay S. Experience-based design, co-design and experience-based co-design in palliative and end-of-life care. BMJ Support Palliat Care. 2017;0:1–7.
22. Bowen DJ, Kreuter M, Spring B, Cofta-Woerpel L, Linnan L, Weiner D, et al. How we design feasibility studies. Am J Prev Med. 2009;36(5):452–7.
23. Sanders EB, Stappers PJ. Co-creation and the new landscapes of design. Co-design. 2008;4(1):5–18
24. Benzein EG, Hagberg M, Saveman BI. 'Being appropriately unusual': a challenge for nurses in health-promoting conversations with families. Nurs Inq. 2008;15(2):106–15.
25. Wilkinson S, Perry R, Blanchard K, Linsell L. Effectiveness of a three-day communication skills course in changing nurses' communication skills with cancer/palliative care patients: a randomised controlled trial. Palliat Med. 2008;22(4):365–75.
26. Clayton J, Butow P, Tattersall M, Chye R, Noel M, Davis J, et al. Asking questions can help: development and preliminary evaluation of a question prompt list for palliative care patients. Br J Cancer. 2003;89(11):2069.
27. Knowles MS, Holton IIIEF, Swanson RA. The adult learner: the definitive classic in adult education and human resource development: Routledge; 2014.
28. Blackwell RW, Lowton K, Robert G, Grudzen C, Grocott P. Using experience-based co-design with older patients, their families and staff to improve palliative care experiences in the emergency department: a reflective critique on the process and outcomes. Int J Nurs Stud. 2017;68:83–94.
29. Sansoni JE, Grootemaat P, Duncan C. Question prompt lists in health consultations: a review. Routledge: Patient Educ Couns. 2015;98(12):1454–64.
30. Martinali J, Bolman C, Brug J, van den Borne B, Bar F. A checklist to improve patient education in a cardiology outpatient setting. Patient Educ Couns. 2001;42(3):231–8.
31. Bolman C, Brug J, Bär F, Martinali J, van den Borne B. Long-term efficacy of a checklist to improve patient education in cardiology. Patient Educ Couns. 2005;56(2):240–8.
32. Fluur C, Bolse K, Strömberg A, Thylén I. Patients' experiences of the implantable cardioverter defibrillator (ICD); with a focus on battery replacement and end-of-life issues. Heart & Lung: The Journal of Acute and Critical Care. 2013;42(3):202–7.
33. Skarman G. Handledning för professionell utveckling: Liber; 2011.
34. Barrows HS. Problem-based learning: an approach to medical education. New York: Springer publishing company; 1980.
35. Aidemark J, Askenäs L, Nygårdh A, Strömberg A. User involvement in the co-design of self-care support systems for heart failure patients. Stockhom: Procedia Computer Science. 2015;64:118–24.

Comparing unplanned and potentially planned home deaths: a population-based

Camilla Kjellstadli[1,2*], Bettina Sandgathe Husebø[2,3], Hogne Sandvik[4], Elisabeth Flo[5] and Steinar Hunskaar[1,4]

Abstract

Background: There is little research on number of planned home deaths. We need information about factors associated with home deaths, but also differences between planned and unplanned home deaths to improve end-of-life-care at home and make home deaths a feasible alternative. Our aim was to investigate factors associated with home deaths, estimate number of potentially planned home deaths, and differences in individual characteristics between people with and without a potentially planned home death.

Methods: A cross-sectional study of all decedents in Norway in 2012 and 2013, using data from the Norwegian Cause of Death Registry and National registry for statistics on municipal health and care services. We defined planned home death by an indirect algorithm-based method using domiciliary care and diagnosis. We used logistic regressions models to evaluate factors associated with home death compared with nursing home and hospital; and to compare unplanned home deaths and potentially planned home deaths.

Results: Among 80,908 deaths, 12,156 (15.0%) were home deaths. A home death was most frequent in 'Circulatory diseases' and 'Cancer', and associated with male sex, younger age, receiving domiciliary care and living alone. Only 2.3% of home deaths were from 'Dementia'. In total, 41.9% of home deaths and 6.3% of all deaths were potentially planned home deaths. Potentially planned home deaths were associated with higher age, but declined in ages above 80 years for people who had municipal care. Living together with someone was associated with more potentially planned home deaths for people with municipal care.

Conclusion: There are few home deaths in Norway. Our estimations indicate that even fewer people than anticipated have a potentially planned home death.

Keywords: Home death, Place of death, Death/epidemiology, Death/statistics and numerical data, Death/classification, Cross-sectional studies, Cause of death, Terminal care, Registries, Retrospective studies

Introduction

Most people wish to spend their last days of life in their own home and die at home [1]. Despite this, the proportion of home deaths in Western countries continues to decline [2]. Exceptions include Canada, the UK and the US, where home deaths have increased the last 15 to 25 years due to implementation of end-of-life programs and policy changes [2–4]. Home deaths increased from 19.3% in 1994 to 29.5% in 2004 in Canada; from 18.3% in 2004 to 20.8% in 2010 in the UK; and from 30.7% in 2000 to 33.5% in 2009 in Medicare beneficiaries aged 66 years and older in the US [2–4].

In Norway, home deaths have been declining, with only 14.3% of deaths taking place at home in 2015 [5, 6]. This is low compared with many other Western countries [7–16]. While home death is not desirable or possible for everyone, we need to know more about who dies at home and influencing factors in order to meet people's preference of dying at home, as well as inform and improve policies. While we know the total number

* Correspondence: camilla.kjellstadli@uib.no
[1]Research Group for General Practice, Department of Global Public Health and Primary Care, University of Bergen, PO box 7804, N-5018 Bergen, Norway
[2]Centre for Elderly and Nursing Home Medicine, Department of Global Public Health and Primary Care, University of Bergen, PO box 7804, N-5018 Bergen, Norway
Full list of author information is available at the end of the article

of home deaths, this does not describe the proportion of people who wished to die at home or the number of deaths that were planned or facilitated to take place at home. We cannot use registry data to estimate people's preferences, but we can differentiate sudden, unplanned home deaths from home deaths where health and care service utilisation implies that resources were allocated to facilitate a home death.

In this study, our aim was first to describe factors associated with home deaths in Norway, and compare them with deaths in other locations. Secondly, we aimed to estimate how many home deaths may have been planned. Lastly, we wanted to analyse differences in individual characteristics between people where home deaths may have been planned, and people where home death did not appear to have been planned.

Method

Data source

We linked data from the Norwegian Cause of Death Registry (NCoDR) and National registry for statistics on municipal health and care services (IPLOS) covering all 83,434 deaths in Norway in 2012 and 2013. Individuals with missing information about place of death or sex ($n = 2526$) were excluded. The final study sample comprised 80,908 individuals.

Information on causes and place of death are registered in NCoDR [17]. In Norway, the doctor who examines the dead body completes the death certificate. This could be the treating general practitioner or institutional doctor, but also a doctor on night duty. The document is sent to the local county court/police, then to the Chief Municipal Medical Officer, before reaching NCoDR. The registry encompasses all residents, irrespective of whether they die in Norway or abroad, and since 2012 also information on deaths for non-residents. NCoDR has a high degree of coverage and completeness, with medical information on more than 98% of all deaths. Three quality assessments have ranked NCoDR in the second best group with "medium" and "medium-high" quality respectively, and lastly in the best group regarding quality. In all these three studies, the extensive use of unspecific codes served to lower the score. Few validation studies have been conducted [17].

IPLOS is a national registry for statistics on municipal health and care services. Since 2007 it has been the main data source for Norwegian municipal health and care statistics. It is compulsory for municipalities to register information on all persons who apply for or receive municipal health and care services, describing the person's resources, need of assistance and services provided. Hospital admissions are also registered, but not used here due to poor data quality. Updates are continuously registered, and sent to the register annually. Data quality is assessed by comparison with information in other official statistics (KOSTRA – Municipality-State-Reporting) and reports returned to the municipalities [18, 19].

Outcome measures

NCoDR provided information regarding cause of death, place of death, age, sex and place of residence (municipality population and centrality). IPLOS provided information regarding municipal services and household. We divided place of death into four categories: home; nursing home; hospital; other (abroad, under transportation to hospital, other). Cause of death was given by the European Shortlist for Causes of Death (EU Shortlist) [20]. Persons missing cause of death, with diagnoses removed due to privacy or with cause of death main diagnosis groups with a frequency of less than 5% of all deaths were labelled "other". We grouped cause of death into eight categories: 'Infectious/parasitic'; 'Symptoms/signs/ill-defined'; 'External'; 'Cancer' (including uncertain malignancy potential); 'Dementia'; 'Circulatory'; 'Respiratory'; 'Other'. Age at time of death was divided into seven groups (0–39, 40–49, 50–59, 60–69, 70–79, 80–89, 90+ years). Municipality centrality was defined as a municipality's geographic location in relation to a centre with important central functions, where 0 is least central (rural) and 3 is most central (urban) [21]. Domiciliary care was coded 'yes' if an individual received practical help or home nursing at any time 0–90 days before death. Nursing home was coded 'yes' if an individual had a stay of any duration in a nursing home or rehabilitation facility 0–90 days before death. Individuals residing in assisted living accommodations with separate apartments were coded as living alone by IPLOS, while individuals in long-term institutional care were coded as cohabiting [18].

Planned and unplanned home deaths

We created an algorithm to estimate potentially planned and unplanned home deaths (Fig. 1). A home death was defined as unplanned if a person did not receive domiciliary care during the last ninety days before death or if a person who died at home with domiciliary care had cause of death 'Symptoms/signs/ill-defined'. 'Symptoms/signs/ill-defined' were labelled unplanned, since people who have a planned home death would most likely have a known diagnosis of life-threatening disease later appearing as underlying cause of death in the death certificate; as opposed to people dying at home suddenly, but not unexpectedly of an unspecific cause. We defined a home death as potentially planned if a person had domiciliary care and a cause of death among the most likely diagnoses to receive palliative care. These were according to the EU Shortlist: 'Cancer' (2.), 'Heart disease' (7.1.2/7.1, 7.2.2, 7.4), 'Chronic pulmonary disease' (8.3.2),

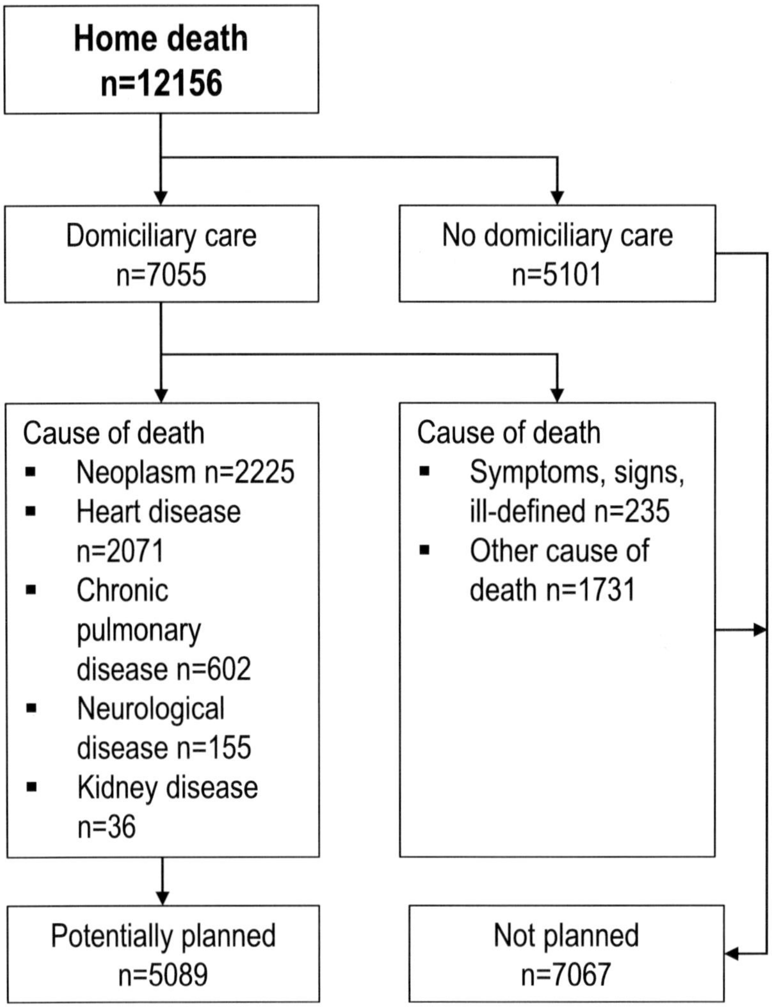

Fig. 1 Algorithm for potentially planned and unplanned home deaths

'Kidney disease' (12.1) and 'Neurological disease' (6.1, 6.3) [20, 22]. Because the majority of people with dementia die in nursing homes, cause of death from 'Dementia' was not included [23]. The remaining home deaths were categorised as unplanned. The age group 0–39 years was given a lower detail level for cause of death than older age groups due to privacy. Cause of death was divided into six categories according to diagnoses most likely to receive palliative care: 'Cancer'; 'Circulatory'; 'Respiratory'; 'Kidney'; 'Neurological'; 'Other'.

Analyses

We used frequency tables and Pearson Chi-square for comparisons. Multinomial logistic regression was used to compare death at home, in nursing home and hospital. Independent variables were sex, age, cause of death, municipality centrality, municipality population and domiciliary care. We did a similar analysis including type of household as explanatory variable in a subpopulation of people who received municipal care at any time (registered in IPLOS). Results are presented as adjusted relative risk ratios (RRRs) with 95% confidence intervals (CI) and *p*-values. xWe used logistic regression to compare potentially planned and unplanned home deaths. Independent variables were sex, age, municipality population, municipality centrality and nursing home stay (model 1). We did a separate analysis for people who received municipal care at any time (registered in IPLOS) with household as an explanatory variable (model 2). Unadjusted and adjusted odds ratios (ORs) with 95% CI and p-values are presented. Significance was accepted at the 5% level ($p < 0.05$) for all analyses. Analyses were conducted with STATA 14 (Stata Corp, College Station, TX).

Results

Describing the population

Among 80,908 deaths 12,156 (15.0%) were classified as home deaths. In total, more women died, with the majority (56.5%) dying in nursing homes (Table 1). While 18.1% of all men died at home, only 12.2% of all women died at home.

Absolute number of home deaths was higher in the older age groups. However, within each age group, home death was more frequent for younger persons (Fig. 2). In people 0–69 years, 26.5% died at home, 19.7% in a nursing home, 44.6% in a hospital and 9.2% in other locations. Only 11.8% of people 70 years or older died at home, while 56.8% died in a nursing home, 30.1% in a hospital and 1.3% in other locations. The most common causes of death were 'Circulatory diseases', 'Cancer', 'Respiratory diseases', 'Infectious diseases' and 'Dementia' (Table 1). 'Circulatory diseases' (34.9%) and 'Cancer' (21.8%) were also the most frequent causes of death within the home death group, while only 2.3% were from 'Dementia'.

A large proportion of deaths had missing information regarding household, largely reflecting people who never received municipal care (Table 1). For those who had services at any time, people living alone (14.2%) died at home more often than those living with others (9.5%). In total, 11.6% had a nursing home stay and 58.0% received domiciliary care in the last 90 days before dying at home. Of all persons who had a nursing home stay in the last 90 days before death, 3.0% died at home, while 17.9% of those receiving domiciliary care died at home.

Comparing home deaths with deaths in nursing homes and hospitals

Multinomial regression showed that women had a lower relative risk than men for dying at home compared with nursing home (Table 2). We found an age gradient with more home deaths in younger age groups, except for people aged 90 years or older who had a higher relative risk for dying at home than in a hospital, but highest relative risk of dying in a nursing home. People who died from 'Cancer' and 'Respiratory disease' had lower relative risk of home death than 'Circulatory disease' compared with nursing home and hospital. People with 'Dementia' had higher relative risk of dying in nursing homes than home, but lower relative risk of dying in hospitals. Recipients of domiciliary care had higher relative risk of dying at home than in nursing homes or hospitals. A similar regression analysis with only persons who at any time had received municipal care (registered in IPLOS), including household as independent variable, did not alter main findings, but showed that people living with others had lower relative risk of home death compared with death in nursing home (RRR 0.77, 95% CI 0.73, 0.82) and hospital (RRR 0.90, 95% CI 0.87, 0.94).

Comparing potentially planned and unplanned home deaths

According to our algorithm for estimating potentially planned and unplanned home deaths (Fig. 1), 56.1% of home deaths and 8.4% of all deaths were potentially planned home deaths when we included everyone with domiciliary care but not 'Symptoms/signs/ill-defined' causes of death. In the full algorithm, including cause of death, 41.9% of home deaths and 6.3% of all deaths were potentially planned home deaths. Men had a higher proportion of both potentially planned and unplanned home deaths than women (Table 3). In people aged 50 years or older 44.5% of home deaths were potentially planned, but only 15.7% in those younger than 50 years. Living alone was more frequent in both potentially planned and unplanned home deaths, but more than half of unplanned home deaths had missing information regarding household, making comparisons uncertain. While 84.0% of 'Cancer' home deaths were potentially planned, this constituted only 10.2% of all 'Cancer' deaths. The proportion of potentially planned home deaths among all home deaths and total number of deaths for each diagnosis were 76.4% and 8.5% in 'Neurological disease', 69.2% and 7.4% in 'Renal disease', 63.2% and 7.3% in 'Respiratory disease' and 48.8% and 8.3% in 'Circulatory disease', respectively. Moreover, 72.1% of all home deaths and 12.9% of all deaths were potentially planned in recipients of domiciliary care.

Table 4 compares two regression models of potentially planned versus unplanned home deaths. In model 1, including all home deaths, women had higher odds than men for having a potentially planned home death, but in model 2, which was restricted to include people who at any time had received municipal care, women had lower odds for having a potentially planned home death. Higher age was associated with more potentially planned home deaths, but in model 2 ages 60–79 years had the highest odds, with declining odds in older age groups. Municipalities with less than 50,000 inhabitants were consistently associated with more potentially planned home deaths, of which municipalities with 5001–10,000 inhabitants had the highest odds. A nursing home stay during the last 90 days before death was associated with higher odds for a potentially planned home death in model 1, but had lower odds in model 2. Living together with someone increased the odds for a potentially planned home death in model 2.

Discussion

Main findings

This population-based registry study showed that home death in Norway was most frequent in 'Circulatory disease' and 'Cancer', and associated with male

Table 1 Distribution of sociodemographic factors and municipal healthcare services by place of death in Norway 2012–2013.*

	Place of death									
	Home		Nursing home		Hospital		Other[a]		Total	
	n	%	n	%	n	%	n	%	n	%
All	12,156	100	39,345	100	26,962	100	2445	100	80,908	100
Sex										
Female	5175	42.6	23,904	60.8	12,613	46.8	598	24.5	42,290	52.3
Male	6981	57.4	15,441	39.2	14,349	53.2	1847	75.5	38,618	47.7
Age (years)										
0–39	549	4.5	70	0.2	796	3.0	426	17.4	1841	2.3
40–49	550	4.5	191	0.5	724	2.7	263	10.8	1728	2.1
50–59	1249	10.3	776	2.0	1877	7.0	389	15.9	4291	5.3
60–69	2381	19.6	2477	6.3	4553	16.9	564	23.1	9975	12.3
70–79	2538	20.9	5917	15.0	6212	23.0	386	15.8	15,053	18.6
80–89	3293	27.1	16,595	42.2	9134	33.9	338	13.8	29,360	36.3
90+	1596	13.1	13,319	33.9	3666	13.6	79	3.2	18,660	23.1
Cause of death										
Infectious/parasitic	1077	8.9	3562	9.1	2131	7.9	264	10.8	7034	8.7
Cancer	2648	21.8	10,728	27.3	8431	31.3	106	4.3	21,913	27.1
Dementia	274	2.3	4951	12.6	211	0.8	11	0.5	5447	6.7
Circulatory	4244	34.9	11,341	28.8	8692	32.2	727	29.7	25,004	30.9
Respiratory	952	7.8	4078	10.4	3117	11.6	65	2.7	8212	10.2
Symptoms/signs/ill-defined	603	5.0	343	0.9	39	0.1	340	13.9	1325	1.6
External causes	754	6.2	416	1.1	788	2.9	657	26.9	2615	3.2
Other	1604	13.2	3926	10.0	3553	13.2	275	11.2	9358	11.6
Household										
Cohabiting	3231	26.6	21,727	55.2	8692	32.2	240	9.8	33,890	41.9
Living alone	4038	33.2	15,341	39.0	8825	32.7	336	13.7	28,540	35.3
Missing[b]	4887	40.2	2277	5.8	9445	35.0	1869	76.4	18,478	22.8
Municipality population										
0–2000	425	3.5	1472	3.7	767	2.8	123	5.0	2787	3.4
2001–5000	1460	12.0	4733	12.0	2508	9.3	271	11.1	8972	11.1
5001–10,000	1795	14.8	5579	14.2	3381	12.5	354	14.5	11,109	13.7
10,001–50,000	4840	39.8	14,844	37.7	10,504	39.0	903	36.9	31,091	38.4
50,001-	3603	29.6	12,632	32.1	9683	35.9	746	30.5	26,664	33.0
Missing[b]	33	0.3	85	0.2	119	0.4	48	2.0	285	0.4
Municipality centrality[c]										
Least central	1531	12.6	5129	13.0	2850	10.6	346	14.2	9856	12.2
Less central	858	7.1	2664	6.8	1859	6.9	201	8.2	5582	6.9
Somewhat central	2431	20.0	7651	19.4	4954	18.4	393	16.1	15,429	19.1
Central	7303	60.1	23,816	60.5	17,180	63.7	1457	59.6	49,756	61.5
Missing[b]	33	0.3	85	0.2	119	0.4	48	2.0	285	0.4
Nursing home[d]										
Yes	1448	11.9	39,945	100.0	7945	29.5	139	5.7	48,877	60.4
No	10,708	88.1	0	0.0	19,017	70.5	2306	94.3	32,031	39.6

Table 1 Distribution of sociodemographic factors and municipal healthcare services by place of death in Norway 2012–2013.* *(Continued)*

	Place of death									
	Home		Nursing home		Hospital		Other[a]		Total	
	n	%	n	%	n	%	n	%	n	%
Domiciliary care[d]										
Yes	7055	58.0	16,455	41.8	15,456	57.3	479	19.6	39,445	48.8
No	5101	42.0	22,890	58.2	11,506	42.7	1966	80.4	41,463	51.2

*Pearson chi-square test: $p < 0.001$ for all categories
[a]Other place of death includes abroad, under transportation to hospital, other specified
[b]Not included in statistical analysis
[c]Classification based on geographical distance to centre with higher functions
[d]Service any time in the period 0–90 days before death

sex, younger age, receiving domiciliary care and living alone. In total, 41.9% of home deaths and 6.3% of all deaths were potentially planned. Potentially planned home deaths were associated with higher age, but declined in ages above 80 years for people who had municipal care. Living together with someone was associated with more potentially planned home deaths for people with municipal care.

Strengths and limitations

To our knowledge, this is the first study to estimate number of potentially planned home deaths by using population-based registry data. The use of routinely collected data, minimises the burden on patients and caregivers, associated with primary data collection in end-of-life care context [24]. The use of death certificates is similar across countries and comparable. NCoDR provides cause of death for more than 98% of all deaths in Norway, but has high use of unspecific cause of death codes increasing the risk of misclassification. Additionally, few diagnoses are verified by autopsy [17]. The study accounts for domiciliary care and nursing home admissions prior to death, but it is a limitation that we do not have information regarding hospital admissions. A methodological limitation is that we have no exact data on planned home deaths, but use an indirect approach by an algorithm. However, there is no registry based information source available as an alternative. A limitation for some analyses is that information regarding whether a person lived alone or together with others was only available for people who had received municipal care. Our definition of a potentially planned home death may also have led to deaths from acute illness being classified as potentially planned. Moreover, we cannot exclude that persons with other

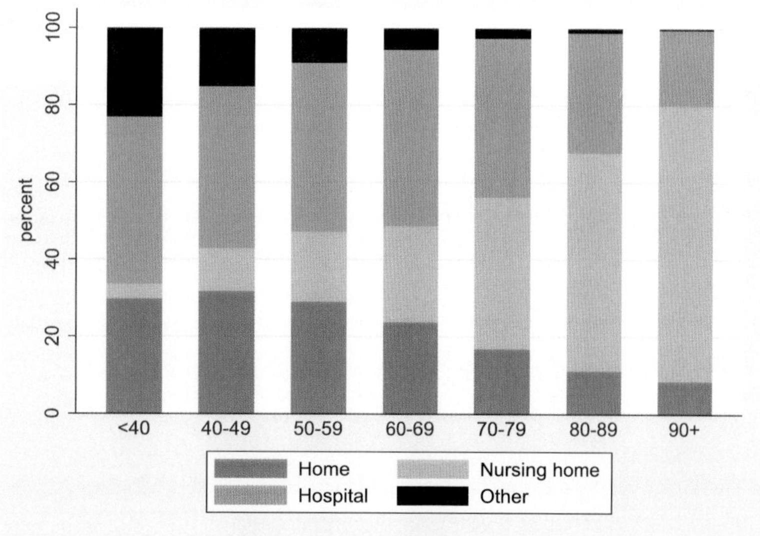

Fig. 2 Distribution of place of death by age groups

Table 2 Adjusted relative risk ratio (RRR) for death at home versus nursing home, and home versus hospital[a]

	Home versus nursing home[a]			Home versus hospital[a]		
	Adjusted RRR	CI	p	Adjusted RRR	CI	p
Sex						
Female	0.67	0.64, 0.71	< 0.001	0.97	0.93, 1.02	0.223
Male	Ref.			Ref.		
Age						
0–39	49.76	38.34, 64.58	< 0.001	2.21	1.94, 2.51	< 0.001
40–49	19.77	16.55, 23.61	< 0.001	2.61	2.31, 2.96	< 0.001
50–59	11.71	10.55, 12.99	< 0.001	2.38	2.18, 2.60	< 0.001
60–69	7.20	6.68, 7.75	< 0.001	1.91	1.78, 2.04	< 0.001
70–79	2.71	2.55, 2.89	< 0.001	1.32	1.24, 1.41	< 0.001
80–89	Ref.			Ref.		
90+	0.55	0.52, 0.59	< 0.001	1.11	1.03, 1.19	0.006
Cause of death						
Infectious and parasitic diseases	0.95	0.88, 1.04	0.267	1.03	0.95, 1.12	0.461
Cancer	0.22	0.21, 0.24	< 0.001	0.48	0.45, 0.51	< 0.001
Dementia	0.23	0.20, 0.26	< 0.001	3.18	2.64, 3.82	< 0.001
Circulatory	Ref.			Ref.		
Respiratory	0.51	0.47, 0.56	< 0.001	0.60	0.55, 0.65	< 0.001
Symptoms/signs/ill-defined	3.84	3.29, 4.48	< 0.001	32.21	23.22, 44.71	< 0.001
External causes	1.92	1.66, 2.21	< 0.001	1.55	1.38, 1.74	< 0.001
Other	0.58	0.54, 0.63	< 0.001	0.76	0.71, 0.82	< 0.001
		Municipality population				
0–2000	1.11	0.97, 1.28	0.135	1.67	1.45, 1.93	< 0.001
2001–5000	1.13	1.03, 1.24	0008	1.73	1.58, 1.93	< 0.001
5001–10,000	1.11	1.02, 1.20	0.014	1.54	1.42, 1.66	< 0.001
10,001–50,000	1.06	1.00, 1.13	0.033	1.30	1.23, 1.37	< 0.001
50,001-	Ref.			Ref.		
Municipality centrality						
Least central	0.95	0.87, 1.03	0.227	0.94	0.86, 1.03	0.198
Less central	1.07	0.97, 1 17	0.190	0.90	0.82, 0.99	0.024
Somewhat central	1.02	0.96, 1.09	0.465	1.01	0.95, 1.07	0.839
Central	Ref.			Ref.		
Domiciliary care						
Yes	2.70	2.58, 2.83	< 0.001	1.35	1.29, 1.42	< 0.001
No	Ref.			Ref.		

[a]Multinomial logistic regression with place of death as dependent variable. Number of observations 78,226

diagnoses than included in our definition may have had planned home deaths.

Few potentially planned home deaths

Our data cannot give information regarding a person's preference for dying at home. However, we will argue that our estimation of potentially planned home deaths in Norway is a valid indication. Planned home death is not feasible without the support of domiciliary care and not probable when cause of death is unknown. Even if there is no preference of dying at home, domiciliary care in itself signals facilitation of more time at home and increases the probability of dying at home [25]. Thus, the highest proportion of home deaths that was not random, and could potentially have been planned, was 56.1% or 8.4% of all deaths in our model. However, it is likely that

Table 3 Comparing potentially planned home deaths with unplanned home deaths and all deaths[a]

	Potentially planned home death		Unplanned home death			All deaths	
	n	%	n	%	p	n	%
All	5089	100	7067	100		80,908	100
Sex					< 0.001		
Female	2458	48.3	2717	38.5		42,290	52.3
Male	2631	51.7	4350	61.5		38,618	47.7
Age (years)					< 0.001		
0–39	60	1.2	489	6.9		1841	2.3
40–49	113	2.2	437	6.2		1728	2.1
50–59	367	7.2	882	12.5		4291	5.3
60–69	887	17.4	1494	21.1		9975	12.3
70–79	1115	21.9	1423	20.1		15,053	18.6
80–89	1673	32.9	1620	22.9		29,360	36.3
90+	874	17.2	722	10.2		18,660	23.1
Cause of death[b]					< 0.001		
Cancer	2225	43.7	423	6.0		21,913	27.1
Circulatory	2071	40.7	2173	30.7		25,004	30.9
Respiratory	602	11.8	350	5.0		8212	10.2
Neurological	155	3.0	48	0.7		1819	2.2
Renal	36	0.7	16	0.2		489	0.6
Other	0	0.0	4057	57.4		23,471	29.0
Household					< 0.001		
Cohabiting	2273	44.7	958	13.6		33,890	41.9
Living alone	2366	46.5	1672	23.7		28,540	35.3
Missing[c]	450	8.8	4437	62.8		18,478	22.8
Municipality population					< 0.001		
0–2000	175	3.4	250	3.5		2787	3.4
2001–5000	651	12.8	809	11.4		8972	11.1
5001–10,000	826	16.2	969	13.7		11,109	13.7
10,001–50,000	2092	41.1	2748	38.9		31,091	38.4
50,001-	1337	26.3	2266	32.1		26,664	33.0
Missing[c]	8	0.2	25	0.4		285	0.4
Municipality centrality					< 0.001		
Least central	647	12.7	884	12.5		9856	12.2
Less central	377	7.4	481	6.8		5582	6.9
Somewhat central	1071	21.0	1360	19.2		15,429	19.1
Central	2986	58.7	4317	61.1		49,756	61.5
Missing[c]	8	0.2	25	0.4		285	0.4
Nursing home[d]					< 0.001		
Yes	860	16.9	549	7.8		46,638	57.6
No	4229	83.1	6518	92.2		34,270	42.2
Domiciliary care[d]					< 0.001		
Yes	5089	100.0	1966	27.8		39,445	48.8
No	0	0.0	5101	72.2		41,463	51.2

[a]P Pearson chi-square test for planned and unplanned home deaths
[b]Cause of death was divided into five categories according to diagnoses most likely to receive palliative care, the rest were labelled other
[c]Not included in statistical analysis
[d]Service any time in the period 0–90 days before death

Table 4 Odds ratio (OR) for potentially planned home death compared with unplanned home death [a]

	Unadjusted			Model 1			Model 2		
	OR	CI	*p*	Adjusted OR	CI	*p*	Adjusted OR	CI	*p*
Sex									
Female	1.50	(1.39, 1.61)	< 0.001	1.29	(1.20, 1.40)	< 0.001	0.90	(0.81, 0.99)	0.039
Male	Ref.			Ref.			Ref.		
Age									
0–39	0.12	(0.09, 0.16)	< 0.001	0.14	(0.11, 0.18)	< 0.001	0.19	(0.13, 0.26)	< 0.001
40–49	0.25	(0.20, 0.31)	< 0.001	0.29	(0.23, 0.37)	< 0.001	0.41	(0.31, 0.54)	< 0.001
50–59	0.40	(0.35, 0.46)	< 0.001	0.46	(0.40, 0.53)	< 0.001	0.71	(0.59, 0.87)	0.001
60–69	0.57	(0.52, 0.64)	< 0.001	0.65	(0.58, 0.72)	< 0.001	1.26	(1.07, 1.48)	0.005
70–79	0.76	(0.68, 0.84)	< 0.001	0.82	(0.74, 0.91)	< 0.001	1.32	(1.14, 1.52)	< 0.001
80–89	Ref.			Ref.			Ref.		
90+	1.17	(1.04, 1.32)	0.009	1.10	(0.97, 1.25)	0.122	0.80	(0.70, 0.92)	0.002
Municipality population									
0–2000	1.19	(0.97, 1.46)	0.102	1.29	(1.02, 1.64)	0.032	1.40	(1.01, 1.95)	0.043
2001–5000	1.36	(1.21, 1.54)	< 0.001	1.36	(1.17, 1.58)	< 0.001	1.40	(1.15, 1.71)	0.001
5001–10,000	1.44	(1.29, 1.62)	< 0.001	1.46	(1.28, 1.67)	< 0.001	1.47	(1.22, 1.75)	< 0.001
10,001–50,000	1.29	(1.18, 1.41)	< 0.001	1.27	(1.15, 1.40)	< 0.001	1.27	(1.12, 1.44)	< 0.001
50,001-	Ref.			Ref.			Ref.		
Municipality centrality									
Least central	1.06	(0.95, 1.18)	0.321	0.85	(0.74, 0.99)	0.031	0.94	(0.78, 1.15)	0.570
Less central	1.13	(0.98, 1.31)	0.086	0.99	(0.85, 1.16)	0.923	1.02	(0.82, 1.26)	0.868
Somewhat central	1.14	(1.04, 1.25)	0.006	0.99	(0.89, 1.10)	0.877	0.99	(0.86, 1.14)	0.904
Central	Ref.			Ref.			Ref.		
Nursing home									
Yes	2.44	(2.18, 2.73)	< 0.001	2.00	(1.78, 2.25)	< 0.001	0.78	(0.68, 0.88)	< 0.001
No	Ref.			Ref.			Ref.		
Household									
Cohabiting	1.68	(1.52, 1.85)	< 0.001				1.62	(1.46, 1.80)	< 0.001
Living alone	Ref.						Ref.		

[a]unadjusted, adjusted model 1 for all home deaths ($n = 12,123$) and adjusted model 2 for persons who had received municipal care ($n = 7261$)

the proportion of potentially planned home deaths is even lower in Norway than our final estimation (41.9% of home deaths and 6.3% of all deaths), as palliative care is mostly given to people with cancer [22, 26].

Most research regarding planned home deaths are interventions trying to enable more home deaths, with little data on the actual rate of planned home deaths before the intervention [27]. We found that only 49% of home deaths from 'Circulatory disease' were potentially planned, while 84% of home deaths from 'Cancer' were potentially planned. This indicates a large proportion of sudden or unexpected home deaths from 'Circulatory disease', but could also indicate inequality between these groups in recognition of palliative care needs [28, 29].

Comparison with previous research

Previous studies have shown that the proportion of home deaths is associated with low functional status, preferences on place of death, home care and its intensity, living with relatives, extended family support, home palliative care, not living in urban areas, higher socio-economic status and being male [8, 14, 16, 25]. Other factors influencing home death are culture, ethnicity and number of hospital and nursing home beds. The relationship with age is more complicated [8, 14, 16, 25].

We found that living alone was associated with more home death. This should be interpreted with caution as we had a large proportion of missing data, but could indicate a large proportion of unexpected home deaths for people living alone. However, in a subpopulation of people who had received municipal care, potentially planned home deaths were associated with living together with someone.

There is no consensus definition on rurality, but there is consistency in associations with place of death across definitions [30]. We did not find any association with our definition of rural areas [21], but municipalities with fewer inhabitants were associated with more home death compared to hospital and also with more potentially planned home deaths. This indicates that other factors than travelling distance to hospitals influence proportion of home deaths. Home nursing coverage could be a contributing factor, as smaller municipalities in Norway have better home nursing coverage than larger municipalities. The largest cities have higher coverage of long-term care in institutions and the lowest coverage of home nursing, which could shift end-of-life care to nursing homes instead of home [31].

Our results also showed that fewer women died at home than men. The association was significant when compared to nursing home, similar to a Swedish study [9]. A possible explanation could be that women care for their spouses and live longer, but the association was present also after adjusting for age and living together with someone. Another explanation could be that men have more sudden and unexpected home deaths, as only men had home deaths from external causes of death or symptoms/signs/ill-defined and more unplanned home deaths from circulatory disease. Still, men had higher odds of a potentially planned home death in the subpopulation who had received municipal care.

Like many other countries, Norway has experienced declining home death rates and a shift from hospital to nursing home deaths [6, 8, 14] . This is partly due to population aging but also end-of-life care policy [2–4, 6]. Incongruence between preferred and actual place of death is common, especially for people with non-malignant disease [29]. Dying in their preferred place is considered a quality indicator of care, and should together with evidence that a majority of people prefer to die at home, be reflected in future planning of palliative care services [1, 32].

Transitions in the last phase of life is another important factor to consider when evaluating quality of end-of-life care. Transitions in the last months and days before death are common, with more than half of dying people having at least one transition [33, 34]. Transitions are shown to be more common in home-dwelling people, where about half have a final transition from home to hospital [33, 34]. Groff et al. found an inverse relationship between number of days in domiciliary care and days spent at home in the last six months before death, interpreted as doing more of one thing led to doing more in other areas as well, and did not necessarily improve patient-centred goals [35]. Although home death will never be a goal or possible for all dying people, a more person-centred goal like "days spent at home" could change the perspective of both the dying person and caregivers and lead to increased time spent at home in the final phase of life, and together with palliative homecare reduce symptom burden and increase chances of home death according to the person's own wishes [27, 36, 37].

Conclusions

This registry based study from Norway shows that home death is relatively infrequent, and by an indirect algorithm-based definition, we have shown that less than half of them are potentially planned home deaths. Future research should investigate how many deaths that are actually planned to take place at home, and the achievement of this goal. There is also a need to understand the transitions in the last phase of life and whether the place of death corresponds to the patients' wish, and how palliative homecare influences such outcomes.

Abbreviations

EU Shortlist: European Shortlist for Causes of Death; RRR: Relative risk ratio; IPLOS: National registry for statistics on municipal health and care services; NCoDR: Norwegian Cause of Death Registry

Acknowledgements

We thank the NCoDR and IPLOS for providing us with data, and the Centre for Elderly and Nursing Home Medicine, University of Bergen, for providing a scientific environment.

Funding

The author(s) disclosed receipt of the following financial support for the research, authorship and/or publication of this article: *Epidemiology of home death in Norway* is supported by the Department of Global Health and Primary Care at the University of Bergen, the G.C. Rieber Foundation and National Centre for Emergency Primary Health Care, Uni Research Health.

Authors' contributions

CK performed study procedures, analysis of data and was responsible for drafting and editing of the manuscript. SH participated in the conception and design of the study, interpretation of the data, and took part in drafting and editing the manuscript. HS participated in the analysis and interpretation of the data and revising the manuscript. BSH participated in the conception and design of the study and revising the manuscript. EF participated in the conception and design of the study and revising the manuscript. All authors read and approved the final manuscript.

Competing interests
The authors declare that they have no competing interests.

Author details
[1]Research Group for General Practice, Department of Global Public Health and Primary Care, University of Bergen, PO box 7804, N-5018 Bergen, Norway. [2]Centre for Elderly and Nursing Home Medicine, Department of Global Public Health and Primary Care, University of Bergen, PO box 7804, N-5018 Bergen, Norway. [3]Bergen Municipality, Bergen, Norway. [4]National Centre for Emergency Primary Health Care, Uni Research Health, Kalfarveien 31, N-5018 Bergen, Norway. [5]Department of Clinical Psychology, University of Bergen, PO box 7804, N-5018 Bergen, Norway.

References

1. Gomes B, Calanzani N, Gysels M, Hall S, Higginson IJ. Heterogeneity and changes in preferences for dying at home: a systematic review. BMC Palliat Care. 2013;12:7.
2. Gomes B, Calanzani N, Higginson IJ. Reversal of the British trends in place of death: time series analysis 2004–2010. Palliat Med. 2012;26:102–7.
3. Wilson DM, Truman CD, Thomas R, Fainsinger R, Kovacs-Burns K, Froggatt K, Justice C. The rapidly changing location of death in Canada, 1994-2004. Soc Sci Med. 2009;68:1752–8.
4. Teno JM, Gozalo PL, Bynum JW, et al. Change in end-of-life care for medicare beneficiaries: site of death, place of care, and health care transitions in 2000, 2005, and 2009. JAMA. 2013;309:470–7.
5. Norwegian Institute of Public Health. Table D3 - Deaths by place of death. In: Norwegian Cause of Death Registry. 2015. http://statistikkbank.fhi.no/dar/. Accessed 11 Aug 2017.
6. Kalseth J, Theisen OM. Trends in place of death: the role of demographic and epidemiological shifts in end-of-life care policy. Palliat Med. 2017;31:964–74.
7. Morin L, Aubry R, Frova L, MacLeod R, Wilson DM, Loucka M, et al. Estimating the need for palliative care at the population level: a cross-national study in 12 countries. Palliat Med. 2017;31:526–36.
8. Dasch B, Blum K, Gude P, Bausewein C. Place of death: trends over the course of a decade: a population-based study of death certificates from the years 2001 and 2011. Dtsch Arztebl Int. 2015;112:496–504.
9. Hakanson C, Ohlen J, Morin L, Cohen J. A population-level study of place of death and associated factors in Sweden. Scand J Public Health. 2015;43:744–51.
10. Jarlbaek L. Dødssted i Danmark 2012–2014 – relateret til dødsårsager, alder, køn, regioner og kommuner. Report no. 4. In: REPHA, Videncenter for Rehabilitering og Palliation. 2017. http://www.rehpa.dk/wp-content/uploads/2017/06/2017-4_D%C3%B8dssted-DK-2012-2014-final.pdf. Accessed 28 Nov 2017.
11. Cohen J, Pivodic L, Miccinesi G, Onwuteaka-Philipsen BD, Naylor WA, Wilson DM, et al. International study of the place of death of people with cancer: a population-level comparison of 14 countries across 4 continents using death certificate data. Brit J Cancer. 2015;113:1397–404.
12. Houttekier D, Cohen J, Surkyn J, Deliens L. Study of recent and future trends in place of death in Belgium using death certificate data: a shift from hospitals to care homes. BMC Public Health. 2011;11:228.
13. Reich O, Signorell A, Busato A. Place of death and health care utilization for people in the last 6 months of life in Switzerland: a retrospective analysis using administrative data. BMC Health Serv Res. 2013;13:116.
14. Black H, Waugh C, Munoz-Arroyo R, Carnon A, Allan A, Clark D, et al. Predictors of place of death in south West Scotland 2000-2010: retrospective cohort study. Palliat Med. 2016;30:764–71.
15. Gisquet E, Julliard S, Geoffroy-Perez B. Do social factors affect the place of death? Analysis of home versus institutional death over 20 years. J Public Health (Oxf). 2016;38:e472–9.
16. Cohen J, Houttekier D, Onwuteaka-Philipsen B, Miccinesi G, Addington-Hall J, Kaasa S, et al. Which patients with cancer die at home? A study of six European countries using death certificate data. J Clin Oncol. 2010;28:2267–73.
17. Pedersen AG, Ellingsen CL. Data quality in the causes of death registry. Tidsskr Nor Laegeforen. 2015;135:768–70.
18. Norwegian Directorate of Health. IPLOS-registeret. Veileder for personell i kommunale helse- og omsorgstjenester. In: Guideline IS-1112. 2015. https://helsedirektoratet.no/retningslinjer/iplos-veileder-for-personell-i-kommunale-helse-og-omsorgstjenester. Accessed 2 Jun 2017.
19. Mørk EB, S; Haugstveit, FV; Sundby, B; Karlsen, H; Wettergreen, J. Kommunale helse- og omsorgstjenester 2016. In: Report Statistics Norway. Statistikk om tjenester og tjenestemottakere. 2017. https://www.ssb.no/helse/artikler-og-publikasjoner/kommunale-helse-og-omsorgstjenester-2016. Accessed 1 Des 2017.
20. Infrastructre Knowledge Base in Europe (INSPIRE). European shortlist for causes of death. In: 2012; 2012. http://inspire.ec.europa.eu/document/CoD. Accessed 9 Aug 2017.
21. Statistics Norway. Variabeldefinisjon: Sentralitet. 1994. https://www.ssb.no/a/metadata/conceptvariable/vardok/927/nb. Accessed 17 Oct 2017.
22. Melby L, Das A, Halvorsen T, Steihaug S. Evaluering av tjenestetilbudet til personer med behov for lindrende behandling og omsorg in: report for the Norwegian Directorate of Health. Report no. A27799. In: SINTEF; 2017. http://www.sintef.no/globalassets/sintef-teknologi-og-samfunn/avdelinger/helse/20.3.17-rapport-lindrende-behandling_revidert-i-versjonsbeskrivelse-og-i-5.2-002.pdf. Accessed 13 Oct 2017.
23. Norwegian Institute of Public Health. Halvparten av oss dør i sykehjem. 2016. https://www.fhi.no/nyheter/2016/halvparten-av-oss-dor-i-sykehjem/. Accessed 17 Oct 2017.
24. Maetens A, De Schreye R, Faes K, Houttekier D, Deliens L, et al. Using linked administrative and disease-specific databases to study end-of-life care on a population level. BMC Palliat Care. 2016;15:86.
25. Higginson IJ, Sarmento VP, Calanzani N, Benalia H, Gomes B. Dying at home–is it better: a narrative appraisal of the state of the science. Palliat Med. 2013;27:918–24.
26. Cohen J, Beernaert K, Van den Block L, Morin L, Hunt K, Miccinesi G, et al. Differences in place of death between lung cancer and COPD patients: a 14-country study using death certificate data. NPJ Prim Care Respir Med. 2017;27:14.
27. Gomes B, Calanzani N, Curiale V, McCrone P, Higginson IJ. Effectiveness and Cost-effectiveness of home palliative care services for adults with advanced illness and their caregivers. Cochrane Database Syst Rev. 2013;6:CD007760.
28. Gadoud A, Kane E, Macleod U, Ansell P, Oliver S, Johnson M. Palliative care among heart failure patients in primary care: a comparison to cancer patients using English family practice data. PLoS One. 2014;9:e113188.
29. Billingham MJ, Billingham SJ. Congruence between preferred and actual place of death according to the presence of malignant or non-malignant disease: a systematic review and meta-analysis. BMJ Support Palliat Care. 2013;3:144–54.
30. Rainsford S, MacLeod RD, Glasgow NJ. Place of death in rural palliative care: a systematic review. Palliat Med. 2016;30:745–63.
31. Otnes BH, Haugstveit FV. Kommunal variasjon i omsorgstjenester. In Report Statistics Norway Report no 2015/44. 2015. https://www.ssb.no/helse/artikler-og-publikasjoner/kommunal-variasjon-i-omsorgstjenester. Accessed 1 April 2018.
32. De Roo ML, Miccinesi G, Onwuteaka-Philipsen BD, Van Den Noortgate N, Van den Block L, Bonacchi A, et al. Actual and preferred place of death of home-dwelling patients in four European countries: making sense of quality indicators. PLoS One. 2014;9:e93762.
33. Van den Block L, Pivodic L, Pardon K, Donker G, Miccinesi G, Moreels S, et al. Transitions between health care settings in the final three months of life in four EU countries. Eur J Pub Health. 2015;25:569–75.
34. Abraham S, Menec V. Transitions between care settings at the end of life among older homecare recipients: a population-based study. Gerontol Geriatr Med. 2016;2:2333721416684400.
35. Groff AC, Colla CH, Lee TH. Days spent at home - a patient-centered goal and outcome. N Engl J Med. 2016;375:1610–2.
36. Sayer C. NEJM Catalyst. In: "Time spent at home" - a patient-defined outcome; 2016. https://catalyst.nejm.org/time-spent-at-home-a-patient-defined-outcome/. Accessed 10 Nov 2017.
37. Costa V, Earle CC, Esplen MJ, Fowler R, Goldman R, Grossman D, et al. The determinants of home and nursing home death: a systematic review and meta-analysis. BMC Palliat Care. 2016;15:8.

Use of hospital palliative care according to the place of death and disease one year before death in 2013

Claire Poulalhon[1], Laureen Rotelli-Bihet[2], Sébastien Moine[3], Anne Fagot-Campagna[1], Régis Aubry[4] and Philippe Tuppin[1*]

Abstract

Background: Only limited data are available concerning the diseases managed before death and hospital palliative care (HPC) use according to place of death in France. We therefore conducted an observational study based on administrative health data in a large population to identify the diseases treated one year before death in 2013, the place of stay with or without hospital palliative care, and the place of death.

Methods: French health insurance general scheme beneficiaries were identified in the National Health data Information System (Snds) with a selection of information. Diseases were identified by algorithms from reimbursement data recorded in the Snds database.

Results: 347,253 people were included in this study (61% of all people who died in France). Place of death was short stay hospital for 51%, Rehab (7%), hospital at home (3%), skilled nursing home (13%) and other (26%). Chronic diseases managed in 2013 before death were cardiovascular/neurovascular diseases (56%), cancers (42%), and neurological and degenerative diseases (25%). During the year before death, 84% of people were hospitalized at least once, and 29% had received HPC. HPC was used by 52% of cancer patients (lung cancer: 62%; prostate cancer: 41%). In the absence of cancer, the use of HPC varied according to the disease: acute stroke: 24%, heart failure: 17%, dementia: 17%, multiple sclerosis: 23%.

Conclusions: Health administrative data can refine the knowledge of the care pathway prior to death and the HPC utilisation and can be useful to evaluate heath policies and improve monitoring and assessment of HPC use.

Keywords: Palliative care, Hospital, Death, Health status, Administrative health data, Place of death, Cancer, End-of-life care

Background

By improving survival, technical and scientific progress in the field of medicine has resulted in a growing burden of chronic diseases and has modified the temporality of the end of life, which may involve the use of palliative care earlier in the course of the disease [1]. In France, one in four people were over the age of 60 years in 2013 for a population of 65.6 million inhabitants, and people over the age of 60 will represent almost one-third of the population in 2060 [2]. This ageing population will lead to an increased number of people with chronic fatal diseases requiring palliative care [3]. Three types of end-of-life pathways have been distinguished: rapid decline, gradual decline with episodes of decompensation, and slow and progressive decline [4]. End of life care is therefore not confined to the last instants of life, but corresponds to a longer period with a high level of health care consumption designed to relieve psychological distress, the patient's symptoms and provide support to caregivers.

* Correspondence: philippe.tuppin@cnamts.fr
[1]National sickness insurance fund, 26-50, avenue du Professeur André Lemierre, 75986 Paris cedex 20, France
Full list of author information is available at the end of the article

In France, a new national plan for the development of end-of-life palliative care and supportive care was launched in 2015 [5]. The previous plan (2008–2012) revealed deficiencies concerning the possibility of maintaining people at home at the end of life with differences in terms of access according to age, place of residence and disease [6]. However, only limited data are available, for France and other countries, concerning the place of death, palliative care needs, palliative care use and end-of-life care pathways according to the patient's characteristics and diseases. These data are derived from studies based on samples or subgroups determined according to the place of management or, more often, causes of death. Hospital diagnoses are less frequently studied using national healthcare administrative databases [7–19]. People needing palliative care in France have been estimated to represent 44% or 69% of deaths on the basis of causes of death associated with a theoretical indication for palliative care [7–9].

The objective of this observational study using administrative health data for a large population was to identify the diseases treated one year before death in 2013, the place of stay with and without hospital palliative care (HPC) and the place of death according to the characteristics of this population.

Methods

Population and settings

This observational study concerned all French national health insurance general scheme beneficiaries (77% of the French population) who died in 2013. The study was confined to this scheme because it systematically records the vital status of its beneficiaries. Individuals without at least one healthcare refund in 2012 and 2013, allowing identification of diseases, and children born in 2013, were excluded. The national health database (Snds) was used to study the various types of hospitals or institutions: short-stay hospitals with acute wards and palliative care facilities (specific wards, mobile teams providing palliative care advice and expertise to other healthcare professionals) and specific beds; rehabilitation (rehab) hospitals, to which people are usually admitted after an acute hospital stay and which are devoted to rehabilitation as well as palliative care depending on their rehabilitation specialization; and hospital at home (HaH) care delivered by hospital teams. Information on skilled nursing home (SNH) stays is available, but not for all retirement homes [20]. Information is not available for mobile teams not specifically attached to HaH units or for ambulatory palliative care provided by general practitioner. Palliative care is provided by specialists in hospital and mainly by general practitioners in SNH. Guidelines on specific pathways and best practices are published by the French National Authority for Health (Haute Autorité de santé, www.has-sante.fr) [21].

Data sources

Data concerning the beneficiaries are collected in the Snds database, which comprises comprehensive, anonymous, individual data concerning all prescriptions, examinations and procedures reimbursed [22]. The Snds database does not contain information on clinical results related to visits, prescriptions or examinations. Nevertheless, it includes information on the presence of certain long-term diseases (LTD) eligible for 100% reimbursement of healthcare. All these data are linked to data concerning hospital stays provided by the French hospital discharge database (PMSI), and residence in SNH. LTD and hospital diagnoses are coded according to the international classification of diseases, 10th edition (ICD-10). There is no data on causes of death.

Data and frequency analysis

HPC in short stay hospitals, Rehab and HaH was identified through palliative care diagnostic codes, specific palliative care beds or classification of the palliative care stay according to the various types of hospitalization. Use of HPC was calculated over the year preceding death including the date of death and at the date of death only. The totals indicated in the tables refer to people receiving HPC during the year before death or at the date of death during the last hospital stay. Information on place of death is available for deaths occurring during hospital stays (short stay hospitals, Rehab or HaH) or in a SNH. Nevertheless, among the "other places" of death, it is not possible to distinguish death at home and death outside home: in a retirement home, in public places, etc. The *Caisse Nationale d'Assurance Maladie* (Cnam) general health scheme fund has developed a tool based on Snds data with algorithms designed to identify beneficiaries reimbursed for chronic diseases and common, serious or expensive diseases and treatments, in order to study these diseases in terms of numbers, prevalence rates, expenditure and annual growth [23]. Information concerning the patients' diseases in 2012 and in 2013 was derived from this tool (Additional file 1). Algorithms identify 56 non-exclusive groups of diseases, classified into 13 main categories, based on principal diagnoses, related or significant associated diagnoses in short-stay hospitals and psychiatric hospitals coded according to ICD-10; long-term disease diagnoses (LTD); dispensing of specific drugs; and specific procedures. Schematically, the term "acute" refers to hospitalization during the year with an appropriate ICD-10 code and the chronic phase is defined by attribution of LTD status during the year and/or hospitalization with specific codes during the last 5 years. The acute episode always takes precedence to a chronic phase and these two groups are mutually exclusive for a given disease. Cancer is defined by short-stay hospitalizations over a 5-year period (specific cancer diagnoses and chemotherapy and radiotherapy codes) and/or LTD status attributed over the previous

2 years. In Tables 2 and 3, two groups were selected: patients with at less a diagnosis of a cancer and patients without diagnosis of cancer but with one or more other diseases. These definitions were submitted to sensitivity analyses concerning the numbers of subjects and the expenditure incurred, and a critical review was conducted by an independent partner, allowing improvement of these algorithms [24].

Characteristics of people died in 2013 were described including age, gender, residence in a SNH, diseases identified by algorithms, and the presence of at least one admission the year before death in each type of hospital and/or on the day of death. Rates of subjects with HPC among all the subjects died in each type of hospital were also calculated according to subject characteristics and diseases. Figure 1 represents the place of stay of beneficiaries on a given day during the year preceding death.

All frequencies were calculated with SAS Enterprise Guide software (version 4.3; SAS Institute Inc., Cary, NC, USA).

Results

Characteristics

A total of 347,253 general scheme beneficiaries who died in 2013 were included (49.7% men and 50.3% of women) (Table 1). The mean age of death was 77 years (73 years for men, 81 years for women). Deaths before the age of 85 years predominantly concerned men, with a particularly marked sex difference between the ages of 15 and 35 years.

Globally, the diseases most commonly managed before death were cardiovascular/neurovascular diseases (56%), especially heart failure (24%), particularly in women and the oldest people, and coronary heart disease (20%), which was more frequent in men. Deceased people had been managed for cancer in 42% of cases (close to 60%

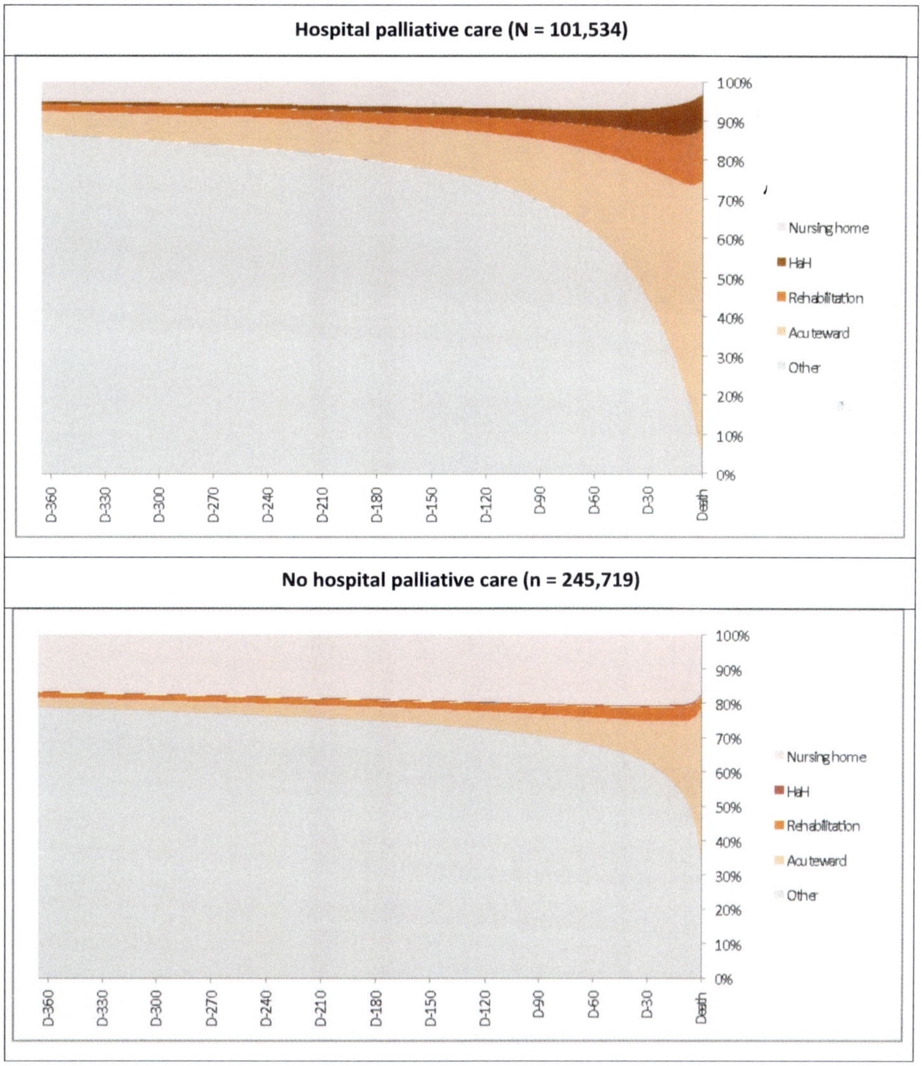

Fig. 1 Setting on a given day the year preceding death and hospital palliative care use

Table 1 Diseases managed of general scheme beneficiaries who died in 2013, according to sex and age

	Total	Sex		Age								
		Men	Women	< 15	15–34	35–44	45–54	55–64	65–74	75–84	85–94	≥ 95
N	347,253	172,591	174,662	1066	4409	7030	18,860	39,656	50,638	89,933	114,652	21,009
%	100.0	49.7	50.3	0.3	1.3	2.0	5.4	11.4	14.6	25.9	33.0	6.1
	%	%	%	%	%	%	%	%	%	%	%	%
Women	50.3	–	–	42.6	32.3	37.2	37.2	34.0	35.6	46.7	63.4	80.9
Age (mean years)	77.0	73.2	80.7	–	–	–	–	–	–	–	–	–
Skilled nursing home resident	21.1	12.8	29.3	–	–	–	–	1.8	5.1	14.0	30.4	42.5
At least one hospitalisation during the year	83.5	85.4	81.6	81.1	59.1	70.6	80.2	85.5	88.5	87.6	82.8	66.5
Short stay hospitals	82.8	84.9	80.7	80.9	58.8	70.1	79.7	85.1	88.1	86.9	81.9	65.3
Rehabilitation	22.6	21.3	24.0	8.4	5.8	8.9	12.9	16.0	19.9	26.4	27.2	17.8
Hospital at home	6.6	7.0	6.2	12.7	6.1	8.2	9.5	10.1	9.3	6.8	4.1	2.6
Diseases managed												
Cardiovascular/neurovascular diseases	56.5	58.4	54.6	16.5	11.4	16.3	24.6	37.9	50.8	63.2	68.8	62.4
Coronary heart disease	20.5	24.6	16.4	0.5	1.2	3.6	7.8	13.9	20.4	24.3	24.0	20.3
Acute stroke	4.9	4.2	5.7	1.3	1.6	2.9	2.9	3.1	4.0	5.9	6.0	3.8
Stroke sequelae	9.5	9.6	9.4	5.1	2.7	2.8	4.0	5.9	8.4	10.8	11.7	10.4
Heart failure	24.3	23.0	25.7	5.3	3.5	4.5	6.5	10.5	17.2	26.7	34.2	32.0
Peripheral artery disease	10.7	13.8	7.6	0.5	0.5	1.1	4.1	9.7	12.5	12.6	11.2	9.0
Arrhythmia	27.5	28.0	27.0	4.0	3.1	4.6	6.9	12.3	21.1	32.5	37.4	28.0
Valvular disease	6.8	6.5	7.0	0.3	0.8	1.5	1.7	3.0	5.4	8.5	9.0	5.4
Pulmonary embolism	1.1	1.0	1.2	0.2	0.5	0.9	1.1	1.4	1.5	1.2	1.0	0.5
Diabetes	21.1	23.5	18.7	0.2	2.1	5.3	10.6	19.5	28.5	27.6	18.9	10.3
Cancers	42.1	48.7	35.6	20.6	17.5	31.2	47.1	58.3	58.7	46.6	31.1	17.9
Female breast	4.8	–	9.5	0.0	1.6	5.8	6.7	5.7	5.5	4.9	4.0	3.1
Colon	5.8	6.4	5.2	0.2	1.0	3.0	4.1	6.0	7.5	7.3	5.0	3.1
Lung	6.5	9.5	3.5	0.0	0.9	5.0	11.5	15.7	12.6	5.8	1.8	0.4
Prostate	5.1	10.2	–	0.1	0.0	0.2	0.6	2.2	5.7	7.6	5.6	2.2
Other cancers	26.3	30.4	22.3	20.6	14.9	20.3	29.2	36.2	37.1	29.4	19.0	10.7
Psychiatric disorders	9.7	9.7	9.8	4.8	21.7	27.1	22.6	15.2	10.0	8.0	6.5	4.4
Psychotic disorders	1.8	1.9	1.8	0.1	6.7	7.3	5.1	3.2	2.2	1.4	0.8	0.5
Manic disorders	0.8	0.65	1.0	0.0	1.5	2.5	1.7	1.4	1.0	0.8	0.4	0.2
Depression	2.9	2.3	3.4	0.1	4.8	7.1	6.1	4.1	2.7	2.5	2.2	1.6
Addictive disorders	2.0	3.0	0.9	0.0	8.2	12.2	10.1	5.1	1.9	0.6	0.2	0.1
Psychotropic treatments[a]	27.2	23.9	30.5	4.4	10.1	16.0	20.3	22.9	24.9	27.9	31.2	30.6
Neurological or degenerative diseases	24.6	19.7	29.4	18.6	10.5	10.4	9.7	8.8	11.8	25.7	37.1	33.1
Dementias (Alzheimer)	18.7	13.3	24.1	0.2	0.3	0.4	0.8	1.8	5.6	19.6	32.6	30.3
Parkinson's disease	3.9	4.1	3.7	0.1	0.1	0.0	0.2	0.7	2.4	5.8	5.3	2.8
Multiple sclerosis	0.2	0.2	0.3	0.0	0.3	0.6	0.6	0.6	0.4	0.2	0.1	0.0
Paraplegia	0.4	0.5	0.3	1.2	1.3	1.1	0.7	0.6	0.5	0.3	0.2	0.1
Myopathy, myasthenia	0.2	0.3	0.2	2.5	1.3	0.6	0.5	0.4	0.3	0.2	0.1	0.1
Epilepsy	2.8	3.0	2.6	11.5	5.6	6.6	5.9	4.1	2.9	2.4	2.0	1.2
Chronic respiratory diseases	20.5	24.2	16.8	19.0	7.0	10.4	16.0	22.6	25.1	24.0	18.3	12.3
Inflammatory or rare diseases or HIV or AIDS	4.3	3.9	4.6	9.4	3.9	5.0	5.4	4.4	4.6	4.8	3.9	2.0
Treated renal failure	1.4	1.8	1.1	0.1	0.6	1.1	1.3	1.5	2.4	2.0	0.9	0.2

Table 1 Diseases managed of general scheme beneficiaries who died in 2013, according to sex and age *(Continued)*

	Total	Sex		Age								
		Men	Women	< 15	15–34	35–44	45–54	55–64	65–74	75–84	85–94	≥ 95
N	347,253	172,591	174,662	1066	4409	7030	18,860	39,656	50,638	89,933	114,652	21,009
%	100.0	49.7	50.3	0.3	1.3	2.0	5.4	11.4	14.6	25.9	33.0	6.1
Diseases of the liver or of pancreas	8.9	11.5	6.4	9.2	7.7	15.0	20.6	17.9	14.7	7.9	3.2	1.3
Other long-term diseases	10.8	9.0	12.6	15.6	7.1	6.6	6.8	7.9	9.0	10.6	12.9	15.6
Maternity	0.05	–	0.1	–	1.6	1.1	0.1	–	–	–	–	–
None of health states above	4.4	4.9	3.9	34.4	38.2	19.2	10.0	5.1	2.7	2.1	2.8	6.7

[a]with or without psychiatric disorders

between the ages of 55 and 74 years, men: 49%; women: 36%), dementia in 19% of cases (men: 13%; women: 24%) , and chronic respiratory disease in 20% of cases (men: 24%: women: 18%).

Hospitalizations and place death

During the year preceding death, 83% of people were hospitalized at least once (short stay hospitals: 83%, Rehab: 23%, HaH: 7%) (Table 1). These proportions were slightly higher for men except for hospitalizations in rehabilitation units (men: 21%; women: 24%). Analysis according to age revealed a high hospitalization rate before the age of 15 years (81%), lower rates between the ages of 15 and 34 years (59%), followed by rates that gradually increased with age until the 75 to 84 years age-group (88%). Although the frequency of at least one Rehab admission to a rehabilitation unit increased regularly with age, the frequency of HaH decreased from the 65–74 years age-group. Fig. I present a dynamic view of the proportion of people in each place of residence on a given day during the year before death. The proportion of people receiving HPC at least once during the year and admitted to a short stay hospital on a given day rapidly increased over the months preceding death: 9% six months before death, 16% three months before death, 34% one month before death and 69% on the day of death. An increased admission rate was also observed for rehabilitation units (one month before death: 9%, on the day of death: 13%) and HaH (6% vs 9%). Inversely, the proportion of people not hospitalized and not living in a SNH decreased markedly (one month before death: 44%, 14 days before death: 29%, on the day of death: 6%). The proportion of people living in a SNH started to decrease three weeks before death (6%) to reach 3% on the day of death. These variations differed or were less marked in the absence of HPC during the year before death, with a moderate increase for short stay hospital admissions (six months before death: 4%, three months before death: 6%, one month before death: 13%, on the day of death: 44%), stable Rehab admissions (4%), and a moderate reduction for "other places" of residence (one month before death: 63%, 14 days before death: 55%, on the day of death: 35%) and SNH (three weeks before death: 21%, on the day of death: 17%).

Overall, death occurred in hospital for 58% of deceased people (51% in short stay hospitals, 7% in Rehab), in HaH for 3%, in SNH for 13% and in "other places" for 26% (public place, home, retirement home, etc.) (Table 2). A higher proportion of women died in SNH (19% vs 7% for men), but with a different mean age. A higher proportion of men died in short stay hospitals (55% vs 47% for women) and in "other places" (29% vs 24%). The proportion of deaths in SNH increased markedly after the age of 85 years, while the proportion of deaths in "other places" reached a peak of 60% between the ages of 15 and 34 years and the proportion of deaths in short stay hospitals reached a peak of 60% between the ages of 55 and 74 years. The proportion of deaths in rehabilitation units increased slightly with age and the proportion of deaths in HaH decreased after the age of 74 years. Sixty-four per cent of people managed for cancer died in a short stay hospital, 7% died in a SNH and 16% died outside of a hospital, HaH or a SNH. The proportions of deaths in SNH (16%) and outside of a hospital, HaH or a SNH (23%) were higher among people with cardiovascular diseases (other than cancer) than for the overall population. These proportions were even higher for people with neurological or degenerative diseases: death in a NSH: 35% and death outside of a hospital or a NSH: 23%.

Use of hospital palliative care

Twenty-nine per cent of all deceased people received hospital palliative care at the date of death or during the year preceding death (Table 3). This proportion varied little according to sex (men: 30%; women: 28%), but more markedly according to age, with 30% for people under the age of 15 years and a peak around 39% between the ages of 55 and 74 years; and also according to CMU-C status (presence: 28%; absence: 34%). People managed for cancer received HPC in 52% of cases (lung cancer 62%; prostate cancer: 41%), while people with other diseases, excluding cancer, received HPC in 24% of cases for acute stroke, 17% of cases for heart failure, 23%

Table 2 Place of death in 2013 according to the general scheme beneficiaries characteristics and diseases managed

Place of death		Short stay hospital	Rehab	Hospital at home	Skilled nursing home	Other
	n[a]	%	%	%	%	%
Total	347.3	51.0	6.5	2.8	13.3	26.4
Men	172.6	54.8	6.1	2.9	7.3	28.9
Women	174.7	47.1	6.8	2.8	19.3	23.9
Age (years)						
< 15	1.1	59.7	1.4	4.2		34.7
15–34	44	37.6	0.9	1.7		59.7
35–44	70	45.8	1.6	2.3	0.1	50.2
45–54	189	55.4	3.0	2.8	0.2	38.6
55–64	397	60.7	4.5	3.5	1.2	30.2
65–74	506	62.0	5.6	3.6	3.2	25.7
75–84	89.9	55.3	7.7	3.1	9.8	24.1
85–94	1147	43.6	8.0	2.3	23.5	22.6
≥ 95	210	27.5	5.2	1.8	40.2	25.3
Cancers	146.2	63.6	8.3	4.7	7.0	16.4
Female breast	16.5	58.9	8.2	4.5	11.1	17.3
Colon	20.1	62.0	8.9	5.0	8.0	16.1
Lung	22.5	71.1	8.2	5.0	2.3	13.4
Prostate	17.6	56.5	8.3	4.4	8.9	21.9
Other cancers	91.4	64.9	8.4	4.9	6.5	15.4
Other diseases in the absence of cancer						
Cardiovascular/neurovascular diseases	121.4	53.2	6.5	1.6	16.1	22.6
Coronary heart disease	45.0	56.1	6.3	1.4	13.0	23.2
Acute stroke	12.9	75.5	7.9	1.3	9.1	6.1
Stroke sequelae	21.7	46.2	6.3	2.1	21.9	23.4
Heart failure	57.3	59.3	7.1	1.6	13.9	18.1
Diabetes	43.3	48.2	5.7	1.7	12.5	31.9
Psychiatric disorders	23.9	34.8	4.0	0.8	16.2	44.1
Neurological or degenerative diseases	63.4	37.4	6.0	2.3	31.7	22.6
Dementias (including Alzheimer)	50.2	35.4	6.4	2.2	35.8	20.2
Parkinson's disease	10.0	38.9	6.1	2.6	28.0	24.4
Multiple sclerosis	0.6	48.5	1.8	5.0	12.0	32.7
Paraplegia	0.8	51.0	5.1	3.8	10.1	30.0
Myopathy or myasthenia	0.6	58.4	3.1	3.1	5.9	29.4
Epilepsy	6.1	44.5	4.5	2.3	18.0	30.8
Chronic respiratory diseases	39.0	56.2	5.7	1.6	10.4	26.1
Inflammatory or rare diseases, HIV or AIDS	9.0	55.2	6.1	1.7	11.8	25.2
Treated renal failure	3.3	72.2	3.1	1.6	5.1	18.0
Diseases of the liver or pancreas	14.6	70.5	4.5	1.0	4.2	19.9
Other long-term diseases	24.2	42.9	5.6	2.0	19.8	29.7

[a]Thousand

Table 3 Hospital palliative care use at the time of death, during the last year (total), or before death for people died in a skilled nursing home or in another place according to sex, age and disease managed

Place of deaths	All places			Short stay hospital		Rehab		Hospital at home		Skilled nursing home#		Other[b]	
	N[a]	Death°	Total	N[a]	Total	N[a]	Total	N[a]	Total	N[a]	Before death	N[a]	Before death
		%	%		%		%				%		%
Total	347.3	15.7	29.2	176.9	39.3	22.51	60.0	9.82	88.9	46.3	7.6	91.7	6.7
Men	172.6	16.6	30.9	94.6	40.1	10.55	60.9	4.97	90.2	12.6	9.6	49.8	6.5
Women	174.7	14.9	27.6	82.3	38.5	11.96	59.1	4.84	87.5	33.8	6.8	41.8	7.0
Age (years)													
< 15	1.1	11.5	30.3	0.6	38.2	0.02	93.3	0.05	95.6		–	0.4	6.2
15–34	4.4	6.6	15.8	1.7	33.3	0.04	58.5	0.08	100		–	2.6	1.6
35–44	7.0	10.7	25.4	3.2	45.4	0.11	68.4	0.16	95	0.0	–	3.5	2.6
45–54	18.9	15.9	34.5	10.4	49.7	0.56	80.0	0.54	96.6	0.0	–	7.3	4.8
55–64	39.7	19.4	39.9	24.1	50.5	1.77	79.4	1.38	95.3	0.5	16.0	12.0	7.3
65–74	50.6	19.8	38.8	31.4	46.5	2.81	71.1	1.81	92.8	1.6	14.0	13.0	8.5
75–84	89.9	17.6	31.7	49.8	38.2	6.92	63.3	2.78	89.1	8.8	10.0	21.6	8.2
85–94	114.7	13.3	22.2	50.0	29.9	9.20	50.9	2.66	81.7	26.9	7.3	25.9	6.6
≥ 95	21.0	8.4	13.2	5.8	25.6	1.09	42.9	0.37	77.8	8.4	3.8	5.3	3.9
Cancers	146.2	25.9	51.9	93.0	57.8	12.19	76.4	6.86	94.5	10.3	18.0	23.9	19.0
Female breast	16.5	24.5	50.1	9.7	59.6	1.35	75.7	0.74	93.9	1.8	15.0	2.9	17.0
Colon	20.1	25.9	52.7	12.5	57.9	1.80	76.8	1.01	94.6	1.6	20.0	3.2	22.0
Lung	22.5	30.5	62.5	16.0	65.5	1.84	84.3	1.12	97	0.5	35.0	3.0	25.0
Prostate	17.6	20.8	40.9	9.9	48.0	1.46	67.2	0.78	92.2	1.6	14.0	3.8	13.0
Other cancers	91.4	26.4	53.3	59.3	58.5	7.68	77.1	4.47	94.7	5.9	19.0	14.0	20.0
Other diseases in the absence of cancer													
Cardiovascular/neurovascular diseases	121.4	10.7	15.9	64.6	19.0	7.88	40.3	1.96	74.9	19.5	6.4	27.5	4.0
Coronary heart disease	45.0	*10.0*	14.9	25.3	17.4	2.82	38.3	0.63	76.5	5.9	6.3	10.4	3.6
Acute stroke	12.9	*18.2*	24.3	9.7	22.6	1.02	51.6	0.17	77.9	1.2	16.0	0.8	11.0
Stroke sequelae	21.7	*11.5*	18.0	10.0	24.2	1.37	41.5	0.46	76.6	4.8	6.0	5.1	5.3
Heart failure	57.3	*11.5*	17.3	34.0	19.1	4.07	39.3	0.90	78	8.0	7.0	10.4	5.2
Diabetes	43.3	9.2	14.1	20.9	18.3	2.45	40.2	0.76	75.8	5.4	6.1	13.8	2.9
Psychiatric disorders	23.9	6.6	10.5	8.3	19.1	0.96	36.9	0.20	76.2	3.9	5.1	10.6	1.9
Neurological or degenerative diseases	63.4	10.9	17.4	23.7	27.1	3.83	44.9	1.44	75.4	20.1	5.3	14.3	5.0
Dementias (including Alzheimer)	50.2	*11.0*	17.2	0.0	27.4	3.21	44.7	1.10	75	0.0	5.4	0.0	5.4
Parkinson's disease	10.0	*11.6*	17.7	17.8	27.4	0.61	46.8	0.26	71.7	18.0	4.6	10.1	4.0
Multiple sclerosis	0.6	*10.2*	23.2	3.9	28.9	0.01	63.6	0.03	80	2.8	8.3	2.4	9.2
Paraplegia	0.8	*10.4*	20.6	0.3	26.2	0.04	44.2	0.03	62.5	0.1	5.9	0.2	6.7
Myopathy or myasthenia	0.6	*14.2*	21.2	0.4	27.4	0.02	55.6	0.02	72.2	0.1	2.9	0.3	3.6
Epilepsy	6.1	*11.3*	18.4	0.3	26.3	0.27	52.8	0.14	75.5	0.0	7.2	0.2	4.4
Chronic respiratory diseases	39.0	10.4	16.5	2.7	19.9	2.24	37.7	0.61	77.4	1.1	7.1	1.9	4.4
Inflammatory or rare diseases, HIV or AIDS	9.0	11.0	17.3	21.9	20.9	0.55	44.2	0.15	81.3	4.1	6.3	10.2	3.8
Treated renal failure	3.3	12.4	20.4	4.9	22.2	0.10	46.0	0.05	80.8	1.1	14.0	2.3	5.3
Diseases of the liver or pancreas	14.6	10.7	16.7	2.3	17.5	0.65	47.2	0.15	86.4	0.2	11.0	0.6	4.7
Other long-term diseases	24.2	9.7	15.1	10.3	21.5	1.36	40.0	0.48	74.5	0.6	5.3	2.9	3.7

[a]Thousand
° Death: hospitalization in which death occurred; Total: hospital palliative care during the last year including hospitalization in which death occurred
[b] No hospital palliative care identifiable in the database at the date of death

of cases for multiple sclerosis, 18% of cases for Parkinson's disease, 17% of cases for dementia, 16% of cases for chronic respiratory disease and 20% of cases for treated renal failure. In more than one-half of cases, HPC was only provided during the stay associated with death (13% of people received HPC before the stay resulting in death, while 16% only received HPC during the stay resulting in death, for a total of 29% of people receiving HPC). Access to HPC during the year before death decreased with age and was less frequent in the absence of cancer. Among the people who died in a NSH, not equipped with a palliative care unit identified in the Snds database, 8% had previously received HPC, especially between the ages of 65 and 84 years and in the presence of a cancer (17%). HPC before death was also observed in the "Other places" category (7%), with higher rates for older people, in the presence of a cancer (19%) and, to a lesser extent, in the presence of multiple sclerosis (9%) or acute stroke (11%). Thirty-five per cent of people who died during other types of hospitalization than short stay hospitals (in rehabilitation units or HaH) had received HPC before death and 69% had received HPC at the date of death.

Discussion

In a large population of deceased people, 60% died in a hospital setting and one-half died in a short stay hospital. The proportion of people hospitalized in a short stay hospital increased rapidly over the three months prior to death. The main chronic diseases managed one year before death were cardiovascular/neurovascular diseases (56%), cancers (42%), and neurological and degenerative diseases (25%). During the year before death, 84% of people were hospitalized at least once, and 29% received HPC. HPC was more frequently used by cancer patients, and, in the absence of cancer, by patients with stroke: 24%, heart failure: 17%, dementia: 17%, multiple sclerosis: 23%.

Comparisons of places of death and diagnosis with French mortality statistics

This study was based on very comprehensive administrative and hospital reimbursement data and a large national study population [22]. The results can be compared with the national population and mortality statistics. Characteristics of deceased general scheme beneficiaries are relatively similar to those of all people who died in France in 2013, but with a smaller proportion of older people compared to the overall population (mean age: men: 73 years vs 79 years, women: 81 vs 85 years) [25]. General scheme beneficiaries are globally younger than beneficiaries of other schemes, which explain why this study included only 61% of all deaths in France, for 77% of the population.

In all deaths in 2013 in France, 57% occurred in hospital, 12% in retirement homes, 25% at home and 6% in a public place or in "Other places" [25]. These figures are similar to those reported in this study: 58% of people died in hospital, 13% died in a SNH and 29% died in "other places" (including 3% in HaH). However, SNH do not include all retirement homes and the proportion of SNH is unknown. This study was unable to directly estimate the proportion of deaths at home, but 29% of deaths occurred outside of hospitals and SNH and therefore theoretically at home (including HaH) or in a public place. As reported in other countries, a very great majority of French people (85%), free of any serious diseases, prefer to die at home [26]. However, in this study, only 42% of people died at home if SNH and "Other places" were considered to be home. This proportion decreased to 36% after subtracting the 6% of nationwide deaths in a public place [25].

End of life can be associated with a context of multiple diseases that cannot be reflected by a single leading cause of death. The distribution of diagnoses identified by subject in our study does not correspond to all causes of death in 2013: tumours (42% in this study for 29% as the leading cause of death), cardiovascular disease (56% for 25%), respiratory tract disease (20% for 7%), and dementia (19% for 4%) [25]. However, some causes of death were not included in the diagnoses because they could not be identified using the Snds database algorithms.

Hospital palliative care use

Twenty-nine per cent of all deceased people received HPC at the date of death or during the year preceding death (16% at the date of death only, and 13% at least before death). These rates were 39% for deaths in short stay hospitals and 44% for all deaths in health care institutions. These rates correspond to a first estimate of HPC use in a large population in France and few data on this subject using hospital diagnosis are available in the international literature (15–17, 19). The results of published studies correspond more to HPC needs, than HPC use, estimated by algorithms using causes of death likely to benefit from palliative care. HPC needs vary according to the causes of death eliminated or included in the algorithm and their specific distributions in different populations [8]. Hospital diagnoses matched with causes of death were also used in an Australian study [19]. The number of people with palliative care needs in France in 2008 was estimated to be 41% of all deaths according to the method of Rosenwax et al. and 69% according to the method of Murtagh et al., which includes more causes of death [8, 27], such as chronic cardiovascular / neurovascular diseases other than heart failure, non-Alzheimer's dementia and respiratory diseases other than chronic obstructive pulmonary disease. Thus, considering available data, estimation of palliative care need by health policymakers could be over or underestimated when national institution. Hospital diagnosis and multiple cause-of-deaths must be considered because cancer diagnosis may not be notified as the main or primary cause of death. While it is recommended to initiate palliative care earlier before death, the rate of palliative care use before death is relatively low in this study, except in rehabilitation units and HaH, which can constitute a short-stay alternative providing more specialized services in this field.

The frequency of palliative care before and at the date of death varies according to the type of disease, as well as their age and sex distributions, such as the classical high proportion of external causes in young boys. The type of palliative care can also vary according to age and type of disease. Analysis of HPC use by disease therefore appears to be more relevant than by causes of death, although other characteristics can also influence management, such as gender, age, and comorbidities.

Strength and limits

Use of palliative care in France is probably underestimated because this study does not take into palliative care managed by the general practitioner at home or palliative care provided in NSH, as no specific markers, such as drug reimbursements, are available due to the lack of specificity. However, 5% of deceased people received HPC before death in a NSH or in "other places", suggesting return or continued management of the patient at home or in a NSH, but the intensity of this care cannot be assessed.

The diseases managed can be identified by multisource algorithms such as those used in this study. These algorithms have been submitted to sensitivity analyses and expert reviews [24]. However, they depend on the use, offer and access to care. The data analyzed in this study were derived from administrative databases with their classical limitations concerning their primary objective, i. e. data collection and coding.

As part of the process of reflection on the end of life, the Snds can be used to describe end-of-life pathways and places of death and will soon be linked to causes of death. In the context of the new national palliative care plan in France, the Snds could be used to monitor several indicators focusing on HPC use, place of death but also to conduct more specific analyses in order to improve or evaluate specific subgroups (people with cancers, younger or older people, treatments and drugs used before death according to the disease).

Conclusion

This study suggests a relatively high level of HPC use in France, especially for certain diseases and in HaH and rehab hospitals. Few people were hospitalized with HPC care recorded in the database before the last hospitalization before death or before return home. In the context of a reflection on the end of life, these results must be refined in order to elucidate various specific aspects (diseases, disparity of use, etc.) based on Snds data, but also with the help of healthcare professionals and patients, in order to guide end-of-life health policies and evaluate heath policies and improve monitoring, such as the national plan, and assessment of HPC use.

Abbreviations

Cnam: *Caisse Nationale d'Assurance Maladie* general health scheme fund; HaH: Hospital at home; HPC: Hospital palliative care; ICD-10: International classification of diseases, 10th edition; LTD: Long-term diseases; PMSI: Programme de médicalisation des systèmes d'information (PMSI) [Medical Information System Programme]; Rehab: Rehabilitation unit; SNH: skilled nursing homes; Snds Système National des données de santé [National Health data Information System]

Authors' contributions

CP, AFC, PT and RA designed the study. LRB, CR drafted the article or revised it critically for important intellectual content. CP carried out data analysis. All authors made a substantial contribution to analysis or interpretation of data and approved the version to be published. All authors read and approved the final manuscript.

Competing interests

The authors declare that they have no competing interest.

Author details

[1]National sickness insurance fund, 26-50, avenue du Professeur André Lemierre, 75986 Paris cedex 20, France. [2]National Palliative care and end of life center, 75020 Paris, France. [3]Health Education and Practices Laboratory, Paris XIII University EA 3412, 93017 Bobigny cedex, France. [4]Pain and palliative Care Department, Teaching Hospital, 25030, Besançon, France.

References

1. Parikh RB, Kirch RA, Smith TJ, Temel JS. Early specialty palliative care–translating data in oncology into practice. N Engl J Med. 2013;369(24):2347–51.
2. Blanpain N, l'horizon COP d p à. Un tiers de la population âgé de plus de 60 ans. Institut national de la statistique et des études économiques (Insee). Insee Première. 2060;2010:1320. www.insee.fr
3. Gilles Pison, Laurent Toulemon. Le nombre de décès va augmenter en France dans les prochaines années. Institut national des études démographiques (INED). Population et Sociétés 2016;531. https://www.ined.fr/
4. Murray SA, Kendall M, Boyd K, Sheikh A. Illness trajectories and palliative care. BMJ. 2005;330(7498):1007–11.
5. Plan triennal 2015-2018 pour le développement des soins palliatifs et l'accompagnement en fin de vie. Ministère des Affaires sociales. In: de la Santé et des Droits des femmes; 2014. www.social-sante.gouv.fr

6. Aubry R. Comité national de suivi du développement des soins palliatifs et de l'accompagnement. Bilan du Programme national de développement des soins palliatifs 2008-2012. Ministère des Affaires sociales. In: de la Santé et des Droits des femmes; 2013. www.social-sante.gouv.fr.
7. Pivodic L, Pardon K, Morin L, et al. Place of death in the population dying from diseases indicative of palliative care need: a cross-national population-level study in 14 countries. J Epidemiol Community Health. 2016;70(1):17–24.
8. Murtagh FE, Bausewein C, Verne J, Groeneveld EI, Kaloki YE, Higginson IJ. How many people need palliative care? A study developing and comparing methods for population-based estimates. Palliat Med. 2014;28(1):49–58.
9. Morin L, Aubry R, Frova L, et al. Estimating the need for palliative care at the population level: a cross-national study in 12 countries. Palliat Med. 2016; 31(6):526–36.
10. Sarmento VP, Higginson IJ, Ferreira PL, Gomes B. Past trends and projections of hospital deaths to inform the integration of palliative care in one of the most ageing countries in the world. Palliat Med. 2016;30(4):63–73.
11. Scholten N, Günther AL, Pfaff H, Karbach U. The size of the population potentially in need of palliative care in Germany–an estimation based on death registration data. BMC Palliat Care. 2016;15:29.
12. Kane PM, Daveson BA, Ryan K, McQuillan R, Higginson IJ, Murtagh FE; BuildCARE. The need for palliative care in Ireland: a population-based estimate of palliative care using routine mortality data, inclusive of nonmalignant conditions. J Pain Symptom Manage 2015;49(4):726–733.e1.
13. Gómez-Batiste X, Martínez-Muñoz M, Blay C, Amblàs J, Vila L, Costa X, Espaulella J, Espinosa J, Constante C, Mitchell GK. Prevalence and characteristics of patients with advanced chronic conditions in need of palliative care in the general population: a cross-sectional study. Palliat Med. 2014;28(4):302–11.
14. Brameld K, Spilsbury K, Rosenwax L, Murray K, Semmens J. Issues using linkage of hospital records and death certificate data to determine the size of a potential palliative care population. Palliat Med. 2016;31(6):537–43.
15. Reich O, Signorell A, Busato A. Place of death and health care utilization for people in the last 6 months of life in Switzerland: a retrospective analysis using administrative data. BMC Health Serv Res. 2013;13:116.
16. Tanuseputro P, Budhwani S, Bai YQ, Wodchis WP. Palliative care delivery across health sectors: a population-level observational study. Palliat Med. 2017;31(3):247–57.
17. Teno JM, Gozalo PL, Bynum JP, et al. Change in end-of-life care for Medicare beneficiaries: site of death, place of care, and health care transitions in 2000, 2005, and 2009. JAMA. 2013;309(25):470–7.
18. Bekelman JE, Halpern SD, Blankart CR, et al. Comparison of site of death, health care utilization, and hospital expenditures for patients dying with Cancer in 7 developed countries. JAMA. 2016;315(3):272–83.
19. Goldsbury DE, O'Connell DL, Girgis A, et al. Acute hospital-based services used by adults during the last year of life in new South Wales, Australia: a population-based retrospective cohort study. BMC Health Serv Res. 2015;15: 537.
20. Atramont A, Rigault A, Chevalier S, Leblanc G, Fagot-Campagna A, Characteristics TP. Diseases and mortality of people admitted to nursing homes for dependent seniors during the first quarter of 2013 in France. Rev Epidemiol Sante Publique. 2017;65(3):221–30.
21. Scotté F, Hervé C, Leroy P, et al. Supportive Care Organization in France: a national in-depth survey among patients and oncologists. Support Care Cancer. 2017;25(7):2111–8.
22. Tuppin P, Rudant J, Constantinou P, Gastaldi-Ménager C, Rachas A, de Roquefeuil L, et al. Value of a national administrative database to guide public decisions: from the Système national d'Information Interrégimes de l'Assurance Maladie (SNIIRAM) to the Système national des Données de Santé (SNDS) in France. Rev Epidemiol Sante Publique. 2017;65(Suppl 4): S149–67.
23. Améliorer la qualité du système de santé et maîtriser les dépenses. Propositions de l'Assurance Maladie pour 2017. CNAMTS. 2016:224. www. ameli.fr.
24. Quantin C. Etude des algorithmes de définition des pathologies dans le Sniiram. CNAMTS;2015. www.ameli.fr
25. Centre d'épidémiologie sur les causes médicales de décès (CépiDc). www. cepidc.inserm.fr
26. Institut français d'opinion publique (IFOP) et ADREA mutuelle. Les attentes et les besoins des Français vis-à-vis de la fin de vie. 2016. www.adrea.fr/ assets/documents/DOCS-FONDATION/Diapo-rsum-IFOP.pdf.
27. Rosenwax LK, McNamara B, Blackmore AM, Holman CD. Estimating the size of a potential palliative care population. Palliat Med. 2005;19(7):556–62.

The degree of social difficulties experienced by cancer patients and their spouses

Takashi Takeuchi[1*], Kanako Ichikura[2,5], Kanako Amano[2], Wakana Takeshita[2,3] and Kazuho Hisamura[4]

Abstract

Background: Although recent studies have increasingly reported physical and psychological problems associated with cancer and its treatment, social problems of cancer patients and their families have not been sufficiently elucidated. The present study aimed to identify cancer-associated social problems from the perspectives of both patients and their spouses and to compare and analyze differences in their problems.

Methods: This was a cross-sectional internet-based study. Subjects were 259 patients who developed cancer within the previous five years and 259 patients' spouses; the data were derived from two surveys in 2010 (patients) and 2016 (spouses) whose participants were not part of the same dyad but matched by propensity scores, estimated for age, sex, and the presence or absence of recurrence. We investigated the social difficulties of cancer patients and patients' spouses. Regarding social difficulties experienced by cancer patients and spouses, the 60 patient survey items were categorized into 14 labels by the Jiro Kawakita (KJ) method, which is a qualitative synthesis method developed by Kawakita to classify categorical data.

Results: Although patients had higher scores on most subcategories, young spouses aged 39 or younger and female spouses had difficulty scores as high as the corresponding patients on many subcategories.

Conclusion: Health care providers should show sufficient concern for both patients and their spouses, particularly young and female spouses.

Keywords: Social problems, Cancer, Patients, Spouses, Difficulties, Internet survey

Background

The diagnosis and treatment of cancer often not only impose physical and mental distress on patients, but also substantially change their daily lives. Consequently, patients often face problems in various aspects of social life, such as family life, relationships with people around them, work, income, leisure activities, and relationships with health care providers [1–5]. Because of current advances in medical technology and availability of outpatient care, the length of hospital stay has been reduced for cancer patients. Because terminal home care is expected to be further promoted in the future, it is assumed that the main site of cancer patient care will increasingly be shifted from hospitals to homes. Under these circumstances, cancer patients and their families are required to deal with various social problems arising as the disease and treatment progress.

Recent studies have increasingly reported on physical problems associated with cancer and its treatment and psychological problems, such as anxiety and depression. As several studies have indicated that social problems experienced by cancer patients have an important impact on their mental health and quality of life [6–10], the need for support for their social problems, as well as the mental care of patients, has been increasingly recognized. However, the reality of the social problems experienced by the families who support cancer patients has not yet been sufficiently understood. Spouse caregivers provide the most extensive and comprehensive care, maintain the caregiver role longer, tolerate greater levels of disability than other

* Correspondence: okashi@bf6.so-net.ne.jp
[1]Section of Psychiatry and Behavioral Sciences, Graduate School of Medical and Dental Sciences, Tokyo Medical and Dental University, 1-5-45 Yushima, Bunkyo-ku, Tokyo 113-8519, Japan
Full list of author information is available at the end of the article

caregivers, and experience more severe lifestyle adjustments [11]. The spouse is the primary informal caregiver for cancer patients, and can experience high levels of stress, potential burnout, depressive symptoms, marital distress, poor health, and unmet needs [12, 13].

Thus, the present study aimed to investigate the degree of social difficulties experienced by cancer patients and their spouses, to identify cancer-associated social problems from the perspectives of both patients and their spouses, and to compare and analyze differences in their problems.

Methods

Study design and subjects

This is a cross-sectional study using internet-based surveys. The internet survey company we used is a Japanese company specializing in academic research. For the patient survey, in January 2010, we screened all registered members of the panel of internet-survey company A and selected those who developed cancer within the previous 5 years and experienced social problems. For the spouse survey, in the same manner in November 2016, we selected spouses of patients who developed cancer within the previous 5 years. Subjects were 259 patients and 259 patients' spouses and all cancer types were selected.

Assessment indicators

The degree of social difficulties experienced by cancer patients and spouses

The list of social difficulties experienced by cancer patients and spouses was prepared based on a list of patients' problems developed from the results of a qualitative survey asking, "What bothers you as a cancer patient?" in our previous study [14]. In this previous study, the list of social difficulties of patients was developed through discussion between an oncology social worker and a psychiatrist who reviewed articles published in Japan and other countries on social problems, distress, stressors, and patients' unmet needs. This list contains 60 items, on which patients are asked to answer the question, "Have you ever experienced any difficulty concerning the following matters at home, at work, or in your community because of your disease and treatment?" by choosing one of the following 6 options: It has been very difficult; it has been fairly difficult; it has not been very difficult; it has never been difficult; I do not know; and not applicable (Table 1). In the present study, to investigate difficulty perceived by spouses regarding the social problems of patients, we asked spouses to answer the question, "Have you ever experienced any difficulty concerning the following matters at home, at work, or in your community because of the disease (cancer) and treatment of the patient (your spouse)?" on the 60 items in the same manner. To use the 60 items for the spouse survey, the word "you" was replaced with "the patient," and "your family" with "you." For both the patient and spouse surveys, the options, "It has never been difficult," "I do not know," and "not applicable," were combined as "It has never been difficult," and the survey results were statistically analyzed as those of a four-choice survey: "It has never been difficult (0 points)," "It has not been very difficult (1 point)," "It has been fairly difficult (2 points)," and "It has been very difficult (3 points)." Furthermore, in the present study, these 60 items were first classified by the Jiro Kawakita (KJ) method (Affinity Diagram). The KJ method is a qualitative synthesis method developed to classify categorical data by Kawakita [15, 16]. Specifically, two clinical psychologists independently classified the 60 items. Then, items with mismatched labels were labeled through discussion between the psychologists. Next, a group led by a psychiatrist that included clinical psychologists routinely involved in supporting cancer patients reviewed the list of labeled items, made corrections to the arrangement of items and wording of the labels, and finalized the labels. Second, these labels were used as the subcategories of this list. For each subcategory, α coefficient was calculated to evaluate internal consistency. Finally, scores on each subcategory were calculated by dividing the total score by the number of items in each subcategory. This research was not a qualitative study. To adjust the scale of the social problems created by Hisamura et al., we used the KJ method which is a qualitative synthesis method. We chose this approach because we study social systems and social problems peculiar to Japan that cannot be measured by existing social problem scales.

Demographic and clinical variables of the patients

The demographic and clinical data were collected from self-administered surveys of all the study subjects. Specifically, the cancer patients were asked to answer multiple-choice questions on their sex, age, the presence or absence of recurrence, cancer sites, treatment, treatment regimens, state of treatment, academic background, and occupation.

Analysis methods

First, sex, age group, and presence or absence of recurrence were selected as covariates that should be adjusted based on clinical judgment, and propensity scores for these covariates were estimated using logistic regression models. Based on the calculated propensity scores, the patient and spouse groups were matched in a 1:1 ratio using nearest neighbor matching by sampling without replacement. Frequency distributions of the matched data were generated for background factors in each group to assess the balance among the covariates.

Second, differences in the degree of social difficulties experienced by the patient and spouse group were analyzed by independent two-sample *t*-tests. Furthermore,

Table 1 Classification of difficulties according to the Jiro Kawakita method

Label	Item
1. Difficulty in performing activities of daily living	Outpatient examinations and regular hospital visits
(α = .847)	Going out and transportation methods (including the use of public transportation systems)
	Taking care of myself (e.g., eating, bathing, toileting, and dressing)
	Household chores (e.g., house cleaning, laundry, meal preparation, and grocery shopping)
	Sex life
	Your disease and treatment have made hobbies, pastimes, and social activities less enjoyable.
2. Difficulty in seeking expert advice on the disease state and treatment	Admission to, discharge from, and transfer from a hospital
(α = .909)	Consulting a specialist other than your attending physician about your disease state and treatment
	You and your family cannot receive necessary psychological counseling.
	In case of sudden deterioration of your physical condition, there is no guarantee that you can immediately consult any doctors at the hospital where you are currently treated (or your neighborhood hospitals or clinics).
	Neither you nor your family have any primary care physicians at hospitals or clinics whom you can consult whenever necessary.
	Selection of a hospital (or a physician) that will provide treatment and examinations to you
3. Complaints with health care providers	Health care providers (e.g., physicians and nurses) do not promptly deal with your physical problems.
(α = .932)	Health care providers do not recognize your emotional problems or show any concern.
	Health care providers (e.g., your attending physician, physicians at other departments, your primary care physician, and nurses) do not sufficiently communicate with each other to arrange your treatment and care.
	Before you choose treatment, health care providers do not sufficiently explain the beneficial and adverse effects of each treatment strategy.
	Health care providers do not sufficiently explain the policy or plan of future treatment.
	You cannot talk frankly with your attending physician.
4. Lack of information on treatment and disease state	You cannot obtain enough information on the methods and contents of tests.
(α = .937)	You do not know how to collect information on the treatment of your disease.
	You cannot obtain enough information on various treatment methods.
	You cannot obtain enough information on complementary and alternative medicine (methods that are not regarded as standard treatment at present, such as health food, hot springs, and Qigong).
	You cannot obtain enough information on palliative medicine and care that alleviates pain and distress.
	You cannot obtain enough information on your current disease state and prognosis.
	You cannot obtain enough information on how to treat adverse effects of treatment that you receive and symptoms of your disease.
5. Lack of information on self-care	You cannot obtain enough information on what to keep an eye on in future life.
(α = .909)	You cannot obtain enough information on appropriate nutrition and dietary patterns.
	You cannot obtain enough information on how to deal with anxiety and depression.
6. Conflict over family relationships	Your family do not understand your disease or treatment well and sufficiently cooperate with you.
(α = .898)	Your views on your disease and treatment differ from the views of your family.
	Talking with your family about your disease
	Relationship and communication with your spouse
7. Concerns for family members	Care of your family (e.g., care of your parents, child-rearing, and nursing by your spouse)
(α = .897)	Burden on your family
	You cannot sufficiently take care of anxiety or concerns that your family have.
	Support offered to your family (e.g., help from people around you or public services) is insufficient.

Table 1 Classification of difficulties according to the Jiro Kawakita method *(Continued)*

Label	Item
	You cannot sufficiently perform your role at home.
	Your family are overly worried about you.
8. Difficulty in planning life	Planning future life of you and your family
(α = .594)	Developing your plans for marriage, pregnancy, and delivery
9. Conflict over relationships with non-family members	Relationships and communication with your friends and people close to you
(α = .902)	Relationships and communication with your neighbors
	Talking about your disease with people at work or in other social occasions
10. Difficulty in adapting to changes in the social environment	You have been discriminated because of your disease.
(α = .804)	The attitudes of people around you have changed after the onset of your disease.
	Your looks (appearance) have changed.
11. Lack of local support services	You do not have any opportunity to talk with people with similar experiences.
(α = .902)	You are lonely.
	You do not have anyone with whom you can consult or have access to services that offer consultation for the disease and medical care.
12. Difficulty in solving work-related issues	It is difficult to return to and continue work (or study if you are a student).
(α = .892)	It is difficult to take a day off from work (or school if you are a student) for treatment.
	Your disease has adversely affected your promotion at work.
	You have been demoted or transferred to an unimportant position at work.
	You have been asked to retire or fired at work (In case of being self-employed, you have closed your business).
13. Difficulty in making financial arrangements	Medical and living expenses during treatment
(α = .824)	The use of financial services (e.g., loan, medical insurance, and life insurance)
	Management of the properties of yours and your family
14. Lack of information on welfare services available during treatment	You cannot obtain enough information on available welfare services and systems (e.g., nursing-care insurance and welfare services for people with disabilities).
(α = .925)	You cannot obtain enough information on available home-based medical care services (e.g., home-visit medical treatment and nursing).
	You cannot obtain enough information on support for your medical care (e.g., wig, elastic stocking, wheelchair, and special bed).

t-tests were also performed to analyze differences in the degree of the difficulties for the following combinations of subgroups: between the younger generation (≤39 years) and middle-aged and older generation (≥40 years), and between male patients/female spouses and female patients/male spouses.

The significance level was set at 5%. SPSS for Windows 23 was used to perform statistical analyses.

Results

Subcategories of social difficulties experienced by cancer patients and spouses according to the KJ method (affinity diagram)

According to the KJ method, social difficulties were classified into 14 labels. Specifically, the 60 items were classified into the following subcategories: "difficulty in performing activities of daily living," "difficulty in seeking expert advice on the disease state and treatment," "complaints with health care providers," "lack of information on treatment and disease state," "lack of information on self-care," "conflict over family relationships," "concerns for family members," "difficulty in planning life," "conflict over relationships with non-family members," "difficulty in adapting to changes in the social environment," "lack of local support services," "difficulty in solving work-related issues," "difficulty in making financial arrangements," and "lack of information on welfare services available during treatment." The α coefficients for the internal consistency of the subcategories are shown in Table 1.

Matching for the characteristics and propensity scores of the subjects

When the patients and spouses were matched based on the propensity scores calculated from logistic regression models, 259 subjects were selected from each of the patient and spouse groups (Fig. 1). Table 2 shows the frequency distributions of the covariates and other background factors for each group. Regarding the covariates, the frequency distributions of sex, age group, and presence or absence of recurrence were completely matched between the patient and spouse groups, confirming that the groups were well balanced and matched. Regarding other background factors, cancer sites varied in both the patient and spouse groups, while most participating patients and patients of most participating spouses were being treated or followed up after the completion of treatment.

Differences in the degree of social difficulties experienced by the patient and spouse groups

The *t*-test results showed that the degree of "difficulty in seeking expert advice on the disease state and treatment" was comparable between the patient and spouse groups ($t = .75$, $p = .45$), whereas the degree of difficulty for all the other subcategories was higher in the patient than the spouse group (Table 3).

Meanwhile, in the younger subgroups (≤39 years), the mean difficulty scores in the spouses increased for all subcategories except "difficulty in adapting to changes in the social environment." The degree of difficulty was comparable between patients and spouses (Table 4).

In the male patient/female spouse subgroups, the mean difficulty scores in the spouses increased for the following subcategories: "difficulty in seeking expert advice on the disease state and treatment," "complaints with health care providers," "lack of information on treatment and disease state," "lack of information on self-care," "concerns for family members," "lack of local support services," "difficulty in making financial arrangements," and "lack of information on welfare services available during treatment." The degree of difficulty for these subcategories was comparable between patients and spouses (Table 5).

Discussion

In the present study, difficulty for cancer patients and their spouses in dealing with social problems was investigated and compared. Because there have been few studies that directly examined these problems, we would like to discuss them in associations with their consequences, such as depression, distress, morbidity, burden, unmet need, and decreased quality of life.

Comparison of difficulty between patients and spouses

The degree of difficulty was higher in the patient than the spouse group for all subcategories except "difficulty in seeking expert advice on the disease state and treatment (lack of opportunities to consult for patient transfer arrangement, hospital selection, second opinion, psychological counseling, etc.)." Patients and partners are interdependent in that cancer impacts on their shared life, both emotionally and practically. However, no conclusion has been reached on whose distress is more severe because there are conflicting reports. While some reports indicate that distress severity is comparable between patients and their spouses or partners, other reports indicate that patients' distress is more severe than that of their spouses or partners, and there are even reports indicating that distress of spouses or partners is more severe than that of patients [17]. Hodges et al. [18] investigated mental distress of spouses or partners of patients over the

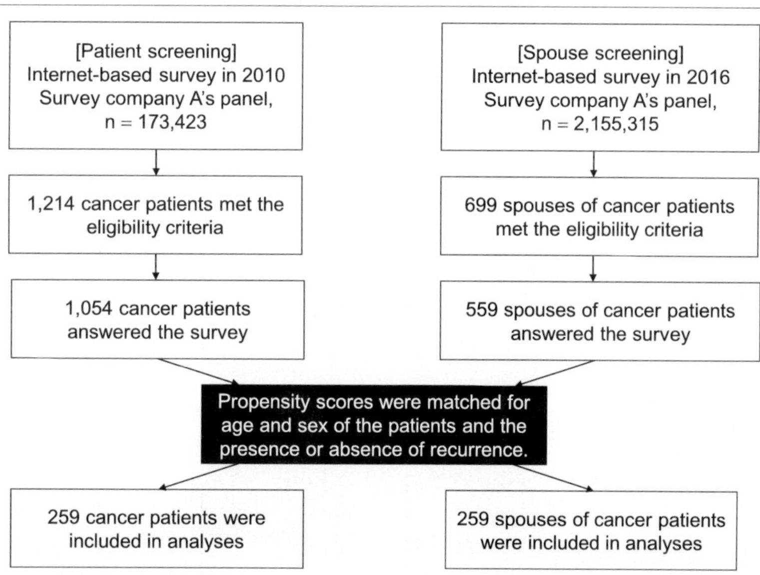

Fig. 1 Trial profile

Table 2 Demographic and clinical data

	Patients n (%)	Spouses n (%)
Patients' sex		
Men	128 (49.4)	128 (49.4)
Women	131 (50.6)	131 (50.6)
Patients' age		
20–29 years	11 (4.2)	11 (4.2)
30–39 years	44 (17.0)	44 (17.0)
40–49 years	67 (25.9)	67 (25.9)
50–59 years	85 (32.8)	85 (32.8)
60- years	52 (20.1)	52 (20.1)
The presence or absence of recurrence		
Primary occurrence	62 (23.9)	62 (23.9)
Recurrence	197 (76.1)	197 (76.1)
Cancer site (including duplicates)		
Lung cancer	34 (13.1)	29 (11.2)
Prostate cancer	25 (9.7)	13 (5.0)
Renal cancer	19 (7.3)	6 (2.3)
Bladder cancer	19 (7.3)	5 (1.9)
Testicular cancer	15 (5.8)	5 (1.9)
Gastric cancer	48 (18.5)	31 (12.0)
Esophageal cancer	20 (7.7)	5 (1.9)
Colorectal cancer	49 (18.9)	50 (19.3)
Liver cancer	17 (6.6)	6 (2.3)
Gallbladder cancer	13 (5.0)	2 (0.8)
Pancreatic cancer	12 (4.6)	3 (1.2)
Breast cancer	79 (30.5)	63 (24.3)
Thyroid cancer	20 (7.7)	6 (2.3)
Head and neck/oral cancer	11 (4.2)	7 (2.7)
Uterine cancer	27 (10.4)	12 (4.6)
Ovarian cancer	18 (6.9)	3 (1.2)
Leukemia	17 (6.6)	8 (3.1)
Malignant lymphoma	18 (6.9)	15 (5.8)
Malignant bone tumor	10 (3.9)	1 (0.4)
Brain tumor	17 (6.6)	1 (0.4)
Skin cancer	14 (5.4)	2 (0.8)
Cancer of unknown primary	5 (1.9)	0 (0.0)
Others	18 (6.9)	24 (9.3)
Treatments (including duplicates)		
Surgery	217 (83.8)	208 (80.3)
Radiation therapy	92 (35.5)	95 (36.7)
Chemotherapy	147 (56.8)	101 (39.0)
Patients' treatment status		
Patients are currently under cancer treatment	138 (53.3)	118 (45.6)
Cancer was cured, and treatment was completed.	90 (34.7)	120 (46.3)
Cancer is not cured, but aggressive treatment has been completed.	12 (4.6)	12 (4.6)
Others	19 (7.3)	9 (3.5)
Academic background		
Junior high-school graduates	8 (3.1)	10 (3.9)
High-school graduates	68 (26.3)	73 (28.2)
Vocational school/junior college graduates	53 (20.5)	65 (25.1)
Four-year college graduates	130 (50.2)	111 (42.9)
Work		
Full-time employment	98 (37.8)	140 (54.1)
Part-time employment	28 (10.8)	35 (13.5)
Full-time housewife	37 (14.3)	55 (21.2)
Leave of absence because of the disease	15 (5.8)	1 (0.4)
Voluntary retirement because of the disease	21 (8.1)	6 (2.3)
Dismissal (closure of business) because of the disease	11 (4.2)	0 (0.0)
Mandatory retirement	23 (8.9)	12 (4.6)
Unemployed	11 (4.2)	6 (2.3)
Others	15 (5.8)	4 (1.5)

course of disease and confirmed that the distress of spouses or partners significantly correlated with that of patients. Then, they indicated that the mental distress of spouses or partners gradually increases after diagnosis and becomes more strongly correlated with that of patients. Because currently treated patients and spouses of such patients accounted for 50% of the subjects in the present study, the degree of difficulty perceived by the spouses might not have been as high as that of difficulty perceived by the patients. However, we assume that the degree of "difficulty in seeking expert advice on the disease state and treatment" in the spouses was as high as that in the patients because spouses were greatly involved in treatment of patients soon after diagnosis.

Difficulty perceived by the young spouses

In the young subgroup, the degree of difficulty perceived by the spouses was as high as that of difficulty perceived by the patients for all subcategories except "difficulty in adapting to changes in the social environment (I feel that my appearance has changed or that I am treated differently)." People aged 39 years or younger, who were classified as the younger generation in the present study, are called "adolescents and young adults (AYA)." Cancer

Table 3 Differences in difficulty between the patients and spouses (patients, $n = 259$; spouses, $n = 259$)

	Patients		Spouses			
	M	SD	M	SD	t	p
1. Difficulty in performing activities of daily living	2.14	.74	1.80	.66	5.48	.00*
2. Difficulty in seeking expert advice on the disease state and treatment	1.87	.82	1.82	.68	.75	.45
3. Complaint with health care providers	1.89	.81	1.71	.66	2.67	.01*
4. Lack of information on treatment and disease state	1.99	.80	1.76	.70	3.40	.00*
5. Lack of information on self-care	2.02	.86	1.77	.76	3.45	.00*
6. Conflict over family relationships	1.88	.82	1.72	.70	2.36	.02*
7. Concerns for family members	2.04	.80	1.86	.70	2.72	.01*
8. Difficulty in planning life	2.04	.85	1.78	.76	3.67	.00*
9. Conflict over relationships with non-family members	1.92	.82	1.71	.79	3.03	.00*
10. Difficulty in adapting to changes in the social environment	2.05	.80	1.68	.73	5.46	.00*
11. Lack of local support services	2.08	.92	1.81	.84	3.47	.00*
12. Difficulty in solving work-related issues	1.84	.85	1.67	.73	2.41	.02*
13. Difficulty in making financial arrangements	2.16	.90	1.87	.81	3.86	.00*
14. Lack of information on welfare services available during treatment	1.80	.91	1.63	.76	2.31	.02*

*$p < 0.05$

patients in the AYA generation experience, after diagnosis and treatment, not only difficulties associated with social relationships, work, academic background, property, etc., but also many physical and psychosocial problems, such as interruptions to romantic and/or intimate relationships, reconsideration of family planning, infertility, and body image dissatisfaction [19, 20]. For this reason, young caregivers in this generation often seem to feel burdened [21, 22] and to perceive a high degree of difficulty.

Difficulty perceived by female spouses

For the combination of a male patient and a female spouse, the degree of difficulty perceived by the spouses was as high as that of difficulty perceived by the patients for "difficulty in seeking expert advice on the disease

Table 4 Differences in difficulty between the patients and spouses in the adolescents' and young adults' generation (patients, $n = 55$; spouses, $n = 55$)

	Patients		Spouses			
	M	SD	M	SD	t	p
1. Difficulty in performing activities of daily living	2.37	.88	2.21	.84	.94	.35
2. Difficulty in seeking expert advice on the disease state and treatment	2.07	1.06	2.18	.82	−.64	.53
3. Complaints with health care providers	2.08	1.02	2.10	.75	−.90	.93
4. Lack of information on treatment and disease state	2.17	1.02	2.10	.84	.41	.68
5. Lack of information on self-care	2.26	1.10	2.08	.90	.92	.36
6. Conflict over family relationships	2.09	.99	2.06	.89	.15	.88
7. Concerns for family members	2.26	.92	2.22	.80	.26	.80
8. Difficulty in planning life	2.57	.96	2.31	1.00	1.41	.16
9. Conflict over relationships with non-family members	2.24	.99	2.10	.95	.79	.43
10. Difficulty in adapting to changes in the social environment	2.42	.95	1.95	.91	2.67	.01*
11. Lack of local support services	2.30	1.10	2.19	.94	.53	.60
12. Difficulty in solving work-related issues	2.17	1.03	2.12	.91	.26	.80
13. Difficulty in making financial arrangements	2.44	.93	2.22	.95	1.22	.23
14. Lack of information on welfare services available during treatment	1.99	1.09	1.93	.94	.34	.73

*$p < 0.05$

Table 5 Differences in difficulty between male patients and female spouses (patients, n = 128; spouses, n = 128)

	Patients		Spouses			
	M	SD	M	SD	t	p
1. Difficulty in performing activities of daily living	2.15	.78	1.75	.70	4.34	.00*
2. Difficulty in seeking expert advice on the disease state and treatment	1.84	.80	1.81	.72	.33	.74
3. Complaints with health care providers	1.86	.81	1.70	.70	1.70	.09
4. Lack of information on treatment and disease state	1.94	.79	1.77	.77	1.81	.07
5. Lack of information on self-care	1.92	.86	1.79	.83	1.26	.21
6. Conflict over family relationships	1.88	.82	1.73	.70	1.60	.11
7. Concerns for family members	2.06	.79	1.88	.74	1.84	.07
8. Difficulty in planning life	2.05	.83	1.76	.74	2.99	.00*
9. Conflict over relationships with non-family members	1.91	.80	1.62	.79	2.99	.00*
10. Difficulty in adapting to changes in the social environment	2.04	.87	1.66	.79	3.65	.00*
11. Lack of local support services	1.98	.88	1.82	.91	1.52	.13
12. Difficulty in solving work-related issues	1.94	.86	1.66	.70	2.90	.00*
13. Difficulty in making financial arrangements	2.24	.93	2.01	.92	1.96	.05
14. Lack of information on welfare services available during treatment	1.80	.91	1.66	.82	1.30	.19

*$p < 0.05$

state and treatment (lack of opportunities to consult for patient transfer arrangement, hospital selection, second opinion, psychological counseling, etc.)," "complaint with health care providers," "lack of information on treatment and disease state," "lack of information on self-care (lack of knowledge on nutritional needs of patients or how to deal with anxiety)," "concerns for family members," "lack of local support services," "difficulty in making financial arrangements," and "lack of information on welfare services available during treatment (lack of knowledge on the nursing-care insurance system or nursing-care facilities and equipment)." Generally, compared to men who take care of their wives with cancer, women who take care of their husbands with cancer have higher mental morbidity (high levels of distress, depression, and anxiety, and a low level of mental health), physical morbidity (low physical health score, decreased physical function, and loss of physical fitness), and social morbidity (low satisfaction in marriage and limited social support) [12, 23, 24]. Ussher et al. [25] attributed this to the fact that women caregivers are positioned as all-encompassing expert careers, expected to be competent at decision-making, a range of physical caring tasks, and provision of emotional support for the person with cancer. The consequences of this positioning are over-responsibility and self-sacrifice, physical costs and overwhelming emotions. Men caregivers positioned caring as a competency task which they had mastered, and which provided them with satisfaction.

Limitations

The present study has several limitations. First, the results may have been affected by measurement bias because of the use of data from internet-based surveys. Data reliability is limited by the facts that the participants in these surveys determined whether they met the eligibility criteria and that data on diagnosis, treatment regimens, etc., were self-reported. Thus, in future studies, more accurate medical data need to be collected by conducting questionnaire or interview surveys at medical institutions in combination with review of medical records. However, a merit of an internet-based survey is that it guarantees anonymity and allows participants to respond without worrying about health care providers. Second, because of arrangements for this study and funding issues, several years passed between the patient and spouse surveys, and we were unable to collect data from patient-and-spouse pairs. These facts may also have contributed to measurement bias. The degree of social difficulties differed between the patients and spouses in the present study because both groups might have had different underlying problems. Thus, in future studies, patient-and-spouse pairs need to be targeted and surveyed around the same time. However, in this study, comparison was made while the differences in background problems were minimized as much as possible by matching propensity scores for data on sex, age group, and presence or absence of recurrence. Third, an analysis of non-responder or cancer patients who did not experience social difficulties is key to gaining information about a possible sample bias that might impact study results. This was not done in this study. Fourth, an unstandardized scale was used in this study. That is why we prepared the scale using the KJ method and confirmed the reliability with an α coefficient.

Conclusions

Health care providers should show sufficient concern for both patients and their spouses, particularly young and female spouses. In other words, it was considered important to change the approach method based on age and sex, and to intervene at the time of diagnosis rather than when the cancer was more advanced.

Abbreviation

AYA: Adolescents and young adults

Acknowledgements

The authors want to thank all cancer patients and their spouses who participated in this study.

Funding

The authors received no financial support for the research, authorship, and/or publication of this article.

Authors' contributions

Data were collected by KA, WT, KH, analyzed by KI, and interpreted by TT and KI. The work was drafted by TT and KI, and the manuscript was reviewed and edited by TT and KI. All authors read and approved the final manuscript.

Competing interests

The authors declare that they have no competing interests.

Author details

[1]Section of Psychiatry and Behavioral Sciences, Graduate School of Medical and Dental Sciences, Tokyo Medical and Dental University, 1-5-45 Yushima, Bunkyo-ku, Tokyo 113-8519, Japan. [2]Section of Liaison Psychiatry and Palliative Medicine, Graduate School of Medical and Dental Sciences, Tokyo Medical and Dental University, Tokyo, Japan. [3]Graduate School of Human Sciences, Waseda University, Saitama, Japan. [4]Department of Medical Oncology, Kanazawa Medical University, Ishikawa, Japan. [5]Department of Health Science, School of Allied Health Sciences, Kitasato University, Kanagawa, Japan.

References

1. Wright EP, Kiely MA, Lynch P, et al. Social problems in oncology. Br J Cancer. 2002;87:1099–104.
2. Muzzatti B, Annunziata MA. Assessing the social impact of cancer: a review of available tools. Support Care Cancer. 2012;20:2249–57.
3. Duijts SF, van Eqmond MP, Spelten E, et al. Physical and psychosocial problems in cancer survivors beyond return to work: a systematic review. Psychooncology. 2014;23:481–92.
4. Yabroff KR, Dowling EC, Guy GP Jr, et al. Financial hardship associated with cancer in the United States: findings from a population based sample of adult cancer survivors. J Clin Oncol. 2016;34:259–67.
5. Catt S, Starkings R, Shilling V, Fallowfield L. Patient-reported outcome measures of the impact of cancer on patients' everyday lives: a systematic review. J Cancer Surviv. 2017;11:211–32.
6. Cull A, Stewart M, Altman DG. Assessment of and intervention for psychosocial problems in routine oncology practice. Br J Cancer. 1995;72:229–35.
7. Kobayashi K, Morita S, Shimonagayoshi M, et al. Effects of socioeconomic factors and cancer survivors' worries on their quality of life (QOL) in Japan. Psychooncology. 2008;17:606–11.
8. Dapueto JJ, Servente L, Francolino C, Hahn EA. Determinants of quality of life in patients with cancer. Cancer. 2005;103:1072–81.
9. Hisamura K, Matsushima E, Tsukayama S, et al. An exploratory study of Soc Probl experienced by ambulatory cancer patients in Japan: Frequency and association with perceived need for help. Psychooncology. 2018; https://doi.org/10.1002/pon.4703. Epub ahead of print
10. Wright P, Downing A, Morris EJ, et al. Identifying social distress: a cross-sectional survey of social outcomes 12 to 36 months after colorectal cancer diagnosis. J Clin Oncol. 2015;33:3423–30.
11. Siegel K, Raveis VH, Houts P, Mor V. Caregiver burden and unmet patient needs. Cancer. 1991;68:1131–40.
12. Li QP, Mak YW, Loke AY. Spouses' experience of caregiving for cancer patients: a literature review. Int Nurs Rev. 2013;60:178–87.
13. Rhee YS, Yun YH, Park S, et al. Depression in family caregivers of cancer patients: the feeling of burden as a predictor of depression. J Clin Oncol. 2008;26:5890–5.
14. Hisamura K. Problems in social lives cancer patients experience and the importance of social support. Gendai no Esupuri. 2010;517:41–53. (in Japanese)
15. Kawakita J. Hassoho [Aboduction]. Tokyo: Chuokoron-Shinsha; 1967. (in Japanese)
16. Kawakita J. Zoku Hassoho [Aboduction: part two]. Tokyo: Chuokoron-Shinsha; 1970. (in Japanese)
17. Hagedoom M, Sanderman R, Bolks HN, et al. Distress in couples coping with cancer: a meta-analysis and critical review of role and gender effects. Psychol Bull. 2008;134:1–30.
18. Hodges LJ, Humphris GM, Macfarlane G. A meta-analytic investigation of the relationship between the psychological distress of cancer patients and their carers. Soc Sci Med. 2005;60:1–12.
19. Quinn GP, Goncalves V, Sehovic I, et al. Quality of life in adolescent and young adult cancer patients: a systematic review of the literature. Patient Relat Outcome Meas. 2015;6:19–51.
20. Leuteritz K, Friedrich M, Nowe E, et al. Life situation and psychosocial care of adolescent and young adult (AYA) cancer patients – study protocol of a 12-month prospective longitudinal study. BMC Cancer. 2017;17:82.
21. Payne S, Smith P, Dean S. Identifying the concerns of informal carers in palliative care. Palliat Med. 1999;13:37–44.
22. Siminoff LA, Wilson-Genderson M, Baker S Jr. Depressive symptoms in lung cancer patients and their caregivers and the influence of family environment. Psychooncology. 2010;19:1285–93.
23. Li Q, Loke AY. A spectrum of hidden morbidities among spousal caregivers for patients with cancer, and differences between the genders: a review of the literature. Eur J Oncol Nurs. 2013;17:578–87.
24. Moser MT, Kunzler A, Nussbeck F, et al. Higher emotional distress in female partners of cancer patients: prevalence and patient-partner interdependencies in a 3-year cohort. Psychooncology. 2013;22:2693–701.
25. Ussher JM, Sandoval M. Gender differences in the construction and experience of cancer care: the consequences of the gendered positioning of cares. Psychol Health. 2008;23:945–63.

Adding a second surprise question triggers general practitioners to increase the thoroughness of palliative care planning: results of a pilot RCT with case vignettes

F. Weijers†, C. Veldhoven†, C. Verhagen, K. Vissers and Y. Engels*

Abstract

Background: In our aging society, palliative care should be a standard component of health care. However, currently it is only provided to a small proportion of patients, mostly to those with cancer, and restricted to the terminal phase. Many general practitioners (GPs) say that one of their most significant challenges is to assess the right moment to start anticipatory palliative care. The "Surprise Question" (SQ1: *"Would I be surprised if this patient were to die in the next 12 months"*?), if answered with "no", is an easy tool to apply in identifying patients in need of palliative care. However, this tool has a low specificity. Therefore, the aim of our pilot study was to determine if adding a second, more specific "Surprise Question" (SQ2: *"Would I be surprised if this patient is still alive after 12 months"*?) in case SQ1 is answered in the negative, prompts GPs to plan for anticipatory palliative care.

Methods: By randomization, 28 GPs in the south-eastern part of the Netherlands were allocated to three different groups. They all received a questionnaire with four vignettes, respectively representing patients with advanced organ failure (A), end stage cancer (B), frailty (C), and recently diagnosed cancer (D). GPs in the first group did not receive additional information, the second group received SQ1 after each vignette, and the third group received SQ1 and SQ2 after each vignette. We rated their answers based on essential components of palliative care (here called RADIANT score).

Results: GPs in group 3 gave higher RADIANT scores to those vignettes in which they would be surprised if the patients were still alive after 12 months. In all groups, vignette B had the highest mean RADIANT score, followed by vignettes A and C, and the lowest on vignette D. Seventy-one percent of GPs in groups 2 and 3 considered SQ1 a helpful tool, and 75% considered SQ2 helpful.

Conclusions: This innovative pilot study indicates that the majority of GPs think SQ2 is a helpful additional tool. The combination of the two "Surprise Questions" encourages GPs to make more specific plans for anticipatory palliative care.

Keywords: Palliative care, Surprise question, Identifying tool, General practitioner, RADIANT

Background

Today most people in the Western world die of chronic, degenerative illnesses and malignancies, rather than of acute lethal diseases [1]. This implies that patients have a longer deteriorating trajectory, with increased symptom burden. For patients, carers, and family members, multidimensional supportive or palliative care is needed, preferably starting during disease-targeted care [1, 2]. The WHO defines palliative care as an early, multidimensional, proactive approach to maintaining or retaining quality of life alongside acceptance of mortality and bereavement. However, a means of demonstrating that a medical professional has fulfilled each of these requirements is not currently available [3].

Temel et al. demonstrated that timely palliative care in patients with metastatic non-small cell lung cancer alongside standard treatment increased their quality of life, reduced depressed mood, and even prolonged survival, as compared

* Correspondence: yvonne.engels@radboudumc.nl
†Equal contributors
Department of Anesthesiology, Pain and Palliative Medicine, Radboud university medical center, Postbox 9101, internal code 549, 6500, HB, Nijmegen, the Netherlands

with standard treatment alone. Bakitas et al. showed that early initiation of palliative care as compared to late initiation led to an increase in life expectancy of cancer patients [4, 5]. Patients with other life-limiting diseases are also in need of early palliative care and may benefit from it [6–8].

Most patients in an advanced stage of a life-limiting disease live at home in the Netherlands, where the general practitioner (GP) acts as a gatekeeper and coordinator of caregiving. This makes the GP the appropriate health care professional to coordinate palliative care [9]. Unfortunately, despite efforts to promote timely palliative care planning and development of tools to identify patients who might benefit from this approach, most GPs only provide terminal, reactive care, mostly to patients with cancer [10]. Consequently, in many patients in an advanced stage of a life-limiting disease, anticipation of future problems, needs, the patient's wishes, and mortality scenarios, does not occur in a timely fashion [3]. One of the barriers to providing anticipatory palliative care is identifying the right moment to start it, particularly in patients with organ failure or frailty [11]. To assist GPs in the identification of patients in need of anticipatory care planning, several tools have been developed [12]. However, most tools contain many items and are time-consuming to apply, when time is at a premium [13–15].

A way to assess the right moment to start palliative care that costs little time is the "Surprise Question" (SQ): *"Would I be surprised if this patient were to die in the next 12 months?"* [16] It appears to be sensitive for predicting 1-year mortality [17–23]. However, it has a low specificity and inadequate predictive value, which means that many identified patients live longer than one year. Therefore, just asking the SQ will identify a patient group that might be too large for a GP to provide structured, anticipatory care to. For that reason, there is a need for an easily applied tool with a higher specificity. Hence, we suggested an additional SQ that reads *"Would I be surprised if this patient is still alive after 12 months?"* when SQ1 is answered in the negative. Up to now, the value of the addition of this second SQ in encouraging proactive palliative care has not been explored, which makes this paper a unique contribution to the international literature.

We pilot tested whether adding SQ2 to SQ1 increases the thoroughness of palliative care planning among GPs and asked whether GPs think the double SQ is useful and applicable in daily practice.

Methods

Study design and participants

Between April and July 2016, we invited a random sample of 140 GPs in the south-eastern part of the Netherlands to participate in our pilot vignette study. Because the second SQ had never been studied before, we performed a pilot RCT. We estimated that about 30% of invited GPs would be willing to participate. Thus, by inviting 140 GPs to participate, we would have about 10 participating GPs per group. This number was expected to be sufficient to answer the research questions, keeping in mind the explorative character of this innovate study. In order to prevent socially desirable answering, we told participating GPs that the purpose of the study was to explore the influence of the type of patient illness on GP's care planning, without mentioning that we were also interested in the influence of the SQs. For the same reason, we did not mention that they would be randomized. Forty-three GPs provided written informed consent, and were randomized to one of the four arms, after stratification for being a "specialized GP" (a GP who has completed an extensive additional course in Palliative care or in Elderly care). In each group, the GPs received a questionnaire with four vignettes [Additional file 1]. Group 1 was used as a control group. Group 2 received only SQ1 after each vignette and in group 3 both SQs (SQ1 and SQ2) were asked after each vignette.

Group 4 received an aid for anticipatory, multidimensional care planning after each vignette in addition to both SQs. However, this concerned another research question; for that reason, in this paper we will only report the results of groups 1–3.

Procedures

All participating GPs received the randomization-assigned questionnaire online through Castor EDC (a valid research database software program), or by mail, according to their preference.

Each questionnaire contained four vignettes representing four different patient cases. Vignette A portrays a patient at an advanced stage of a chronic condition (chronic heart failure and chronic obstructive pulmonary disease), vignette B a patient with terminal metastatic pancreatic cancer, vignette C a frail lady with dementia and vignette D a relatively young patient with a recently diagnosed metastatic colon carcinoma. These vignettes were inspired by real anonymized cases from one of the authors (CV). [Additional file 1].

With each vignette, the respondent was asked if he would plan any kind of care for this particular patient. If so, they were asked to describe what instructions they would give to their young and inexperienced GP-trainee (who therefore needs explicit instructions) and about what kind of care needs to be planned for this patient in the upcoming period. At the end of the questionnaire, GPs in the corresponding groups were asked their opinions about the applicability and usefulness of, respectively, SQ1 and SQ2 [Table 1].

Outcome measures

All invited GPs were asked to provide socio-demographics and palliative care experience-related data [Table 2]. All information provided in the questionnaire was collected anonymously in Castor EDC and blindly evaluated. As a

Table 1 Questions asked to the GPs regarding palliative care provision

1. Which aspects trigger you in general to start palliative care? (groups 1-3)* (2missing)
2. Do you think the Surprise Question, 'Would you be surprised if this patient were to die within 12 months? ' would be helpful to identify patients in need of palliative care? (group 2)* (1 missing)
3. Is this Surprise Question applicable in daily practice? What are your concerns /barriers to apply them? (group 2)* (1 missing)
4. Do you think the second Surprise Question, in addition to the first SQ, would be of use in identifying patients in need of palliative care? (group 3)* (1 missing)
5. Are these two Surprise Questions applicable in daily practice? What are your concerns/barriers to apply them? (group 3) (1 missing)

*study group(s) that received this question

scoring instrument did not exist to assess whether all requirements of the WHO palliative care definition are fulfilled, we created a scoring instrument in order to analyze the open text fields and quantify them, dubbed the RADboud Indicators of ANTicipatory care (RADIANT) score [Table 3]. Therefore, we searched for guidelines from Pallialine (a Dutch website with an evidence and consensus based collection of palliative care guidelines, powered by the Netherlands Comprehensive Cancer Organization; IKNL), requirements from the WHO concerning Palliative Care and information from thuisarts.nl (a Dutch website for patients, powered by the Dutch College of General Practitioners, with clear information about various subjects including treatment limitations and end-of-life preferences) and a list of discussion points about patients' end of life, powered by the Royal Dutch Medical Association [3, 24–26].

The primary outcome was the correlation between answer combinations for SQ1 and SQ2 ("Yes/No I would / would not be surprised if this patient were to die in the next 12 months" and "Yes/No I would / would not be surprised if this patient is still alive after 12 months") and RADIANT scores. If an answer combination of SQ1: "No" and SQ2: "Yes" correlates with higher RADIANT scores than answer combination of SQ1: "No" and SQ2: "No", it suggests that this answer combination prompts GPs to plan anticipatory care more thoroughly.

Secondary outcomes were

a. differences in mean RADIANT scores per vignette A-D between the three GP-groups, particularly between the group with only SQ1 (group 2) and the group with both SQs (group 3). This difference in scores represents the extra value of the double SQ, as compared to SQ1 alone, in prompting GPs to plan anticipatory palliative care and the quality and thoroughness of care they described.

b. differences in mean RADIANT scores of all groups together between the cases in vignettes A-D. (Do the cases (type and progression of disease) influence the time-point, kind, and extent of care planning?)

c. differences between study group 1–3 in how often various aspects of the RADIANT score are mentioned in care plans.

d. Finally, with open questions, we qualitatively explored how GPs evaluated the single SQ and the double SQ.

Statistical analysis

Continuous, normally distributed data were expressed as means and percentages. Because of the small numbers, no effect sizes were calculated.

Table 2 Baseline characteristics

Characteristic	Group 1	Group 2	Group 3	Non participants[a]
N	9	10	9	42[c]
Age mean	48	45	53	59
Male gender n (%)	5 (56)	3 (30)	6 (67)	19 (45)
Type of practice n (%)				
Single-handed practice	1 (11)	0 (0)	3 (33)	4 (10)
Two-man practice	3 (33)	6 (60)	2 (22)	12 (29)
Group practice	5 (56)	4 (40)	4 (44)	26 (62)
Years of working experience as GP, mean	16.7	14.5	22.5	20.5
GP trainer n (%)	2 (22)	6 (60)	6 (67)	15 (36)
Specialised GP[b] n (%)	0 (0)	1 (10)	0 (0)	1 (2)
Estimated number of palliative patients / year, mean	5.1	6.4	6.7	5.7
Interest in palliative care (0: not at all; 10 extremely interested), mean	7.9	8.3	7.9	8.0
Self-assessed expertise in palliative care (0: no expertise; 10 extremely high expertise), mean	6.7	7.1	7.7	7.3

[a]GPs who were invited to participate in the study, but did not give informed consent (97) or gave informed consent but did not complete the vignette questionnaire (5)
[b]A GP that has followed an extensive additional course in palliative care or in elderly care
[c]GPs who provided socio-demographics and palliative care related data

Table 3 RADIANT scoring table

Item	Score	Provenance[a]
1. Discusses patient's personal aspects of quality of life	1	x, y
2. Discusses how to achieve patient's personal goals	1	q, x, y
3. Adheres to the patient's preferences	1	q, y
Provides attention to the following dimensions:		q, x, y
4. Somatic problems		
5. Social context and finances		
6. Caregiving and activities of daily living		
7. Existential and psychological issues		
8. Involves other disciplines, including consultation team palliative care	1	y
9. Provides palliative care alongside disease-oriented care	1	x
Discusses advance care planning aspects:		
10. Hospital admissions	1	q, z
11. Antibiotics use	1	q, z
12. CPR policy	1	q, y, z
13. Mechanical ventilation	1	q, z
14. Treatment limitations – not specified	1	q, y
15. Dying scenario's	1	q, y
16. Life prolonging treatments (e.g. artificial feeding and i.v. fluids)	1	q, z
17. Preferences for end-of-life care (e.g. palliative sedation, euthanasia)	1	q, y, z
18. Preferred place of death	1	q, y, z
19. Writes assignment for the out-of-hours GP cooperative	1	q
20. Involves family and loved-ones in care planning	1	q, x, y
21. Provides care to family and loved-ones	1	x, y
Maximum score	21	

[a]provenance, q Royal Dutch Medical Association [26], x WHO definition of palliative care [3], y Pallialine [24], z Thuisarts [25]

Ethical justification

The study was approved by the research ethics committee of Radboud university medical center in accordance with the Medical Research Involving Human Subjects Acts (WMO), case number 2016–2716. We obtained written consent from all participants to report individual anonymized data.

Results

Study participants

Of the 140 GPs approached, 57 did not want to participate and 40 never answered our invitation; thus in total 97 GPs did not provide informed consent [Fig. 1]. Fourty-three GPs agreed to participate and were randomized into groups 1–4 and sent the corresponding questionnaire. Of those 33 were in groups 1–3. Twenty-eight GPs completed the questionnaire and 5 did not, mostly due to high workload or personal circumstances [Fig. 1]. Of these 28 GPs, nine were in group 1, ten in group 2, nine in group 3. Their characteristics are included in Table 2.

Characteristics of participants in the different groups were mostly similar. However, the percentage of males in group 2 was lower and the percentage of GP-trainers in group 1 was lower. The mean age was 49 (SD 9.2) and they had an average GP work experience of 18 (SD 9.4) years. Four GPs worked in an individual practice (14%), 11 GPs (39%) in a two-man practice and 13 (46%) in a group practice. Only one of them (4%) completed an additional course in palliative care or in elderly care and 14 (50%) were GP-trainers. Participants treated a mean of six palliative patients a year, and GPs rated their interest in palliative care as an 8.0 (scale 0–10; 0: not at all-10: extremely interested) and their self-assessed expertise in palliative care as a 7.2 (scale 0–10; 0: no expertise-10: extremely high expertise).

Primary outcome measure: Correlation between answer combinations on SQ1 and SQ2 and RADIANT scores

In group 3, GPs who answered that they would not be surprised if this patient were to die in 12 months, and would be surprised if this patient is still alive after 12 months, had higher RADIANT scores than GPs in the same group who answered that they would not be surprised if this patient were to die in 12 months but they would also not be surprised if this patient is still alive after 12 months [Table 4].

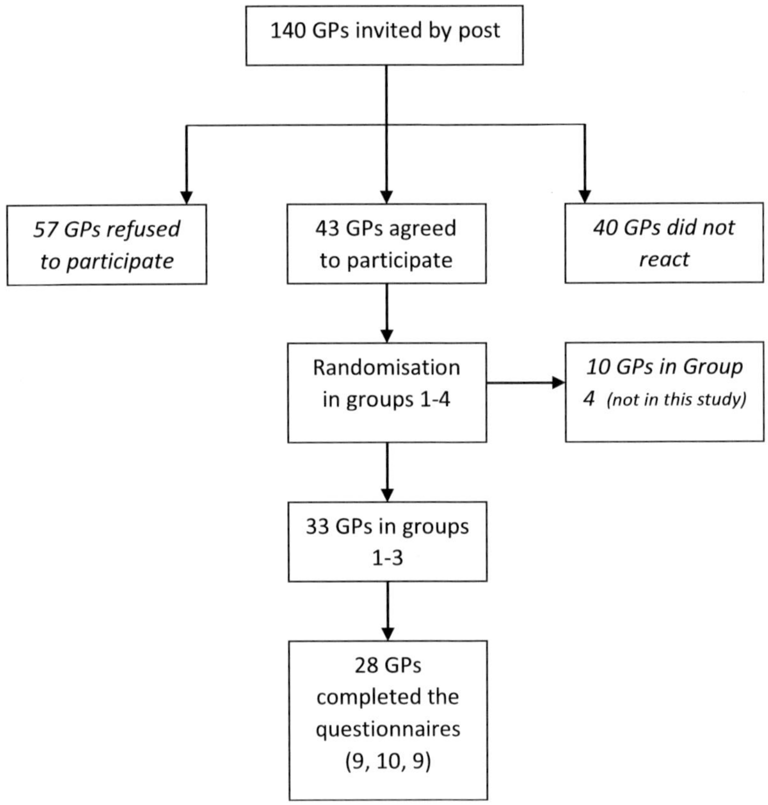

Fig. 1 Flowchart study participants. Legend: -

Secondary outcome measures

We did not find differences between GPs groups 1–3 in Radiant scores. Regarding vignettes A, B and D, group 3 has lower scores than group 1 and 2 [Table 5]. In all groups, vignette B (end-stage metastatic pancreatic cancer) had the highest mean score, followed by vignettes A (advanced organ failure) and C (frailty), and the lowest on vignette D (recently diagnosed metastatic colon carcinoma). In group 3, those vignettes of whom the GPs would be surprised if they were still alive after one year had mostly higher Radiant scores than the others. [Table 5].

GPs mentioned specific treatment limitations least often in their care plans and in only three care plans (3%) GPs mentioned that they would discuss how to achieve patients' personal goals. There were no striking differences between groups 1–3, except for involving other disciplines (50% of the case vignettes in group 1, compared to 20% for groups 2 and 3) and involving family and loved ones in planning care (36% of the case vignettes in group 1, compared to 22% and 25% in groups 2–3 respectively).

GPs' opinion about triggers to start palliative care

Many GPs mentioned that, in general, the diagnosis of a disease without curative options prompts them to start a palliative care approach. Their intuition, or information from a medical specialist, that death is approaching are considered important triggers. They also mentioned that they are prompted by frailty, complex situations, or when a patient suddenly or gradually has increased care needs. These latter situations give a GP the feeling of lagging behind events and of no longer being able to act proactively: "the feeling of being overtaken by events." Also, the absence of a family caregiver or lack of a social network prompts them to initiate palliative care. Some GPs especially want to adhere to the patient's wishes and start palliative care when the patient himself asks for it or gives other signals of being open to a conversation about palliative care: "the tangibility of the finiteness of life and the patient's capacity to feel this too." One GP in group 1 described SQ1 as an important trigger, another GP in group 1 mentioned SQ2, although they were not offered these questions and SQ2 has not been described before.

In the groups that received it, 12 out of 17 GPs who answered SQ1 (71%) considered it a helpful tool. However, GPs mentioned the inadequate specificity: "for anyone over 85, this could be their last year, but I will not start a palliative approach for all of them." Regarding SQ2, 6 out of 8 GPs who answered it (75%) considered it helpful. Some of them already were familiar with SQ1 and found it helpful to determine the right moment to start anticipatory palliative care planning. One GP in group 3 noted: "I use the first surprise question on a regular basis, but the

Table 4 Answers on SQ1[a] and SQ2[b] and RADIANT scores[c] per group[d] and per vignette

Vignette	Group 2[e] n = 10	RADIANT score group 2 mean	Group 3[f] n = 9	RADIANT score group 3 mean
A[g]	10 SQ1 'no'	6.0	5 SQ1 'no' & SQ2 'yes'	5.0
			4 SQ1 'no' & SQ2 'no'	1.5
B[h]	10 SQ1 'no'	5.8	9 SQ1 'no' & SQ2 'yes'	5.0
C[i]	9 SQ1 'no'	4.0	5 SQ1 'no' & SQ2 'yes'	4.6
	1 missing		3 SQ1 'no' & SQ2 'no'	4.0
			1 missing	
D[j]	5 SQ1 'no'	3.0	2 SQ1 'no' & SQ2 'yes'	3.0
	4 SQ1 'yes'	1.8	3 SQ1 'no' & SQ2 'no'	2.3
			3 SQ1 'yes' & SQ2 'no'	0
			1 missing	

[a]SQ1: Would I be surprised if this patient were to die in the next 12 months?
[b]SQ2: Would I be surprised if this patient is still alive after 12 months?
[c]RADIANT score: see Table 3
[d] only group 2 and group 3 are represented here, as group 1 did not receive any SQ
[e]group 2: received only SQ1 after each vignette
[f]group 3: received SQ1 and SQ2 after each vignette
[g]vignette A: advanced organ failure
[h]vignette B: end-stage metastatic pancreatic cancer
[i]vignette C: frailty
[j]vignette D: recently diagnosed metastatic colon cancer

second one is new to me. They seem to be the same, but surely there is a nuanced difference. When the answer to SQ1 is 'No' and to SQ2 is 'Yes', it is clearer to me that the palliative phase has begun. The only objection is that these questions are subjective and therefore a physician can make a very inaccurate estimation. So I suggest answering these two SQs over again when the situation changes."

Discussion

Up to now, the classical SQ(1) alone was used and has proven to have low specificity as a tool to predict death, which may lead to a large and unselected group of patients for whom a GP should plan multidimensional, proactive, palliative care. Some participating GPs in this study underlined this shortcoming. Furthermore, its performance is insufficient in non-cancer patients [23]. Adding SQ2 to SQ1 may improve specificity as prognostic tool, but more meaningfully, combining the two SQs will help a medical professional to select a smaller, more accessible group of patients in need of anticipatory palliative care. The GP can then focus on these patients and plan palliative care more thoroughly.

Many tools have recently been developed to identify patients in need of palliative care in general practice, e.g. RADPACT, SPICT, NEPCAL, GSF [12]. These tools require more time investment and availability of indicators and are therefore less suitable for screening of patients in a GP's daily practice. Also, most tools are focused on

Table 5 Mean cumulative RADIANT scores[a] per group, per vignette and per SQ answer combination

Vignette	Group 1 n = 9	Group 2 n=10[b]		Group 3 n=9[b]		Mean n = 28
		SQ1[c] all answers	SQ1 'no'	SQ1 all answers	SQ1 'no' & SQ2[d] 'yes'	
A[e]	4.6	6.0	6.0	3.4	5.0	4.7
B[f]	5.9	5.8	5.8	5.0	5.0	5.6
C[g]	4.6	4.0	4.0	4.4	4.6	4.3
D[h]	2.9	2.7	3.0	1.6	3.0	2.4
Mean	4.5	4.6	4.7	3.6	4.4	

[a]RADIANT score: see Table 3
[b]some missing data: in both group 2 and group 3 one GP did not fill out vignettes C and D
[c]SQ1: Would I be surprised if this patient were to die in the next 12 months?
[d]SQ2: Would I be surprised if this patient is still alive after 12 months?
[e]vignette A: advanced organ failure
[f]vignette B: end-stage metastatic pancreatic cancer
[g]vignette C: frailty
[h]vignette D: recently diagnosed metastatic colon cancer

the palliative patient in the terminal phase, which implies that after identification there will be less time for proactive and anticipatory care planning. However, all of these tools are useful for meeting patients' wishes, needs, and possible future scenarios and should be used in combination during conversations with the patient.

We did not study the prognostic value of the SQs. Already in 2005 Lynn suggested using the SQ to identify "whether the person is in a fragile enough condition that relatively minor worsening or intercurrent illnesses could lead to mortality. Some of the patients identified by the surprise question will end up living for years in a fragile state, and some will die soon, but all typically need the services that are priorities in the last phase of life: advance care planning, comfort measures, assistance for daily activities, family support, and so forth" [27]. Also Downar et al. noted the importance of using the SQ as a screening test for patients who might benefit from a palliative care approach [28]. Recognizing the patient in need is a prerequisite to starting proactive palliative care [29], not the prognosis.

Most participating GPs considered the already-known SQ1 and also the new SQ2 helpful.

As one of the triggers to start palliative care, some GPs mentioned "if a patient himself asks for it". However, De Vleminck et al. demonstrated that patients, and particularly patients with disease trajectories other than cancer, are very unlikely to start discussing anticipatory care planning on their own initiative [30].

Strengths and limitations

This is the first study in which the SQ is used in combination with case vignettes to see whether it prompts GPs to thoroughly plan proactive palliative care, instead of studying its prognostic value, which has been questioned before [31]. Adding a more specific trigger, SQ2, is also innovative.

However, the study also has several limitations. In this pilot study, the number of included GPs was limited and not sufficient to discover statistical significance. It was meant as a first exploration and therefore all results should be interpreted with caution. Although we aimed to use the results for a full-scale study, the relatively small percentage of GPs that wanted to participate in this vignette study led us to abandon this plan. Instead, we have started a prospective study in which GPs screened their patient list with both SQs. One year later, a retrospective medical record review will take place to determine sensitivity and specificity of both SQs and whether the different answers to these SQs are related to anticipatory care planning and care needs.

The response rate of 22% is about the same as in Schnakenberg et al.'s study (27.5%). In that study, GPs in Germany and Sweden were sent surveys about palliative care, which took no more than ten minutes to fill out [32]. Although we consider 22% fairly low, given the time required to complete the questionnaire (30–40 min) and Dutch GPs' high workload, it is satisfactory.

Vignette 4, concerning the patient with recently diagnosed metastatic colon carcinoma, was not completed by two GPs and also had the lowest RADIANT score. We think that mainly the case itself will have influenced the score, but maybe the order in which the vignettes were presented might have influenced this outcome as well.

Although the RADIANT score is not a validated tool, it enabled us to quantify the open text fields and thus to compare groups not only qualitatively but also quantitatively. We chose anticipatory care to have a high share of the total RADIANT score, because we believe a medical professional can only provide good palliative care when, in addition to addressing actual problems, he also anticipates possible future problems. Besides, a medical professional can only be proactive when he is made aware of his patient's condition, which is what we aimed to achieve with the SQs.

Whether the RADIANT score is related to the quality of a palliative care plan (the obtained scores are a fraction of the total possible score per vignette of 21 points) still needs to be studied in real patient care, as well as the validity and specificity of the tool.

Finally, we do not know whether all GPs in group 3 have understood the subtle but essential difference between SQ1 and SQ2. After all, we did not provide any explanation about the intention or use of this new SQ2.

Recommendations

This simple, additional SQ2 was considered helpful by GPs and showed promising pilot results. In four prospective studies in, respectively, general practice, a medical oncology outpatient clinic, the Intensive Care Unit and nursing homes, we will further explore its usefulness and validity.

Conclusions

In our pilot study, SQ2 in addition to SQ1 seems to contribute to more extensive and anticipatory palliative care planning for those patients of whom GPs would be surprised if they were still alive after 12 months, and to less extensive and anticipatory care planning when they would not be surprised if a patient were still alive after 12 months. Most GPs who received it considered SQ2 a useful addition to SQ1.

Abbreviations

GP: General Practitioner; RADIANT: Radboud Indicators of Anticipatory care; SQ1: Would I be surprised if this patient were to die within the next 12 months?; SQ2: Would I be surprised if this patient is still alive after 12 months?

Acknowledgements
We thank all GPs for participation in our vignette study.

Funding
No funding.

Authors' contributions
CV developed SQ2 and the vignettes. FW has developed the questionnaire, sent invitations to GPs, collected data and drafted the manuscript. YE wrote the project proposal and led the project. CV, CV, KV and YE revised the manuscript critically for important intellectual content. All authors read and approved the final manuscript.

Authors' information
F. Weijers; MD, special interest in Palliative Care.
C. Veldhoven; MD General Practitioner in Berg en Dal, the Netherlands, palliative care specialist; Department of Anesthesiology, Pain and Palliative Medicine.
C. Verhagen; MD PhD Medical Oncologist and palliative care specialist; Department of Anesthesiology, Pain and Palliative Medicine and department of Medical Oncology.
K. Vissers; MD PhD FIPP Professor in Pain and Palliative Medicine; Department of Anesthesiology, Pain and Palliative Medicine.
Y. Engels; PhD Associate professor in timely palliative care and member of Department of Anesthesiology, Pain and Palliative Medicine.

Competing interests
The authors declare that they have no competing interests.

References
1. Seale C. Changing patterns of death and dying. Social science & medicine (1982). 2000;51(6):917–30.
2. Thoonsen B, Groot M, Engels Y, Prins J, Verhagen S, Galesloot C, van Weel C, Vissers K. Early identification of and proactive palliative care for patients in general practice, incentive and methods of a randomized controlled trial. BMC Fam Pract. 2011;12:123.
3. World Health Organisation (WHO) Definition of Palliative Care.http://www.who.int/cancer/palliative/definition/en/. Accessed 29 October 2017.
4. Temel JS, Greer JA, Muzikansky A, Gallagher ER, Admane S, Jackson VA, Dahlin CM, Blinderman CD, Jacobsen J, Pirl WF, et al. Early palliative care for patients with metastatic non-small-cell lung cancer. N Engl J Med. 2010; 363(8):733–42.
5. Bakitas MA, Tosteson TD, Li Z, Lyons KD, Hull JG, Li Z, Dionne-Odom JN, Frost J, Dragnev KH, Hegel MT, et al. Early versus delayed initiation of concurrent palliative oncology care: patient outcomes in the ENABLE III randomized controlled trial. Journal of clinical oncology : official journal of the American Society of Clinical Oncology. 2015;33(13):1438–45.
6. Evangelista LS, Lombardo D, Malik S, Ballard-Hernandez J, Motie M, Liao S. Examining the effects of an outpatient palliative care consultation on symptom burden, depression, and quality of life in patients with symptomatic heart failure. J Card Fail. 2012;18(12):894–9.
7. Wong FK, Ng AY, Lee PH, Lam PT, Ng JS, Ng NH, Sham MM. Effects of a transitional palliative care model on patients with end-stage heart failure: a randomised controlled trial. Heart. 2016;102(14):1100–8.
8. Brannstrom M, Boman K. Effects of person-centred and integrated chronic heart failure and palliative home care. PREFER: a randomized controlled study. Eur J Heart Fail. 2014;16(10):1142–51.
9. Gomes B, Calanzani N, Curiale V, McCrone P, Higginson IJ. Effectiveness and cost-effectiveness of home palliative care services for adults with advanced illness and their caregivers. The Cochrane database of systematic reviews. 2013;6:Cd007760.
10. Abarshi EA, Echteld MA, Van den Block L, Donker GA, Deliens L, Onwuteaka-Philipsen BD. Recognising patients who will die in the near future: a nationwide study via the Dutch sentinel network of GPs. The British journal of general practice : the journal of the Royal College of General Practitioners. 2011;61(587):e371–8.
11. De Vleminck A, Houttekier D, Pardon K, Deschepper R, Van Audenhove C, Vander Stichele R, Deliens L. Barriers and facilitators for general practitioners to engage in advance care planning: a systematic review. Scand J Prim Health Care. 2013;31(4):215–26.
12. Maas EA, Murray SA, Engels Y, Campbell C. What tools are available to identify patients with palliative care needs in primary care: a systematic literature review and survey of European practice. BMJ Support Palliat Care. 2013;3(4):444–51.
13. Thoonsen B, Engels Y, van Rijswijk E, Verhagen S, van Weel C, Groot M, Vissers K. Early identification of palliative care patients in general practice: development of RADboud indicators for PAlliative care needs (RADPAC). The British journal of general practice : the journal of the Royal College of General Practitioners. 2012;62(602):e625–31.
14. Claessen SJ, Francke AL, Engels Y, Deliens L. How do GPs identify a need for palliative care in their patients? An interview study. BMC Fam Pract. 2013;14:42.
15. Gómez-Batiste X, Murray SA, Thomas K, Blay C, Boyd K, Moine S, Gignon M, Van den Eynden B, Leysen B, Wens J, Engels Y, Dees M, Costantini M. Comprehensive and integrated palliative care for people with advanced chronic conditions: An update from several European initiatives and recommendations for policy. J Pain Symptom Manage. 2017;53:509–17.
16. Pattison M, Romer AL. Improving care through the end of life: launching a primary care clinic-based program. J Palliat Med. 2001;4(2):249–54.
17. Moroni M, Zocchi D, Bolognesi D, Abernethy A, Rondelli R, Savorani G, Salera M, Dall'Olio FG, Galli G, Biasco G, et al. The 'surprise' question in advanced cancer patients: a prospective study among general practitioners. Palliat Med. 2014;28(7):959–64.
18. Moss AH, Lunney JR, Culp S, Auber M, Kurian S, Rogers J, Dower J, Abraham J. Prognostic significance of the "surprise" question in cancer patients. J Palliat Med. 2010;13(7):837–40.
19. Moss AH, Ganjoo J, Sharma S, Gansor J, Senft S, Weaner B, Dalton C, MacKay K, Pellegrino B, Anantharaman P, et al. Utility of the "surprise" question to identify dialysis patients with high mortality. Clin J Am Soc Nephrol. 2008; 3(5):1379–84.
20. Pang WF, Kwan BC, Chow KM, Leung CB, Li PK, Szeto CC. Predicting 12-month mortality for peritoneal dialysis patients using the "surprise" question. Perit Dial Int. 2013;33(1):60–6.
21. Da Silva Gane M, Braun A, Stott D, Wellsted D, Farrington K. How robust is the 'surprise question' in predicting short-term mortality risk in haemodialysis patients. Nephron Clin Pract. 2013;123(3–4):185–93.
22. Cohen LM, Ruthazer R, Moss AH, Germain MJ. Predicting six-month mortality for patients who are on maintenance hemodialysis. Clin J Am Soc Nephrol. 2010;5(1):72–9.
23. Downar J, Goldman R, Pinto R, Englesakis M, Adhikari NK. The "surprise question" for predicting death in seriously ill patients: a systematic review and meta-analysis. CMAJ. 2017;189(13):E484–93.
24. Palliaine: General principles of palliative care. [http://palliaine.nl/algemene-principes-van-palliatieve-zorg] Accessed 14 Apr 2018.
25. Information for patients about end-of-life decisions and treatment limitations [http://www.thuisarts.nl/levenseinde] Accessed 14 Apr 2018.
26. Talk timely to your patient about end of life issues [https://www.knmg.nl/web/file?uuid=0b6dabe5-bbac-49ea-82ef-7a5262e0c6f6&owner=5c945405-

d6ca-4deb-aa16-7af2088aa173&contentid=1217&elementid=147756]
Accessed 14 Apr 2018.

27. Lynn J: Living long in fragile health: the new demographics shape end of life care. Hastings Cent Rep 2005, Spec No:S14–S18.
28. Downar JGR, Pinto R, Englesakis M, Adhikari NK. The "surprise question" for predicting death in seriously ill patients: a systematic review and meta-analysis. CMAJ. 2017;189(13):484–93.
29. Highet G, Crawford D, Murray SA, Boyd K. Development and evaluation of the supportive and palliative care indicators tool (SPICT): a mixed-methods study. BMJ Support Palliat Care. 2014;4(3):285–90.
30. De Vleminck A, Pardon K, Beernaert K, Deschepper R, Houttekier D, Van Audenhove C, Deliens L, Vander Stichele R. Barriers to advance care planning in cancer, heart failure and dementia patients: a focus group study on general practitioners' views and experiences. PLoS One. 2014;9(1): e84905.
31. Janssen DJA, Van de Beuken-Van Everdingen, MHJ, Schols, MGA: Suprised by the 'surprise question' Ned Tijdschr Geneeskd 2015:159:A8427.
32. Schnakenberg R, Goeldlin A, Boehm-Stiel C, Bleckwenn M, Weckbecker K, Radbruch L. Written survey on recently deceased patients in Germany and Switzerland: how do general practitioners see their role? BMC Health Serv Res. 2016;16:22.

"It doesn't exist…": negotiating palliative care from a culturally and linguistically diverse patient and caregiver perspective

Emma Kirby[1*], Zarnie Lwin[2,3], Katherine Kenny[1], Alex Broom[1], Holi Birman[1] and Phillip Good[3,4,5]

Abstract

Background: The end of life represents a therapeutic context that acutely raises cultural and linguistic specificities, yet there is very little evidence illustrating the importance of such dynamics in shaping choices, trajectories and care practices. Culture and language interplay to offer considerable potential challenges to both patient and provider, with further work needed to explore patient and caregiver perspectives across cultures and linguistic groups, and provider perspectives. The objective of this study was to develop a critical, evidence-based understanding of the experiences of people from Culturally and Linguistically Diverse (CALD) backgrounds, and their caregivers, in a palliative care setting.

Methods: A qualitative study, using semi-structured interviews to explore key experiences and perspectives of CALD patients and caregivers currently undergoing treatment under oncology or palliative care specialists in two Australian hospitals. Interviews were digitally audio recorded and transcribed in full. A thematic analysis was conducted utilising the framework approach.

Results: Sixteen patients and fourteen caregivers from a range of CALD backgrounds participated in semi-structured interviews. The research identified four prevalent themes among participants: (1) Terminology in the transition to palliative care; (2) Communication, culture and pain management; (3) (Not) Talking about death and dying; and, (4) Religious faith as a coping strategy: challenging the terminal diagnosis.

Conclusions: CALD patients and caregivers' experiences are multifaceted, particularly in negotiating linguistic difficulties, beliefs about treatment, and issues related to death and dying. Greater attention is needed to develop effective communication skills, recognise CALD patients' particular cultural, linguistic and spiritual values and needs, and acknowledge the unique nature of each doctor-patient interaction.

Keywords: Palliative care, Cultural and linguistic diversity, Qualitative, Australia

Background

The transition to palliative care is challenging for patients and their loved ones [1, 2]. Culturally and linguistically diverse (CALD) populations may need extra support [3], as their experience of transition may entail additional complications around language and cultural values, including barriers to communication and isolation from the broader community. While doctor-patient-caregiver communication around transitions to palliative care has been shown to be complex and prone to interpersonal difficulties [1, 4, 5], cultural and linguistic diversity further complicates doctor-patient communication and treatment options, and the decision to cease potentially life-prolonging treatment [4, 6–9]. In the transition to palliative care, and cultural expectations around death and dying more broadly, CALD patients and families must navigate a range of challenges across the domains of formal and informal care. This study aimed to explore the experiences and perspectives of both CALD patients and family caregivers, revealing various implications for practice for oncologists and palliative care specialists treating CALD

* Correspondence: Emma.kirby@unsw.edu.au
[1]Practical Justice Initiative, Faculty of Arts and Social Sciences, University of New South Wales, Level 3 Goodsell Building, University of New South Wales, Sydney, NSW 2052, Australia
Full list of author information is available at the end of the article

patients in the Australian hospital system. Specifically, we focus on the transition to palliative care.[1] to explore attitudes towards, and understandings and experiences of, end-of-life care among CALD patients and their caregivers.

Cultural and linguistic diversity when approaching the end of life

Australia is culturally and linguistically diverse, with a range of cultural values and beliefs shaping illness experiences, access to care and interactions with healthcare providers [10]. CALD populations face particular challenges when it comes to accessing healthcare in Australia and in most western nations, including issues related to language and communication, cultural preferences, and isolation [10–12]. In relation to end of life care, patients and caregivers from CALD backgrounds have varying preferences regarding the disclosure of diagnosis and prognosis and the management decision-making in health/care [13, 14]. Internationally, there have been some attempts to understand the particular needs of diverse populations in end-of-life care [15, 16], yet further in-depth, patient-focused work still remains necessary [17, 18].

Cultural expectations, decision-making and care

Although full disclosure of diagnosis and prognosis is not uniformly practiced in all cultures, it is central to the Western biomedical system [19]. In Australia, doctors are trained in breaking 'bad news' to patients and families, particularly when transitioning patients to palliative care [20, 21]. This system is based on the principles of medical ethics, with the notion of 'patient autonomy' at its centre [22, 23]. As such, the right of the patient to know their health status and make decisions about treatment options is considered a key facet of medical care. However, some CALD patients and caregivers – particularly those who are older or less 'acculturated' to western biomedical contexts – may prioritise a family decision-making model when it comes to treatment decisions [22, 24], or indeed, may defer decisions to their doctors who may be afforded significant cultural authority [7, 25, 26]. As such, Western biomedical notions of patient-centred care may not resonate with patients and caregivers from different cultural backgrounds who have considerably different expectations of medical systems [26–28].

Communication, culture and palliative care

Doctor-patient communication around diagnosis/prognosis and treatment decision-making is informed by a range of lay and expert interpretations of illness and mortality. Lay interpretations in particular are highly culturally variable and can pose particular challenges for CALD patients and caregivers. For example, the words 'cancer' or 'palliative' are avoided across a number of cultural contexts because of their direct association with death [25, 29]. There are several explanations for this, including: persistent taboos around cancer and mortality, the idea that speaking of cancer will hasten death, and the idea that the timing of death can be known only by god [25]. Diagnostic/prognostic disclosure is thus a culturally-laden form of communication with considerable implications for palliative care. Furthermore, in the palliative care context, communication necessarily extends beyond doctor-patient relations to include the family, which is often viewed as the appropriate 'unit of care'. Yet in CALD contexts, family caregivers may be called upon to perform multiple types of caring roles: It is not unusual, for instance, for family caregivers to take on the role of interpreting during medical examinations [30]. Despite the greater accuracy of professional interpreters in conveying information to patients [31], many patients prefer the familiarity of family caregivers [7]. However, the use of family members as interpreters can also be fraught, with tensions around who controls the actual consultation process, and the information conveyed between doctor and patient as mediated by the interpreting caregiver [25, 30, 32]. As we discuss below, such multifarious and complex factors may result in additional confusion, misunderstandings and frustrations in the transition to palliative care for CALD patients and caregivers.

Methods

This study, while discrete, was part of a broader program of research exploring the lived experience of the end of life. We used qualitative semi-structured interviews to explore the experiences of CALD patients' and caregivers' transition to palliative care. Following local and national ethics approval [HREC approval: HREC/14/MHS/22], potential participants were approached by the clinical members of the research team during routine clinic appointments or during inpatient stays at two metropolitan hospitals in south-east Queensland, Australia. When appropriate, potential participants were approached with the aid of an accredited professional interpreter.[2] Each patient and/or caregiver was given ample opportunity to discuss the study and the context of the interview. Participants who were interested in taking part in the study were then contacted to schedule a convenient time and location for the interview to take place. Eligible participants were people over the age of 18 from CALD communities, defined as those from non-Indigenous ethnic/language groups other than the English-speaking majority in Australia. Patients were approached based on their CALD status as noted in hospital records, who were currently undergoing treatment under oncology or palliative care specialists within the two hospitals. While we did not limit recruitment to specific diagnoses or stage of disease, eligible patients were those who were no longer undergoing potentially curative treatment, and were being transitioned to palliative care. Caregivers were approached based on their provision of care for patients from CALD communities, or based on their own CALD status.

A purposive sampling strategy was used, and coordinated through whole research team meetings, including the clinical members of the research team who approached participants. The process was iterative, and regularly reviewed to update the strategy and facilitate discussion around which patients and carers to approach in order to include participants from a range of backgrounds, including spread across age, sex, languages spoken, inpatient/outpatient status, and public/private care settings. All interviews, conducted during 2014, were digitally audio-recorded and transcribed in full in English.[3] During the interviews we focused on the following domains: experiences and understandings of palliative care; communication, needs and values in the context of hospital care; experiences of being cared for/caring at a time of serious illness; and, experiences and perspectives on formal/institutional support/care for patients and caregivers with CALD backgrounds. The COREQ qualitative research reporting checklist was used to ensure comprehensive reporting [33].

Analysis

Data analysis took place concurrently with the qualitative fieldwork over a period of 7 months. In line with sociological interpretive traditions, our approach to analysis focused on reaching a nuanced understanding of the range of perspectives, within systems of beliefs and life experiences more broadly [34]. We employed the framework approach of qualitative data analysis using NVivo 10 software to systematically analyze the transcripts. We employed the following steps: (1) Familiarization: the researchers reviewed the manuscripts. (2) Identification of framework: key themes were identified around which the data were organized. (3) Indexing: application of themes to text. This stage involved using NVivo 10 to label and arrange each excerpt of text, use of a word or term, or research note related to each participant and transcript. This produced several (complicated and overlapping) lists including data and notes from several participants according to each theme. (4) Charting: use of headings and sub-headings to build up a picture of the data as a whole. Each thematic 'index' was discussed by three research team members, with Author A leading the development of summaries or 'charts' for each thematic area: one 'overall' summary, along with one summary of patient participants and one for caregiver participants. (5) Mapping and interpretation: in which associations were clarified and explanations developed. This involved finding associations between and within themes, moving towards and developing explanations for the findings in line with our research aims [35]. The three research team members participated in all stages of the analysis and independently coded the data, and these separate analyses were then cross-checked to uncover related and/or deviant cases/themes, and to develop an overall interpretation of the data. Once a theme was identified in the transcripts, interviews were searched for related comments using constant comparison in order to further develop themes [36]. In this way the richness of the data was retained, while interrelated associations were uncovered. Analytical rigor was augmented by constant comparison and searching for negative cases during code and theme development [35–37]. Following ongoing concurrent analysis of the interviews, informed by the concept of saturation in qualitative research [38]. the researchers agreed that no new themes relating to the topics of study were likely to be identified from further interviews.

Results

Participants were recruited from 1 public hospital, and 1 private hospital which had provision for public patients through government-funded beds within the private setting. Twenty-two patients and 17 caregivers volunteered to participate, 30 of whom were recruited (16 patients and 14 caregivers[4]). All of the patients had advanced cancer, were no longer receiving potentially curative treatments, 8 of the patients were hospital inpatients at the time of interview, and 8 were outpatients. The caregivers were all family members of the patient for whom they were caring, including daughters ($n = 4$), wives ($n = 4$), husbands ($n = 4$), a granddaughter, and an ex-wife. Several participants spoke multiple languages; the majority of participants spoke some English. Five patients and 5 caregivers were interviewed with the assistance of a professional accredited interpreter. These participants were given a participant information and consent form in a language of their choosing, and were given time to ask any questions about the project and their participation through the interpreter present, prior to giving written consent. Four of the caregiver participants were caring for patients who were also participating in interviews. For these patient-carer dyads, participants were given the option to be interviewed separately or together. Two of patient-carer dyads chose to be interviewed together. Semi-structured interviews lasted up to 60 min (median: 33 min). Table 1 provides a summary of participant characteristics.

Here we report on the emergent themes following our systematic analysis of the interview transcripts. Participants offered varying degrees of information about their experiences and perspectives on their cancer, supportive

Table 1 Characteristics of the sample

Characteristic	Patients (*n* = 16)	Caregivers (*n* = 14)
Age		
20–29	–	1
30–39	1	1
40–49	1	4
50–59	3	1
60–69	7	7
70–79	2	–
80–89	2	–
Sex		
Male	5	4
Female	11	10
Religion		
Baptist	–	1
Buddhist	2	1
Catholic	3	4
Christian	2	1
Greek Orthodox	1	1
Hindu	1	–
Jehovah's Witness	1	–
Latter Day Saints	1	–
Muslim	1	1
None/Not Disclosed	3	5
Pentecostal	1	–
Care type		
Public	12	8
Private	4	4
Not Disclosed	–	2
Regional origin		
Eastern Europe	–	1
European Union	6	2
Oceania	3	1
Asia	5	8
Africa	2	–
Middle East	–	2
Languages spoken		
Afrikaans	1	–
Arabic	–	2
Cantonese	1	2
Dutch	1	–
English	12	11
French	–	1
German	3	–
Greek	1	–
Hindi	1	–

Table 1 Characteristics of the sample *(Continued)*

Characteristic	Patients (*n* = 16)	Caregivers (*n* = 14)
Hungarian	2	–
Italian	2	1
Macedonian	–	1
Mandarin	4	5
Melanesian	1	–
Malay	1	–
Polish	1	–
Somali	1	–
Tagalog	–	1
Taiwanese	1	–

and/or palliative care. What was clear, throughout the participant cohort of both patients and caregivers, was that managing hospital treatment for serious illness had the potential to entail significant physical and emotional vulnerability, compounded by communication problems and cultural divergence. Our analysis revealed four predominant themes: (1) Terminology in the transition to palliative care; (2) Communication, culture and pain management; (3) (Not) Talking about death and dying; and, (4) Religious faith as a coping strategy: challenging the terminal diagnosis.

Terminology in the transition to palliative care

A key theme within the interviews was the variable, or complete lack of, understanding of the concept and meaning of palliative care. Given that there is no equivalent term for 'palliative care' in many languages, the majority of participants experienced difficulties in understanding the meaning of the term, and the consequences of the transition to palliative care for treatment and prognosis. As shown in the indicative quotes in Table 2, the expectation of more traditional forms of home-based care for the dying (provided by family or informal caregivers) meant that hospital-based palliative care was difficult to comprehend for several participants. At times, patients confused in-patient palliative care with ongoing 'active' treatment that would be aimed at prolonging their lives. That is, some patients believed a return home was indicative of the onset of the dying process and thus, in contrast, that remaining in hospital entailed hope for recovery. Many caregivers lacked a working understanding of the meaning of palliative care, and we heard many accounts of caregivers around 'doing homework' in order to understand what 'palliative' meant and what 'palliative care' entailed. Other participants wished to avoid discussions around terminal prognoses and were reluctant to discuss plans for end of life care. In still other cases (and as with diagnosis), patients and caregivers felt that the meaning of palliative care had

Table 2 Indicative quotations: terminology in the transition to palliative care

Participant	Indicative quotation
Caregiver #1	I'm the type that when you tell me something, especially with regards to my parent's health ... I'll go and look it up on the internet and research it so that I understand what's going on so I can help them through it. ... even if I had to try and explain it to him using palliative as the word, I couldn't because it doesn't exist. It doesn't exist.
Caregiver #4	*Interviewer: How did the staff explained palliative care to you?* I find it out from the web. Yeah, I find it out from the web. They have explained, but I was still a little bit puzzled by the explanation.
Caregiver #2	*Interviewer: Looking back, do you recall what your understanding of palliative care was before your husband came to [Palliative care unit]?* Special cancer.
Patient #11	Actually, I don't know. I don't think I really know what the word palliative means.
Patient #1	P1:They've never heard of it [palliative care] ... No. I mean they will give you all the medicines that they can afford and if they can't do anymore then people normally they will just go back to the Island or the village where they come from and just ready to die. They just, just accept it.
Caregiver #3	The thing is, my grandmother, I don't think that she knows what palliative care means. I think my aunties were trying not [to] tell her that she's going to die or something... They don't want her to get upset and stuff like that. She doesn't really know what it means to be in palliative care. That's the main thing. She thought that she's here, I don't know, maybe she'll get better, she said.
Caregiver #9 (via interpreter)	Her understanding is that palliative care is for the patients who can't, at the moment because she can still look after him medicine-wise, can still give him the medications he needs, but because the palliative care is for people out of that, what do you call it, too far gone, I guess. That's her understanding of palliative care.

been explained by clinicians in ways that were not clear. Thus we found a number of difficulties in participants' understandings and comprehension of the notion of 'palliative care', the precise nature of which varied across patients and caregivers. While various cultural 'taboos' around dying played a role, so too did difficulties at the level of translation including the lack of ability to translate and explain the term. What 'palliative' meant was, for many participants, lost in translation. Alternatively, in other cases, where 'palliative' was taken by participants to be synonymous with approaching the end of life, use of the term was consciously withheld by clinicians at the request of family caregivers.

Communication, culture and pain management

A key facet of the transition to palliative care in Australia is the focus on pain and symptom management for patients with advanced cancer [39, 40]. During the interviews with both patients and caregivers, we heard multiple accounts of the difficulties in communicating with clinicians in terms of expectations of treatment, which were shaped by the variable understandings of and meanings attached to palliative care (discussed above). This was most evident in relation to pain and symptom management, with the interviews revealing a variety of different cultural scripts around the expectation of pain and pain relief, as shown in Table 3. As noted above, a significant proportion of the patients we

Table 3 Indicative quotations: Communication, culture and pain management

Participant	Indicative quotation
Caregiver #1	I'm like their nurse, I'll go and look it up on the internet and research it so that I understand what's going on so I can help them through it. I'm the one dealing with the doctors and with medications and all of that.
Caregiver #7	Speaking to that doctor when I went once myself I think there was a communication issue. He sort of said that he didn't feel that he didn't get that she was in as much pain as she was ... I think a lot of people from other parts of the world where medical care isn't so good they seem to have a greater tolerance for pain than people that are used to getting painkillers and whatever. So I think that's part of the problem in that she didn't express to him in a way that he comprehended how much pain she was in.
Patient #8	... I never knew you don't have to pain like you are paining, if that makes sense. I don't think that's good English. The pain that I'm going through [prior to pain medication], you don't have to have that.
Patient #14	When I had this pain in my fingers to start with to get out of that they gave me steroids and morphine... I thought steroids were for horses but they were for me too. In the end I thought, "Why make life more difficult than what you've already had? Why not accept?"
Patient #4 (via interpreter)	What has happened she said, when I was new I used to get interpreted but for sometimes now, each time I come they said, "We couldn't find an interpreter, blah, blah," a bit of excuse that they make...Yeah, it's hard. Because I don't understand what the doctor tells me and the doctor doesn't understand what I tell him what happened if there's no interpreter.
Patient #16	Nobody there to listen to you. So then I spoke to doctor himself and I told him. I said, "Doctor this is very painful." New doctor had come. Now that guy also gave some bloody shitty medicine or something. Then he turns around, 2 days later, he said, "It will take time to go because what I've given you is just a painkiller."

interviewed talked of their belief that by virtue of being in hospital and receiving hospital-based expert medical treatment, they might or would get better and recover. Moreover, the majority of participants (both patients and caregivers) discussed the importance of stoicism and tolerance in the face of physical pain. Thus, participants told us that, when asked about pain by clinicians, patients were likely to down-play the extent of their pain, potentially making it difficult for clinicians to manage pain effectively, or indeed understand the patient experience. One participant provided a poignant anecdote about how this initial hesitation was overcome by a nurse who persisted with their queries until the patient finally felt they could rely on them and fully disclose the extent of their discomfort. For others, communication with clinicians about pain and symptoms was very difficult in the absence of an interpreter. For a few participants, this was experienced as frustrating and isolating, as they felt they could not adequately communicate their needs, nor were their needs well-understood by clinicians. Caregivers discussed similar issues with us, and were often particularly concerned that the Australian medical system was not well equipped to deal with either their cultural or linguistic requirements.

(Not) talking about death and dying

The avoidance of talking about cancer, death and dying was a predominant theme within the participants' accounts, and one that was explicitly linked to cultural background (see Table 4 for indicative quotations). Talking about death and dying, or terminal illness was frequently associated by participants with 'giving up' or hastening death. That is, participants understood death to be more likely to happen, or more likely to happen quickly, if openly acknowledged, verbalised or discussed. As such, participants spoke of strictly limiting talk about cancer or the end of life, as it was in stark contrast to the strong desire to maintain hope. Both patients and caregivers within our sample spoke of their unwillingness to talk about the prospect of dying as part of their culture or underlying belief system. Such discussions were described as being viewed as demoralising and unnecessarily upsetting for those who are already unwell. Such active avoidance of discussing the terminal diagnosis was also linked to issues around disclosure of information, as well as religion, faith and hope, as we discuss below.

Religious faith as a coping strategy: Challenging the terminal diagnosis

Many patients – often with the support of their caregivers – talked about the centrality of their faith and religion as a means of coping, as shown in Table 5. Patients and caregivers frequently commented on their preference to focus on religious faith (which they associated with hope) instead of medical futility (which they associated with 'giving up' and death). As one caregiver noted about the counselling offered to them and their partner, talking about particular problems only made it more difficult to cope. For some patients, religious faith presented a challenge to their doctor's expertise and authority, with implication that God knows better, or that God would intervene and assist their healing. One participant admonished herself for saying the word 'cancer', explaining this this would anger God, and chose instead to attribute any negative wording about her condition to medical reports by prefacing them with 'according to the report'. Faith and religion was a particularly prominent coping strategy among our participants. These belief systems were frequently talked about by participants as part of the cultural fabric with which experiences of illness and care were interwoven.

Table 4 Indicative quotations: (Not) Talking about death and dying

Participant	Indicative quotation
Caregiver #11	It's not in our culture to say you're going to die. I don't even want to accept myself still. I know that she is ill but I'm still thinking you never know. Miracle may happen or something. It's hard but I will never tell her. She doesn't know now. She doesn't know. I don't think I would like her to know because she'll be scared or something. But in our culture you never say to the patient.
Caregiver #1	Sometimes being completely honest and brutal like that is not the right thing to do from a cultural background … I would have told him, "Look dad, there is a tiny little spot that they found there. They're going to investigate it further. We don't know exactly what it is. You're in good hands." … dad thinks that by talking about death or telling him he's dying, that you're going to bring it on, bring on the process a lot quicker.
Caregiver #3	In my culture, they don't really talk about dying. They're scared of it…They don't want to think about my grandma's going to die. They just deal with it day-by-day. They don't really plan and they don't really say, "Oh, yeah, she's going to die soon." They don't want to talk about it.
Patient #16	It's a cultural thing. But cultural thing a lot of sons they would say, "Yes, yes," kind of a thing and not get so involved. But my children are very involved and I presume they love me… I would [be] more content to have my sons have it [knowledge of the details of the patients' prognosis] than to me because, you see, it unnecessarily worries me and it doesn't solve anything. So I would be happy if my sons know everything about it and they gave me information and that's okay with me because I trust them implicitly.
Patient #5	So we could [not] say that "I am sick, I am so unlucky, I'm an idiot" Because that will influence the effect on us. So we all say that "I am happy, I'm fabulous, I'm so beautiful." I have to say like this.
Patient #8	It was on [date] and she actually said, "I think it's cancer." I remember how shocked I was that a doctor could throw a word around word like that…So to hear the word, I was really upset. How can you throw a word around like that?

Table 5 Indicative quotations: Hope and faith: Challenging the terminal diagnosis

Participant	Indicative quotation
Patient #5	So my bone cancer considered very, very dangerous and I shouldn't say my mine bone cancer, sorry God. I cannot say that I have cancer he will give me bad feeling ... I believe God. God say that everything that come out from your mouth, we always have to say positive about us. I'm not sick, I'm healthy, God is healing me. The more we say about negative thing, the more that negativity will come to us.
Patient #16	I believe in God. There's a particular God, that I believe in. I have 100% faith that he is not going to let me down, that everything's going to come through correct.
Patient #8	I'm very positive in my approach to my illness. So I believe God is going to heal me. [...] Even if I might be on my deathbed, I will still believe the manifestation of my healing will come. That's how I prefer to die and pass away... I'm going to not to be a statistic of a carcinoma death, but I will be a miracle.
Patient #3	The doctor can't tell me how many more years or months I have. So I can only sense it myself, feel it myself, I suppose.
Patient #5	I, myself, believe God will heal me. So when Dr. [Name] say, "Nothing we can do." I say to myself, "Yeeha, God will show His power. He will heal me."
Caregiver #14	I'm a spiritual person, as in I believe that there is someone looking out for us. Not so that I go to church. But I have a strong sense of faith and my dad has a strong sense of faith and he is a very positive person and that's what's been helping him throughout his whole illness because he thinks he's just going to get better and he's very positive. So we do, we have a strong sense of faith.

Discussion

A significant body of existing research has revealed multiple cultural factors which can shape experiences of discussing and managing death and dying [6, 13]. The findings presented in this paper have provided additional insight into the experiences of CALD patients and their caregivers, and how they manage the challenging nexus of formal care; beliefs about treatment, death and dying; linguistic difficulties; communication around diagnosis, prognosis, pain and symptoms, with clinicians. For clinicians, understanding these complex dynamics is important for effectively communicating, establishing trust and making decisions with both CALD patients and their families. This requires a nuanced negotiation and understanding of both the broader cultural perspective of the patient and the interpersonal relationships within the family unit of care.

Our findings novel data from during the transition to palliative care, which support previous research highlighting the difficulties of communicating with CALD patients about the meaning of palliative care [4, 9], as understandings of the context and services offered by palliative care were incomplete or absent for the majority of participants. The data highlights the importance of clinicians' ability to identify and remedy misunderstandings about (or lack of understanding of) the meaning and context of palliative care, and what patients and caregivers might expect from this stage in the patient's care plan. Indeed, our findings point to the significance of ensuring the meaning of language is understood, while maintaining a culturally sensitive disposition (though this is no straightforward task). Moreover, given that several participants described their deliberate avoidance of such discussions, our findings provide new insight into the importance of sensitivity to cultural taboos and scripts around cancer, death and dying.

The findings presented here suggest that such cultural taboos are interpreted in a variety of ways with a variety of consequences. While some (sometimes quite specific) cultural taboos exist in relation to discussing cancer or death, the primary reason given by our participants for such avoidance strategies was the desire to maintain hope and, in the case of patients withholding their status from loved ones, to prevent suffering or concern. In many cultures (including in many western contexts) the maintenance of hope is particularly pertinent approaching the end of life [41], where the transition to palliative care may be seen as giving up hope and provides challenges in terms of denial and acceptance [42]. While the majority of participants recounted avoiding talking about the terminal diagnosis, all of the patients we interviewed were receiving treatment and transitioning to palliative care, suggesting difficulties in communicating the full implications of the transition to palliative care (whether because of difficulties of language, conversational reticence, or avoidance as discussed above). That is not to say that patients or their caregivers were ignorant or uninformed about the details of their diagnosis, but rather that they frequently did not wish to verbalise or discuss them. While such accounts at the end of life are hardly exclusive to CALD patients and caregivers [40–43], our findings point to the complex interplay of culture and care in the every day experience of the transition to palliative care for CALD patients and caregivers.

Successfully engaging in discussions with CALD families around palliative care issues, then, is clearly not as straightforward as simply identifying a particular nationality or cultural background and the associated beliefs and norms, which would amount to a form of cultural stereotyping. Instead, a patient or caregiver's willingness (or disinclination) to discuss cancer and dying can be recognised as necessarily influenced by a multitude of factors, including individual biography, family relationships, educational attainment and cultural background including, most notably in this study, elements of faith and hope. This highlights some of the challenges palliative care and oncology clinicians may face when working with CALD patients and caregivers, and the importance of approaching each case as unique, with good communication between clinicians and the patient about their particular cultural, linguistic and spiritual values and needs. A number of researchers have argued the importance of clinicians actively exploring case-by-case cultural preferences for how end of life contexts are approached, in particular around patient and caregiver preferences for decision-making and information about their diagnosis and prognosis [8, 22, 26].

Our study has various limitations which are somewhat similar to those faced by clinicians involved in the transition to palliative care. Given the linguistic barriers, the sensitive topic of the interviews, and the conducting of interviews within a busy hospital setting (albeit in a private room), conversations between the researchers and participants were at times stunted, short, and interrupted. Our participants were recruited from two hospitals in one Australian city. As such, our findings may not be indicative of the experiences of CALD patients and caregivers elsewhere. Participants self-selected by volunteering, and were from a wide range of cultural backgrounds, with varying levels of health-literacy in relation to the Australian health system. It is noteworthy to stress again that our findings should not be generalised to all CALD patients and caregivers. Indeed, we reiterate here the almost infinite spectrum of experience for those within CALD communities, and the use of 'CALD' to describe a static or homogenous group, or indeed as particular categories (e.g. country of birth), as unhelpful. Finally, we note here the complexities of interviews conducted in English with participants for whom English is not their first language, or through an interpreter, and the potential consequences for data collection, analysis and reporting.[5] The process of cross language qualitative research has been shown to be complicated and often flawed [44]. While we engaged with issues around competence (using only accredited interpreters) and style (using consecutive interpreting), as well as strategies for building rapport (including making the interpreter 'visible' and part of the conversation), we acknowledge the limitations of having an interpreter present, and the limitations in terms of translation of data [44, 45].

Conclusions

CALD patients and caregivers' experiences are multifaceted, particularly in negotiating linguistic difficulties, beliefs about treatment, and issues related to death and dying. Greater attention is needed to develop effective communication skills, recognise CALD patients' particular cultural, linguistic and spiritual values and needs, and acknowledge the unique nature of each doctor-patient interaction. Our findings point to some of the shared barriers and challenges experienced by CALD patients and caregivers in the transition to palliative care which can be broadly attributed to a lack of cultural and linguistic concordance with the Australian hospital system, and the clinicians therein, as well as revealing the difficulties in dealing with sensitive topics such as the end of life. Future research focusing on the meanings of various serious, life-limiting or terminal illnesses is needed across a diverse range of CALD patients and caregivers to better understand CALD experiences of the Australian health system and the ways by which culture and biography inflect illness (and care) experience. Further, to explore what can be learned from CALD communities as well as how to include and engage with CALD populations to continue to improve outcomes.

Endnotes

[1]We define the transition to palliative care as the referral and transfer to the care of a palliative care service. This transitional process may entail initial or ongoing consultation with a palliative care specialist within the current clinical setting, and may occur alongside potentially curative treatment, but eventually involves movement to another setting under the care of a palliative care service.

[2]Participants were approached using an interpreter in cases where participating clinician researchers determined the need for an interpreter as part of the patients care/consultations. That is, if a patient requested, or was deemed by clinicians to require an interpreter for their hospital appointments, we also used an interpreter to approach them about participation in the study.

[3]All interviews were conducted by the same research assistant interviewer, a sociologist with experience in conducting qualitative interviews, who was female and from an Anglo-Australian background. The interviewer was supported by the other members of the research team, including regular debriefing, redevelopment of the interview schedule and strategies/approaches to interviewing people within sensitive or vulnerable contexts, and interviewing through interpreters.

[4]Thirty nine potential participants were approached in total, all of whom initially agreed to participate; six dropped out of the study following initial interest and prior to taking part in an interview; three participants were not interviewed due to repeated difficulties in scheduling and availability.

[5]For example, several of our codes and subthemes were clear when getting a 'whole' sense of an interview transcript, but because of differences in linguistic style or proficiency in English among our participants, do not lend themselves straightforwardly

to being depicted through quotations within a paper in a conventional sense. A consequence of this is that some participants' voices are not privileged (or seemingly valued) within this paper, and as a research team we acknowledge the contribution made by all participants, and the value of every participant's data within our analytic process.

Abbreviations
CALD: Culturally and Linguistically Diverse; COREQ: COnsolidated criteria for REporting Qualitative research; HREC: Human Research Ethics Committee

Acknowledgements
The authors thank the study participants who generously offered their time and crucial insight into this research topic.

Funding
The authors gratefully acknowledge the interviewed participants and the financial support of the Australian Research Council (nos. LP120200268 and DE150100285) and the RACP Foundation (Cottrell Research Establishment Fellowship).

Authors' contributions
The project was designed and developed by AB, EK, ZL and PG. Data was collected by a research assistant with support from EK and AB. Data analysis was led by AB and EK with substantial input from ZL, PG, KK and HB. All authors contributed to the drafting and revising of the manuscript, and approved the final version of the manuscript.

Competing interests
The authors declare that they have no competing interests.

Author details
[1]Practical Justice Initiative, Faculty of Arts and Social Sciences, University of New South Wales, Level 3 Goodsell Building, University of New South Wales, Sydney, NSW 2052, Australia. [2]Royal Brisbane and Women's Hospital, Brisbane, QLD, Australia. [3]University of Queensland, Brisbane, QLD, Australia. [4]St Vincent's Private Hospital Brisbane, Brisbane, QLD, Australia. [5]Mater Health Services Brisbane, Brisbane, QLD, Australia.

References
1. Broom A, Kirby E. The end of life and the family: hospice patients' views on dying as relational. Sociology of Health and Illness. 2013;35(4):499–513.
2. Broom A. Dying: a social perspective on the end of life. Surrey, England: Ashgate; 2015.
3. Broom A, Good P, Kirby E, Lwin Z. Negotiating palliative care in the context of culturally and linguistically diverse patients. Intern Med J. 2013b;43(9):1043–6.
4. Broom A, Kirby E, Good P, et al. The art of letting go: referral to palliative care and its discontents. Soc Sci Med. 2013c;78:9–16.
5. Kirby E, Broom A, Good P, et al. Families and the transition to specialist palliative care. Mortality. 2014;19(4):323–41.
6. Kaufert JM, Lavallee M. End-of-life decision making among aboriginal Canadians: interpretation, mediation, and discord in the communication of "bad news". J Palliat Care. 1999;15(1):31–8.
7. Robb N, Greenhalgh T. "You have to cover up the words of the doctor": the mediation of trust in interpreted consultations in primary care. J Health Organ Manag. 2006;20(5):434–55.
8. Barclay JS, Blackhall LJ, Tulsky JA. Communication strategies and cultural issues in the delivery of bad news. J Palliat Med. 2007;10(4):958–77.
9. Kirby E, Broom A, Good P, Bowden V, Lwin Z. Experiences of interpreters in supporting the transition from oncology to palliative care: a qualitative study. Asia Pac J Clin Oncol. 2017;13(5):e497–505.
10. Clark K, Phillips J. End of life care - the importance of culture and ethnicity. Aust Fam Physician. 2010;39(4):210–3.
11. Rao DV, Warburton J, Bartlett H. Health and social needs of older Australians from culturally and linguistically diverse backgrounds: issues and implications. Australas J Ageing. 2006;25(4):174–9.
12. de Graaf FM, Franke AL, van den Muijsenbergh ME, van der Geest S. 'Palliative care': a contradiction in terms? A qualitative study of cancer patients with a Turkish or Moroccan background, their relatives and care providers. BMC Palliat Care. 2010;9:19.
13. de Graaff FM, Francke AL, van den Muijsenbergh ME, van der Geest S. Talking in triads: communication with Turkish and Moroccan immigrants in the palliative phase of cancer. J Clin Nurs. 2012;21:21–2.
14. Xue D, Wheeler JL, Abernethy AP. Cultural differences in truth-telling to cancer patients: Chinese and American approaches to the disclosure of 'bad news'. Progress in Palliat Care. 2011;19(3):125–31.
15. Perkins HS, Cortez JD, Hazuda HP. Cultural beliefs about a Patient's right time to die: an exploratory study. J Gen Intern Med. 2009;24(11):1240–7.
16. Gysels M, Evans N, Meñaca A, et al. Culture is a priority for research in end-of-life care in Europe: a research agenda. J Pain Symptom Manag. 2012;44(2):285–94.
17. Huang YL, Yates P, Prior D. Accommodating the diverse cultural needs of cancer patients and their families in palliative care. Cancer Nurs. 2009;32(1):E12–21.
18. Goodall KT, Newman LA, Ward PR. Improving access to health information for older migrants by using grounded theory and social network analysis to understand their information behaviour and digital technology use. Eur J Cancer Care. 2014;23(6):728–38.
19. Gordon D. Tenacious assumptions in western medicine. In: Lock M, Gordon D, editors. Biomedicine Examined. Dordrecht: Kluwer Academic Publishers; 1988. p. 19–56.
20. Girgis A, Sanson-Fisher RW. Breaking bad news: consensus guidelines for medical practitioners. J Clin Oncol. 1995;13(9):2449–56.
21. Butow P, Tattersall MHN, Clayton J, Goldstein D. Breaking bad news and truth disclosure in Australia. In: Surbone A, Zwitter M, Rajer M, Stiefel R, editors. New challenges in communication with Cancer patients. Boston, MA: Springer US; 2013. p. 377–87.
22. Blackhall LJ, Murphy ST, Frank G, et al. Ethnicity and attitudes toward patient autonomy. J Am Med Assoc. 1995;274(10):820–5.
23. Beauchamp TL, Childress JF. Principles of biomedical ethics. New York: Oxford University Press; 2001.
24. Kwak J, Haley W. Current research findings on end-of-life decision making among racially or ethnically diverse groups. Gerontologist. 2005;45:634–41.
25. Butow P, Lobb E, Jefford M, et al. A bridge between cultures: interpreters' perspectives of consultations with migrant oncology patients. Support Care Cancer. 2012;20(2):235–44.
26. Chiu C, Feuz M, McMahan R, et al. "Doctor, make my decisions": decision control preferences, advance care planning, and satisfaction with communication among diverse older adults. J Pain Symptom Manag. 2016;51(1):33–40.
27. Huang X, Butow P, Meiser B, Goldstein D. Attitudes and information needs of Chinese migrant cancer patients and their relatives. Aust NZ J Med. 1999;29(2):207–13.
28. Mitchison D, Butow P, Sze M, et al. Prognostic communication preferences of migrant patients and their relatives. Psycho-Oncology. 2012;21(5):496–504.
29. Broom A, Kirby E, Good P, et al. The troubles of telling: managing communication about the end of life. Qual Health Res. 2014;24(2):151–62.

30. Gray B, Hilder J, Donaldson H. Why do we not use trained interpreters for all patients with limited English proficiency? Is there a place for using family members? Aust J Prim Health. 2011;17:240–9.
31. Farini F. The pragmatics of emotions in interlinguistic healthcare settings. Res Lang. 2013;11:163.
32. Leanza Y, Boivin I, Rosenberg E. Interruptions and resistance: a comparison of medical consultations with family and trained interpreters. Soc Sci Med. 2010;70(12):1888–95.
33. Tong A, Sainsbury P, Craig J. Consolidated criteria for reporting qualitative research (COREQ): a 32-item checklist for interviews and focus groups. Int J Qual Health Care. 2007;19(6):349–57.
34. Charmaz K. 'Discovering' chronic illness: using grounded theory. Soc Sci Med. 1990;30(11):1161–72.
35. Pope C, Ziebland S, Mays N. Analysing qualitative data. In: Pope C, Mays N, editors. Qualitative research in health care. 3rd ed. Oxford: Blackwell Publishing; 2006. p. 63–81.
36. Ezzy D. Qualitative analysis. Allen and Unwin: Australia; 2002.
37. Fitzpatrick R, Boulton M. Qualitative research in health care: the scope and validity of methods. J Eval Clin Pract. 1996;2:123–30.
38. Malterud K, Siersma VD, Guassora AD. Sample size in qualitative interview studies. Qual Health Res. 2015;26:1753–60.
39. Boström B, Sandh M, Lundberg D, Fridlund B. Cancer-related pain in palliative care: patients' perceptions of pain management. J Adv Nurs. 2004; 45(4):410–9.
40. Mitchell G. Palliative care in Australia. Ochsner J. 2011;11:334–7.
41. Borneman T, Stahl C, Ferrell BR, Smith D. The concept of hope in family caregivers of patients at home. J Hosp Paliat Nurs. 2002;4(1):21–33.
42. Zimmerman C. Death denial: obstacle or instrument for palliative care? An analysis of clinical literature. Sociol Health Illn. 2017;29(2):297–314.
43. Markovic M, Manderson L, Wray N, Quinn M. He's telling us something. Anthropol Med. 2004;11(3):327–41.
44. Squires A. Methodological challenges in cross-language qualitative research: a research review. Int J Nurs Stud. 2009;46:277–87.
45. Temple B. Crossed wires: interpreters, translators, and bilingual workers in cross-language research. Qual Health Res. 2002;12(6):844–54.

The availability and effectiveness of tools supporting shared decision making in metastatic breast cancer care

Inge Spronk[1*], Jako S. Burgers[2], François G. Schellevis[1,3], Liesbeth M. van Vliet[1] and Joke C. Korevaar[1]

Abstract

Background: Shared decision-making (SDM) in the management of metastatic breast cancer care is associated with positive patient outcomes. In daily clinical practice, however, SDM is not fully integrated yet. Initiatives to improve the implementation of SDM would be helpful. The aim of this review was to assess the availability and effectiveness of tools supporting SDM in metastatic breast cancer care.

Methods: Literature databases were systematically searched for articles published since 2006 focusing on the development or evaluation of tools to improve information-provision and to support decision-making in metastatic breast cancer care. Internet searches and experts identified additional tools. Data from included tools were extracted and the evaluation of tools was appraised using the GRADE grading system.

Results: The literature search yielded five instruments. In addition, two tools were identified via internet searches and consultation of experts. Four tools were specifically developed for supporting SDM in metastatic breast cancer, the other three tools focused on metastatic cancer in general. Tools were mainly applicable across the care process, and usable for decisions on supportive care with or without chemotherapy. All tools were designed for patients to be used before a consultation with the physician. Effects on patient outcomes were generally weakly positive although most tools were not studied in well-designed studies.

Conclusions: Despite its recognized importance, only two tools were positively evaluated on effectiveness and are available to support patients with metastatic breast cancer in SDM. These tools show promising results in pilot studies and focus on different aspects of care. However, their effectiveness should be confirmed in well-designed studies before implementation in clinical practice. Innovation and development of SDM tools targeting clinicians as well as patients during a clinical encounter is recommended.

Keywords: Shared decision making, Metastatic breast cancer, Decision aid

Background

Breast cancer is the most commonly diagnosed cancer type among women worldwide and the fifth cause of cancer related deaths [1]. In metastatic breast cancer care many complex decisions need to be made, of which most are preference-sensitive [2, 3]. Important treatment decisions include for example whether or not to start chemotherapy or targeted therapy [4].

Shared decision making (SDM) is an approach in which health care providers and patients share the best evidence when facing decisions, and patients are encouraged to be actively involved in decision making [5, 6]. SDM has been identified as an important element for good advanced cancer care [7]. Most cancer patients prefer to participate in decision making [8, 9]. Among patients with advanced cancer, women with breast cancer in particular wish to be actively involved in decision making [10]. SDM is associated with positive patient outcomes, including knowledge regarding available options, perceived quality of care [11, 12], and quality of life [13].

* Correspondence: ingespronk@gmail.com
[1]NIVEL (Netherlands Institute for Health Services Research), P.O. Box 1568, 3500BN Utrecht, The Netherlands
Full list of author information is available at the end of the article

The use of tools might support active participation of patients in decision-making. Examples of such instruments are 1) decision aids (DAs) which are designed to be used by patients before doctor visits to prepare for decision making [14–16], and 2) tools to be used by both health care providers and patients during clinical encounters [17, 18]. DAs are developed to support patients in decision making by providing an overview of the available (treatment) options and their associated outcomes [15, 19]. There are many types of DAs, such as video or audiotapes, patient letters, computer programs, leaflets, and interactive media [12].

The tools designed to be used during consultation with a health care provider have been developed to facilitate a conversation between health care providers and patients about the relevant (treatment) options. In general, these tools are brief and present a summary of available options. Examples are decision boards, bar charts, option grids and consult decision aids [17, 18, 20–22].

The aims of this study were 1) to make an inventory of instruments and tools, including DAs and tools used during clinical encounters, that are currently available for supporting SDM in metastatic breast cancer care and 2) to evaluate the effectiveness of these tools based on published studies.

Methods

Three strategies were used to identify tools for supporting SDM in metastatic breast cancer. First, a systematic search of relevant databases was undertaken, secondly an internet search was conducted and lastly experts who appeared in the searches were contacted.

Systematic search

Search strategy

A systematic literature search was conducted in Cinahl, Medline, PsychInfo and Pubmed to identify relevant articles published between 1 January 2006 and 18 January 2017. This time frame was chosen as we were looking for tools that are still clinical relevant and up-to-date. If there were instruments developed before 2006 that are still relevant, we would have find them in either later publications, via our internet search, or via the experts that we have approached. The search strategy was developed in collaboration with an experienced librarian and checked by an expert in the field. It combined terms covering the areas of breast cancer (breast cancer; breast carcinoma; breast neoplasms), advanced cancer (advanced cancer, metastatic cancer, palliative care), decision making (decision making, decision support, decision aid, shared decision) (Appendix 1). Hand-searching of reference lists of included articles was conducted to identify additional studies.

Study selection

The search was performed by one reviewer (IS), and after removal of duplicates, irrelevant articles were eliminated on the basis of title and abstract. Ten percent was independently evaluated by two reviewers (IS and JK). There was no disagreement between the reviewers on inclusion. Therefore, the remaining abstracts were evaluated by one reviewer (IS). Screening of full text of relevant articles was independently performed by two reviewers (IS and JK). Disagreements were resolved by discussion with a third reviewer (FS).

Inclusion criteria

Research articles and (systematic) reviews on studies conducted in advanced breast cancer patients, written in any language and published in a peer-reviewed journal were included for review. Studies needed to focus on the development and/or evaluation of an initiative or tool that focused on i) information provision about decisions, ii) decision making process, or iii) eliciting treatment preferences in metastatic breast cancer care. Outcomes included in the studies had to be any i) patient-reported outcome, or ii) health outcome.

Data extraction

Characteristics of tools (name, country, description, target population, type of tool, decision on which tool focusses), study characteristics (first author, year of publication, study size, patients characteristics, study design, outcome measures) and patient-reported and health outcomes were independently extracted by two reviewers (IS and JK).

Study quality

Quality of the studies evaluating the tools was independently assessed by two reviewers (IS and JK) using the Grading of Recommendations Assessment, Development and Evaluation (GRADE) methodology [23]. This methodology classifies evidence into four levels of quality (high to very low). First the studies were classified based on their design, with high quality for randomized control trials and low quality for observational studies. These initial grades can be downgraded or upgraded after assessment of their weaknesses and strengths. The five downgrading criteria are risk of bias, indirectness of evidence, inconsistency of results imprecision of results, and publication bias. The three upgrading criteria are large magnitude of effect, dose-response, and opposing residual confounding or bias. Based on the up- and downgrading criteria, the final evidence grade was determined [23].

Internet search and consultation of experts

An internet search was performed and experts were approached to complement the systematic literature search using the same inclusion criteria. Google searches covering the areas metastatic breast cancer (advanced breast cancer, metastatic breast cancer, palliative breast cancer care) and decision making (decision making, decision support, decision aid, shared decision) were carried out and websites presenting an overview of decision aids were studied (http://www.med-decs.org/, https://decisionaid.ohri.ca/). National and international experts who appeared in the systematic literature and internet searches were approached via email and asked whether they were aware of tools, instruments or initiatives supporting SDM in metastatic breast cancer care. From the tools identified by internet searches and experts the same characteristics were extracted as from those identified by the systematic literature search.

Results

The initial literature search resulted in 687 potentially relevant articles. After removal of duplicates and elimination of non-eligible papers based on title and abstract, 13 full-text articles were considered, of which seven were included for review (Fig. 1). The seven articles described five different tools. In addition, the internet search revealed two relevant tools. All 17 experts approached responded and identified one additional relevant tool (Table 1).

In total, seven tools were identified (Table 1). Three were developed in the USA, three in the Netherlands and one in Canada and Australia. Four tools were specifically designed for metastatic breast cancer, the others for metastatic cancer patients in general. Three tools focused on the decision on whether or not to start chemotherapy [24–27]. The other four focused on all possible decisions during the entire metastatic breast cancer care trajectory. All tools were developed for patients to be used before consultation with their health care provider. Only one tool [28] provided a summary report to the health care provider which could be discussed during a consultation.

The content of five out of seven tools was evaluated in published studies (Table 2). Of four of these, the effectiveness was studied as well. CONNECT, the communication aid from Meropol et al. was tested in a randomized clinical trial [28]. Outcome measures included consultation content, treatment outcome expectations, decisional conflict, patient satisfaction with the content and format of the communication, and satisfaction with the survey and/or communication skills training. CONNECT made it easier for patients to make treatment decisions ($P = 0.003$) and patients were more satisfied with their decision ($P < 0.001$), with physician communication ($P = 0.026$), with discussion regarding support services ($P = 0.029$) and quality of life concerns ($P = 0.042$), but not with discussion of diagnosis/prognosis, treatment options, or support/community services. The DA of Oostendorp et al., [25, 26, 29] was

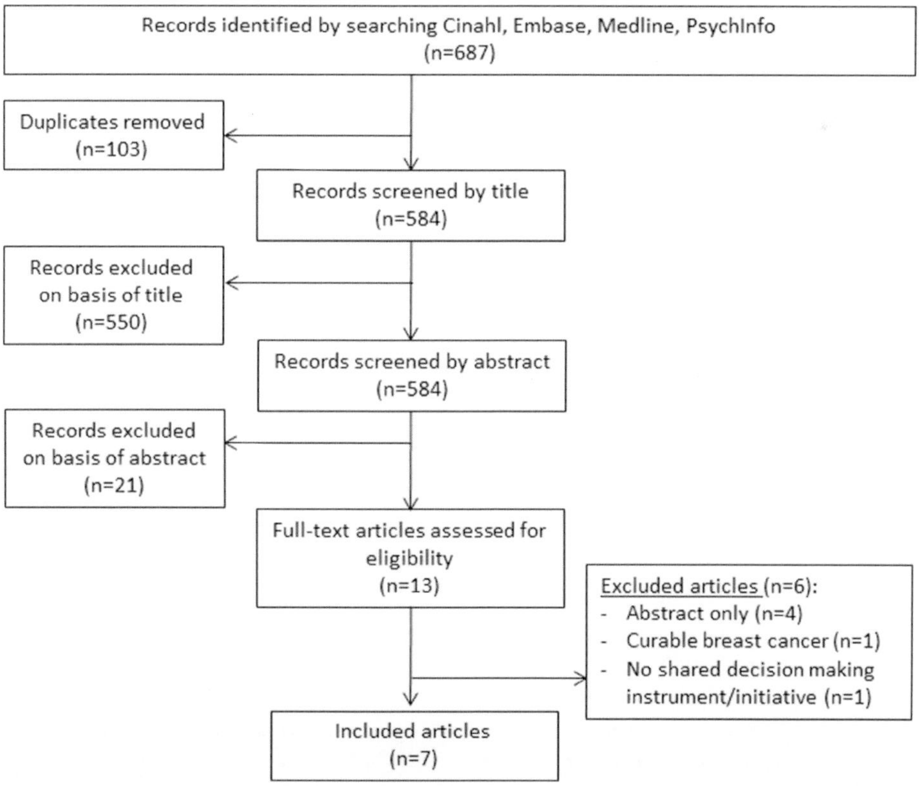

Fig. 1 Flowchart outlining article selection process

Table 1 Overview of tools for shared decision making in metastatic breast cancer

Name tool/short description	Country	Source[a]	Specific for metastatic breast cancer	Description of tool
CONNECT	USA	S	No	A communication aid that assesses patient preferences and values, and includes communication skills training, plus summary report to the physician.
Decision aid on first, second, third and fourth line chemotherapy	USA	S	No	State-of-the-art tables with information for patients with advanced breast, lung, colon, and hormone-refractory prostate cancers
Decision aid on first-line chemotherapy	Australia and Canada	E, S	Yes	A DA presenting options of supportive care, with or without chemotherapy. Potential benefits and side effects of different chemotherapy regimens, and evidence-based prognostic estimates are described, and a values clarification exercise is included.
Decision aid on second-line chemotherapy	The Netherlands	E, I, S	Yes	A DA describing the adverse events, response of the cancer and survival of supportive care with or without second-line palliative chemotherapy.
Decision aid 'metastatic breast cancer'	The Netherlands	I	Yes	A booklet presenting information on therapies and supportive treatment in metastatic breast cancer. It provides information on what characteristics define how metastatic breast cancer can be treated and shows other patients arguments for and against treatment.
Consultation guide	The Netherlands	E	No	A booklet with sample questions and an instrument for value clarification.
Living with Metastatic Breast Cancer: Making the Journey Your Own.	USA	S	Yes	A thirty-minute video/DVD and accompanying booklet depicting the experiences of 4 women living with metastatic breast cancer.

Note. [a]Source: *S* systematic search, *E* experts, *I* internet search
DA decision aid

evaluated in a randomized clinical trial. Primary outcome measures included several measurements on patient's well-being on which the DA had no statistically significant effect. The DA was associated with stronger treatments preferences of patients ($P = 0.030$) and with increased subjective knowledge ($P = 0.022$), but not with any of the other secondary outcomes measures. The two other tools [27, 30] were tested in pilot studies without control groups. The DA of Smith et al. [27] assessed whether patients choose to use the DA, investigated the knowledge of patients about the disease and treatment and examined whether the information of the DA was helpful and if the patient wanted to share the information with the physician. All except one patient used the DA and knowledge about the cure of advanced cancer improved after using the DA ($P = 0.15$). Most patients found the information helpful and almost all patients wanted to share information with their physician after use of these DAs, which might result in SDM. The study on the DA developed by Sepucha et al. [30] evaluated acceptability of the DA and its impact on decisions. The DA was rated acceptable, did not increase distress ($P = 0.34$) and the treatment goal was most often to lengthen life. Most patients (88%) wanted to be involved in shared decision making, however, only 41% found that decision making was shared and 38% achieved their desired level of participation in decision making. The content of the tool and attitudes towards the tool developed by Chiew et al. was evaluated by both patients and medical oncologists [24]. The patients concluded that the DA was acceptable and helpful and the majority recommend the use of this DA to others. Also the oncologists were positive about the DA and found the DA appropriate for all or most patients.

The quality of five evaluation studies could be assessed. According to the GRADE approach, the quality of the studies ranged between moderate and very low (Table 2). All studies had noteworthy shortcomings, mainly because of the study design. Two had a randomized design and the others were observational studies [24, 27, 30]. The quality of the three observational studies was downgraded to 'very low' due to small samples sizes, unclear descriptions of inclusion criteria and lack of information on loss to follow-up. The quality of the studies with a randomised design was downgraded as well [28, 29]. Both studies had a high drop-out rate. And one defined no primary outcome and presented selective results as two of the intervention arms were combined to obtain significant results.

Discussion

This review identified seven tools to support SDM in metastatic breast cancer care. All were designed to be used independently by patients before consulting a physician. None was developed to be used by both a health care provider and patient during a clinical encounter, although one tool

Table 2 Evaluated tools

Name tool/ short description	First author (year)	Study population[a]	Design	Decision aid outcome measures	Outcome	GRADE
CONNECT	Meropol (2013)	Metastatic cancer patients, $n = 629$ (F:48%), mean age: 59 year	Randomized clinical trial with 3 arms	Consultation content, treatment outcome expectations, decisional conflict, patient satisfaction with the content and format of the communication, and satisfaction with the survey and/or communication skills training	• Treatment decisions were easier to reach ($P = 0.003$) • Patients were more satisfied with decisions ($P < 0.001$) • Patients were more satisfied with physician communication ($P = 0.026$) • Patients were more satisfied with discussion regarding support services ($P = 0.029$) and quality of life concerns ($P = 0.042$) • No statistically significant differences in satisfaction regarding discussion of diagnosis/prognosis, treatment options, or support/community services.	Low
Decision aid on first, second, third and fourth line chemotherapy	Smith (2011)	Patients with metastatic breast, colorectal or lung cancer, $n = 27$ (F:56%), mean age: 63 year	Pilot pretest, posttest study	Number of patients who opt for full disclosure once they viewed the DA The amount of information patients have about cure, response rates, and symptom control; the impact of truthful information on hope, whether the information was deemed helpful to the patient; and whether the patient want to share the information with a physician	• 96% of the patients chose to complete the DA • The proportion of patients who thought that advanced cancer could be cured reduced from 52 to 31% ($P = 0.15$) • 87% of the patients overestimated the effect of palliative chemotherapy • No distress was noted and hope did not change • 74% found the information helpful • 93% wanted to share the information with their family and physician	Very low
Decision aid on first-line chemotherapy	Chiew (2008)	Metastatic breast cancer patients, $n = 17$ (F:100%), median age: 58 year Medical oncologists, $n = 7$	Pilot observational study	Patients' attitudes toward the DA, and oncologist feedback regarding attitudes toward the DA.	• The DA was rated acceptable and helpful. • The DA contains an appropriate amount of information, and the length is appropriate • 94% of the patients would recommend use of the DA to others • Oncologists received the DA positively and found it appropriate for all or most patients	Very low
Decision aid on second-line chemotherapy	Oostendorp (2017)	Patients with metastatic breast or colorectal cancer, $n = 128$ (F:63%), median age: 62 year	Randomized clinical trial	Anxiety, depression, general health, cancer worries, health-related quality of life, coping styles, amount of information received, satisfaction with quality of information, subjective knowledge, treatment preference, decision satisfaction and uncertainty, decision control and treatment attitudes.	• The DA had no adverse impact on patient's well-being • Use of the DA was associated with stronger treatment preferences ($P = 0.030$) and increased subjective knowledge ($P = 0.022$) • No statistically significant differences in anxiety, depression, general health, cancer worries, health-related quality of life, coping styles, amount of information received, satisfaction with quality of information, decision satisfaction and uncertainty, decision control and treatment attitudes.	Moderate
						Very low

Table 2 Evaluated tools *(Continued)*

Name tool/ short description	First author (year)	Study population[a]	Design	Decision aid outcome measures	Outcome	GRADE
Living with Metastatic Breast Cancer: Making the Journey Your Own	Sepucha (2009)	Metastatic breast cancer patients, $n = 32$ (F:100%), median age: 55 year	Pilot pretest, posttest study	Use and acceptability of DA, distress, treatment goals, and preference for and actual participation in decision	• The DA was rated acceptable and did not increase distress ($P = 0.34$) • Most patients (88%) desired to share decision making with their physician • 41% of the patients found that decision making was shared • 38% achieved their desired level of participation • The main goal of treatment was most often to lengthen life	

Note. [a]Study population: *n* sample size, *F* female, *NA* not applicable
DA decision aid

provided a summary report for the physician which could be discussed during a consultation. In general, the identified tools had positive effects on patient satisfaction with their treatment decision and on patients' desire to share information with their physician. However, it is unclear whether they encourage SDM during a clinical encounter as this was not studied. The effectiveness of the included tools was barely studied. Evidence from the included studies was in general low due to multiple sources of bias, which may have skewed the results.

The revealed tools to support patients in SDM have some limitations. The effectiveness of only four of them was evaluated [27–30]. Of these, the one with the highest level of evidence was not effective [29]. The other tool with a somewhat higher level of evidence of effectiveness is not available anymore [28] as the tool was not kept up-to-date. The two remaining tools might be useful in clinical practice as their results are promising in pilot studies. These tools could be used next to each other as the DA of Smith et al. [27] focuses on chemotherapy, whereas the DA of Sepucha et al. [30] shows the experiences of four women living with metastatic breast cancer. A limitation of these tools is that they were only tested in a pilot study without a control group. Further testing of these tools in better designed studies is required before they are implemented. The consultation guide presenting information on therapies and supportive treatment in metastatic breast cancer, was not evaluated, but might also be useful for patients with metastatic breast cancer.

Despite the calls for integrating SDM in clinical practice, implementation of SDM into daily care is lacking [31–34]. The lack of available SDM supporting tools and time concerns might be barriers for implementation [6]. Our review shows the availability of a few tools to be used by patients before visiting the physician and the lack of tools to be used during a clinical encounter in metastatic breast cancer care. In general, tools to be used by patients before visiting the health care provider lead to better understanding of choices, however, yet are not enough to guarantee SDM [14, 35]. In order to facilitate SDM during a clinical encounter, SDM tools for both health care providers and patients have been designed [35–37]. For curative breast cancer and other tumour types, such tools are available [17, 18]. These tools make options more visible, enhances patients confidence and involvement, and clinicians find it easier to implement SDM in practice [18]. For decision making in metastatic breast cancer care, there is a pressing need for similar tools as many complex decisions have to be made and alignment of care with patient preferences is necessary.

When developing, testing and implementing tools for SDM during a clinical encounter, several recommendations can be made. First, tools should be based on the best available scientific evidence and being kept up-to-date [25, 38–40]. Second, patients should be included in their development to ensure the tools are user-friendly and understandable [41]. Third, the impact on patient outcomes should be evaluated. Fourth, the conditions for appropriate use of tools in clinical practice should be realized, e.g. clinical teams should recognise the importance of SDM and should be trained in SDM [6, 42], and sufficient time should be available to use a tools for SDM during a clinical encounter [6, 43–45].

Conclusions

Only two tools for SDM in metastatic breast cancer care were positively evaluated on effectiveness and are currently available. These are developed to be used by patients before consulting the physician. None have been tested in well-designed studies. These tools show promising results in pilot studies and focus on different aspects of care. However, their effectiveness should be confirmed in well-designed studies before implementation in clinical practice. Innovation and development of SDM tools targeting clinicians as well as patients during a clinical encounter is recommended.

Appendix 1. Search strategy

Table 3 Search in Pubmed (date: 18 January 2017)

Search strategy		Number of hits
	Breast cancer	
#1	"breast cancer" [tiab]	
#2	breast neoplasms [mesh]	
#3	"breast neoplasm*" [tiab]	
#4	"breast carcinoma" [tiab]	
#5	"breast tumor" [tiab]	
#6	"breast tumour" [tiab]	
#9	#1 OR #2 OR #3 OR #4 OR #5 OR #6 OR #7 OR #8	307,107
	Palliative care	
#10	palliative care [mesh]	
#11	palliative [tiab]	
#12	Hospice Care [mesh]	
#13	hospice [tiab]	
#14	end-of-life [tiab]	
#15	terminal [tiab]	
#16	incurable [tiab]	
#17	Terminal Care [mesh]	
#18	"early palliative care" [tiab]	
#19	"serious illness" [tiab]	
#20	"advanced cancer" [tiab]	
#21	"metastatic cancer" [tiab]	
#22	metastasis [tiab]	
#23	Neoplasm Metastasis [MeSH Terms]	
#24	#10 OR #11 OR #12 OR #13 OR #14 OR #15 OR #16 OR #17	770,461
	Decision making	
#19	"decision making"[tiab]	
#20	"decision support"[tiab]	
#21	"decision aid*"[tiab]	
#22	"choice behavior"[tiab]	
#23	"choice behaviour"[tiab]	
#24	(((((shared)[tiab] OR sharing)[tiab] OR informed[tiab]))) AND ((decision*[tiab]) OR choice*[tiab])	
#25	#19 OR #20 OR #21 OR #22 OR #23 OR #24	116,279
#26	#9 AND #18 AND #25	314
	limit #26 to (humans and yr. = "2006–2017")	181

Note. This initial search strategy was adapted to Cinahl, Medline and PsychInfo

Abbreviations

DA: Decision aid; GRADE: Grading of Recommendations Assessment, Development and Evaluation; SDM: Shared decision-making

Acknowledgements

We thank Prof. dr. Glyn Elwyn for checking our search strategy.

Funding

LvV is funded by a Dutch Cancer Society Young Investigator Grant (Grant number: 10392). The other authors are not funded.

Authors' contributions

All authors contributed to the study concept and design, the data analysis and interpretation, reviewed the final manuscript, and agree to be accountable for all aspects of the work. IS and JK collected and extracted the data, and checked the quality of the data. The manuscript was prepared by IS and edited by JB, FS, LvV and JK.

Competing interests

The authors declare that they have no competing interests.

Author details

[1]NIVEL (Netherlands Institute for Health Services Research), P.O. Box 1568, 3500BN Utrecht, The Netherlands. [2]Dutch College of General Practitioners, Utrecht, The Netherlands. School CAPHRI, Department Family Medicine, Maastricht University, Maastricht, The Netherlands. [3]Department of General Practice & Elderly Care Medicine/ Amsterdam Public Health Research Institute, VU University Medical Center, Amsterdam, The Netherlands.

References

1. GLOBOCAN 2012: Estimated Cancer Incidence, Mortality and Prevalence Worldwide in 2012. 2012. http://globocan.iarc.fr/Pages/fact_sheets_cancer.aspx (2012). Accessed 1 Feb 2017.
2. Lux MP, Bayer CM, Loehberg CR, Fasching PA, Schrauder MG, Bani MR, et al. Shared decision-making in metastatic breast cancer: discrepancy between the expected prolongation of life and treatment efficacy between patients and physicians, and influencing factors. Breast Cancer Res Treat. 2013;139:429–40.
3. Leighl NB, Butow PN, Tattersall MH. Treatment decision aids in advanced cancer: when the goal is not cure and the answer is not clear. J Clin Oncol. 2004;22:1759–62.
4. Partridge AH, Rumble RB, Carey LA, Come SE, Davidson NE, Di Leo A, et al. Chemotherapy and targeted therapy for women with human epidermal growth factor receptor 2–negative (or unknown) advanced breast cancer: American Society of Clinical Oncology clinical practice guideline. J Clin Oncol. 2014;32:3307–29.
5. Elwyn G, Laitner S, Coulter A, Walker E, Watson P, Thomson R. Implementing shared decision making in the NHS. BMJ. 2010;341:c5146.
6. Légaré F, Ratté S, Gravel K, Graham ID. Barriers and facilitators to implementing shared decision-making in clinical practice: update of a systematic review of health professionals' perceptions. Patient Educ Couns. 2008;73:526–35.
7. Institute of Medicine. Delivering high-quality cancer care: charting a new course for a system in crisis. Washington, DC: National Academies Press; 2013.

8. Degner LF, Sloan JA. Decision making during serious illness: what role do patients really want to play? J Clin Epidemiol. 1992;45:941–50.
9. Keating NL, Guadagnoli E, Landrum MB, Borbas C, Weeks JC. Treatment decision making in early-stage breast cancer: should surgeons match patients' desired level of involvement? J Clin Oncol. 2002;20:1473–9.
10. Gaston CM, Mitchell G. Information giving and decision-making in patients with advanced cancer: a systematic review. Soc Sci Med. 2005;61:2252–64.
11. Kehl KL, Landrum MB, Arora NK, Ganz PA, Van Ryn M, Mack JW, et al. Association of actual and preferred decision roles with patient-reported quality of care: shared decision making in cancer care. JAMA Oncol. 2015;1:50–8.
12. Stacey D, Légaré F, Lewis K, Barry MJ, Bennett CL, Eden KB, et al. Decision aids for people facing health treatment or screening decisions. Cochrane Database Syst Rev. 2017;Issue 4. Art. No.: CD001431. https://doi.org/10.1002/14651858.CD001431.pub5
13. Kashaf MS, McGill E. Does shared decision making in cancer treatment improve quality of life? A systematic literature review. Med Decis Mak. 2015; 35:1037–48.
14. Hargraves I, Montori VM. Decision aids, empowerment, and shared decision making. BMJ. 2014;349:g5811.
15. Stacey D, Bennett CL, Barry MJ, Col NF, Eden KB, Holmes-Rovner M, Thomson R. Decision aids for people facing health treatment or screening decisions. Cochrane Database Syst Rev. 2011;10(10).
16. Ozanne EM, Partridge A, Moy B, Ellis KJ, Sepucha KR. Doctor-patient communication about advance directives in metastatic breast cancer. J Palliat Med. 2009;12:547–53.
17. Elwyn G, Lloyd A, Joseph-Williams N, Cording E, Thomson R, Durand M-A, et al. Option grids: shared decision making made easier. Patient Educ Couns. 2013;90:207–12.
18. Stacey D, Légaré F, Lyddiatt A, Giguere AM, Yoganathan M, Saarimaki A, Tugwell P. Translating evidence to facilitate shared decision making: development and usability of a consult decision aid prototype. The Patient. 2016; 9(6):571–82.
19. Elwyn G, O'Connor A, Stacey D, Volk R, Edwards A, Coulter A, et al. Developing a quality criteria framework for patient decision aids: online international Delphi consensus process. BMJ. 2006;333:417.
20. Elwyn G, Edwards A, Hood K, Robling M, Atwell C, Russell I, et al. Achieving involvement: process outcomes from a cluster randomized trial of shared decision making skill development and use of risk communication aids in general practice. Fam Pract. 2004;21:337–46.
21. Whelan T, Gafni A, Charles C, Levine M. Lessons learned from the decision board: a unique and evolving decision aid. Health Expect. 2000;3:69–76.
22. Tang J, Shakespeare T, Lu J, Chan Y, Lee K, Wong L, et al. Patients' preference for radiotherapy fractionation schedule in the palliation of symptomatic unresectable lung cancer. J Med Imaging Radiat Oncol. 2008;52:497–502.
23. Guyatt GH, Oxman AD, Vist GE, Kunz R, Falck-Ytter Y, Alonso-Coello P, et al. GRADE: an emerging consensus on rating quality of evidence and strength of recommendations. BMJ. 2008;336:924–6.
24. Chiew KS, Shepherd H, Vardy J, Tattersall MH, Butow PN, Leighl NB. Development and evaluation of a decision aid for patients considering first-line chemotherapy for metastatic breast cancer. Health Expect. 2008;11:35–45.
25. Oostendorp LJ, Ottevanger PB, van de Wouw AJ, Schoenaker IJ, de Graaf H, van der Graaf WT, et al. Expected survival with and without second-line palliative chemotherapy: who wants to know? Health Expect. 2015;18:2903–14.
26. Oostendorp LJM, Ottevanger PB, van de Wouw AJ, Honkoop AH, Los M, van der Graaf WTA, et al. Patients' preferences for information about the benefits and risks of second-line palliative chemotherapy and their oncologist's awareness of these preferences. J Cancer Educ. 2016;31:443–8.
27. Smith TJ, Dow LA, Virago EA, Khatcheressian J, Matsuyama R, Lyckholm LJ. A pilot trial of decision aids to give truthful prognostic and treatment information to chemotherapy patients with advanced cancer. J Support Oncol. 2011;9:79.
28. Meropol NJ, Egleston BL, Buzaglo JS, Balshem A, Benson AB, Cegala DJ, et al. A web-based communication aid for patients with cancer. Cancer. 2013; 119:1437–45.
29. Oostendorp LJM, Ottevanger PB, Donders ART, Wouw AJ, Schoenaker IJH, Smilde TJ, et al. Decision aids for second-line palliative chemotherapy: a randomised phase II multicentre trial. BMC Med Inform Decis Mak. 2017;17:130.
30. Sepucha KR, Ozanne EM, Partridge AH, Moy B. Is there a role for decision aids in advanced breast cancer? Med Decis Mak. 2009;29:475–82.
31. Department of Health. Equity and excellence: liberating the NHS. London: National Health Service; 2010.
32. United States Federal Statute. The patient protection and affordable care act. Washington: US Government; 2010.
33. Australian Commission on Safety and Quality in Health Care: National Statement on health literacy: taking action to improve safety and quality; 2014.
34. Chow S, Teare G, Basky G. Shared decision making: helping the system and patients make quality health care decisions. Saskatchewan: Health Quality Council; 2009.
35. Stiggelbout AM, Van der Weijden T, De Wit M, Frosch D, Légaré F, Montori VM, et al. Shared decision making: really putting patients at the Centre of healthcare. BMJ. 2012;344:e256.
36. Breslin M, Mullan RJ, Montori VM. The design of a decision aid about diabetes medications for use during the consultation with patients with type 2 diabetes. Patient Educ Couns. 2008;73:465–72.
37. Elwyn G, Frosch D, Volandes AE, Edwards A, Montori VM. Investing in deliberation: a definition and classification of decision support interventions for people facing difficult health decisions. Med Decis Mak. 2010;30:701–11.
38. Joseph-Williams N, Newcombe R, Politi M, Durand M-A, Sivell S, Stacey D, et al. Toward minimum standards for certifying patient decision aids: a modified Delphi consensus process. Med Decis Mak. 2014;34:699–710.
39. Durand M-A, Witt J, Joseph-Williams N, Newcombe RG, Politi MC, Sivell S, et al. Minimum standards for the certification of patient decision support interventions: feasibility and application. Patient Educ Couns. 2015;98:462–8.
40. Montori VM, LeBlanc A, Buchholz A, Stilwell DL, Tsapas A. Basing information on comprehensive, critically appraised, and up-to-date syntheses of the scientific evidence: a quality dimension of the international patient decision aid standards. BMC Med Inform Decis Mak. 2013;13:S5.
41. Montori VM, Breslin M, Maleska M, Weymiller AJ. Creating a conversation: insights from the development of a decision aid. PLoS Med. 2007;4:e233.
42. Lloyd A, Joseph-Williams N, Edwards A, Rix A, Elwyn G. Patchy 'coherence': using normalization process theory to evaluate a multi-faceted shared decision making implementation program (MAGIC). Implement Sci. 2013;8:102.
43. Joseph-Williams N, Elwyn G, Edwards A. Knowledge is not power for patients: a systematic review and thematic synthesis of patient-reported barriers and facilitators to shared decision making. Patient Educ Couns. 2014;94:291–309.
44. O'Brien MA, Ellis PM, Whelan TJ, Charles C, Gafni A, Lovrics P, et al. Physician-related facilitators and barriers to patient involvement in treatment decision making in early stage breast cancer: perspectives of physicians and patients. Health Expect. 2013;16:373–84.
45. Belcher VN, Fried TR, Agostini JV, Tinetti ME. Views of older adults on patient participation in medication-related decision making. J Gen Intern Med. 2006;21:298–303.

Does special education in palliative medicine make a difference in end-of-life decision-making?

Reetta P. Piili[1,2,3*], Juho T. Lehto[1,2], Tiina Luukkaala[4,5], Heikki Hinkka[6] and Pirkko-Liisa I. Kellokumpu-Lehtinen[1,2]

Abstract

Background: Characteristics of the physician influence the essential decision-making in end-of-life care. However, the effect of special education in palliative medicine on different aspects of decision-making in end-of-life care remains unknown. The aim of this study was to explore the decision-making in end-of-life care among physicians with or without special competency in palliative medicine (cPM).

Methods: A questionnaire including an advanced lung cancer patient-scenario with multiple decision options in end-of-life care situation was sent to 1327 Finnish physicians. Decisions to withdraw or withhold ten life-prolonging interventions were asked on a scale from 1 (definitely would not) to 5 (definitely would) – first, without additional information and then after the family's request for aggressive treatment and the availability of an advance directive. Values from chronological original scenario, family's appeal and advance directive were clustered by trajectory analysis.

Results: We received 699 (53%) responses. The mean values of the ten answers in the original scenario were 4.1 in physicians with cPM, 3.4 in general practitioners, 3.4 in surgeons, 3.5 in internists and 3.8 in oncologists ($p < 0.05$ for physicians with cPM vs. oncologists and $p < 0.001$ for physicians with cPM vs. others). Younger age and not being an oncologist or not having cPM increased aggressive treatment decisions in multivariable logistic regression analysis. The less aggressive approach of physicians with cPM differed between therapies, being most striking concerning intravenous hydration, nasogastric tube and blood transfusions. The aggressive approach increased by the family's request ($p < 0.001$) and decreased by an advance directive ($p < 0.001$) in all physicians, regardless of special education in palliative medicine.

Conclusion: Physicians with special education in palliative medicine make less aggressive decisions in end-of-life care. The impact of specialty on decision-making varies among treatment options. Education in end-of-life care decision-making should be mandatory for young physicians and those in specialty training.

Keywords: Decision-making, Terminal care, Education, Palliative medicine, Life support care

Background

Rapid developments in medicine have allowed many interventions for patients with very advanced diseases. At the same time, the difficulty of choosing worthwhile therapies for each patient has led to the use of non-beneficial treatments among dying patients at their end-of-life (EOL) [1]. In contrast, well-timed palliative care improves patients' quality of life and symptom control and reduces invasive procedures and costs [2–8].

Appropriate decision-making is mandatory in high-quality EOL-care to prevent non-beneficial treatments and relieve suffering. The decisions include, but are not limited to, statements on cardiopulmonary resuscitation, parenteral fluids, and diagnostic tests. This decision-making is a challenging process involving many ethical, legal, medical and psychological aspects [9–16].

* Correspondence: piili.reetta.p@student.uta.fi
Abstract of the article has been presented as an oral presentation in the 15th world congress of the European Association for Palliative Care.
[1]Faculty of Medicine and Life Sciences, University of Tampere, Tampere, Finland
[2]Department of Oncology, Tampere University Hospital, Tampere, Finland
Full list of author information is available at the end of the article

Physicians' decisions vary concerning different interventions. In a Scandinavian study, 57% of intensive care physicians would continue intravenous hydration, but only 5% of them measured blood glucose during EOL-care [17]. Physicians also decide to withdraw therapies less frequently than to withhold them, probably because they feel withdrawal is more difficult and ethically problematic [18–21].

In addition to medical facts and personal characteristics, education and specialty of the physician influence the complex decision-making in EOL [11]. Although education in palliative care increases the knowledge and skills needed to perform high-quality EOL-care [22–27], the effectiveness of special training in palliative medicine (PM) on different aspects of decision-making in EOL-care remains unknown.

Most patients wish their closest ones to be involved in EOL decision-making, and discussions with the family are essential [28–30]. The families' opinions are also shown to influence physicians' decisions [12, 31, 32], although discordance between patients' wishes, caregivers' preferences and caregivers' predictions of patients' preferences may exist [28, 33]. Advance directives reinforce patients' participation and help with decision-making [31, 32, 34]. However, there are variations in how advance directives are understood and taken into account [12, 35–37].

The aim of our study was to examine whether special education in PM affects decision-making in EOL-care, as evaluated by a hypothetical patient scenario with different alternatives. The impact of family requests, written advance directives, and physicians' background factors on their decisions were analysed.

Methods

Participants

A postal survey with a questionnaire was provided to 1327 Finnish physicians in autumn 2015. The sample consisted of 500 general health care practitioners (GPs), 300 surgeons, and 300 internists randomly selected from the register of the Finnish Medical Association. The sample size is similar to our previous studies done sixteen years ago and is based on the distribution of different specialities in Finland, which has remained largely unchanged over the years studied [10–12, 38, 39]. In addition, the questionnaire was send to all Finnish oncologists ($n = 158$) and all physicians with a special competency in PM ($n = 82$), excluding those with a mailing proscription ($n = 23$). Two reminders were send to nonrespondents.

A cover letter including an introduction to the study and an assurance of anonymity and voluntariness was mailed together with the questionnaire. This study was approved by the Regional Ethics Committee of Tampere University Hospital, Finland (R15101).

Special competency in palliative medicine

In Finland, postgraduate training in PM leads to a certification for special competency in PM (cPM) awarded by the Finnish Medical Association [40]. Finnish physicians are allowed to start this postgraduate training after working at least 2 years as a physician. This special training consists of 150 h of theoretical education in different aspects of PM, 200 patient interactions in palliative care, 2 years of clinical practice including a working period in a specialized palliative care unit for a minimum of 3 months, and a final written examination.

Questionnaire

The questionnaire has been previously used and validated with Finnish physicians. A pilot study was done in January 1999. The questionnaire was sent to 45 physicians (health care practitioners and specialists) twice at two-week intervals in order to test the reliability of the responses to patient scenarios and the questions on attitudes and values. Thirty physicians returned two acceptable questionnaires. The value of kappa coefficient for an acceptable scenarios or questions was determined to be more than 0.40, which is a commonly accepted limit for reliability. [10–12, 38]

The questionnaire includes seven hypothetical patient scenarios together with questions concerning responders' background, personal features, and attitudes. In this study, we included one of the patient scenarios designed to study doctors' treatment decisions in the EOL-care. In addition, questions about the responders' own advance directives, experience in EOL-care among relatives, treatment of EOL patients within 2 years, availability of professional supervision, chief position and financial responsibility at work together with age and sex were used as background factors. The parts of the questionnaire used in this study are available as an Additional file 1.

Case scenario

The scenario presented a 62-year-old male patient with pulmonary cancer and metastases. He was admitted to hospital ward and received high-dose morphine medication. Due to respiratory weakening, he had become comatose the night before.

He also suffered from severe anaemia and had abundant pleural effusion and fever.

After the presentation of the patient scenario, there was a question about the treatment decision: Which of the following treatments already started (*) or planned would you withhold or withdraw? In the first situation, there was no possibility of discussing the matter with the family and there was no advance directive. The decision responses were expressed on a scale from 1 (I definitely would not) to 5 (I definitely would). The treatments were a) antibiotics (*); b) mechanical ventilation (*); c) blood transfusion; d) pleural drainage; e) chest x-ray examination; f) laboratory tests; g) intravenous hydration (*); h) nasogastric tube (*); i) thrombosis prophylaxis (*); and j) supplementary oxygen (*).

After the original patient scenario, two alternatives with extra information were provided: 1) the patient's daughters come to you distressed and crying, expressing their hope that everything possible will be done to save their father's life; 2) there is a written advance directive in the patient's medical chart in which he expresses his wish that all active treatment should be withdrawn if there is no hope for recovery. After each of these alternatives the same questions (with the same treatment options as in the original scenario) were asked. Questions were asked to be answered in the given order and not to change answers once decided.

Statistical analysis

Different responder groups were compared by t-test for normally distributed continuous variables (Fig. 1) and by chi-square or Fisher's exact tests when appropriate for categorical variables (Tables 2 and 3). The answers on the 5-step Likert scale in the scenarios were converted to a 2-step scale: 1–3, "would not withdraw or withhold and don't know" and 4–5, "would withdraw or withhold". Measured mean distributions of the chronological original scenario, family's appeal and advance directive values were clustered by trajectory analysis [41]. The trajectories were created according to the measurements of mean values in each responder as a continuous outcome measure. The analyses undertaken were latent class mixture models of quadratic trajectories including a random intercept and concomitant variables. Models were fitted

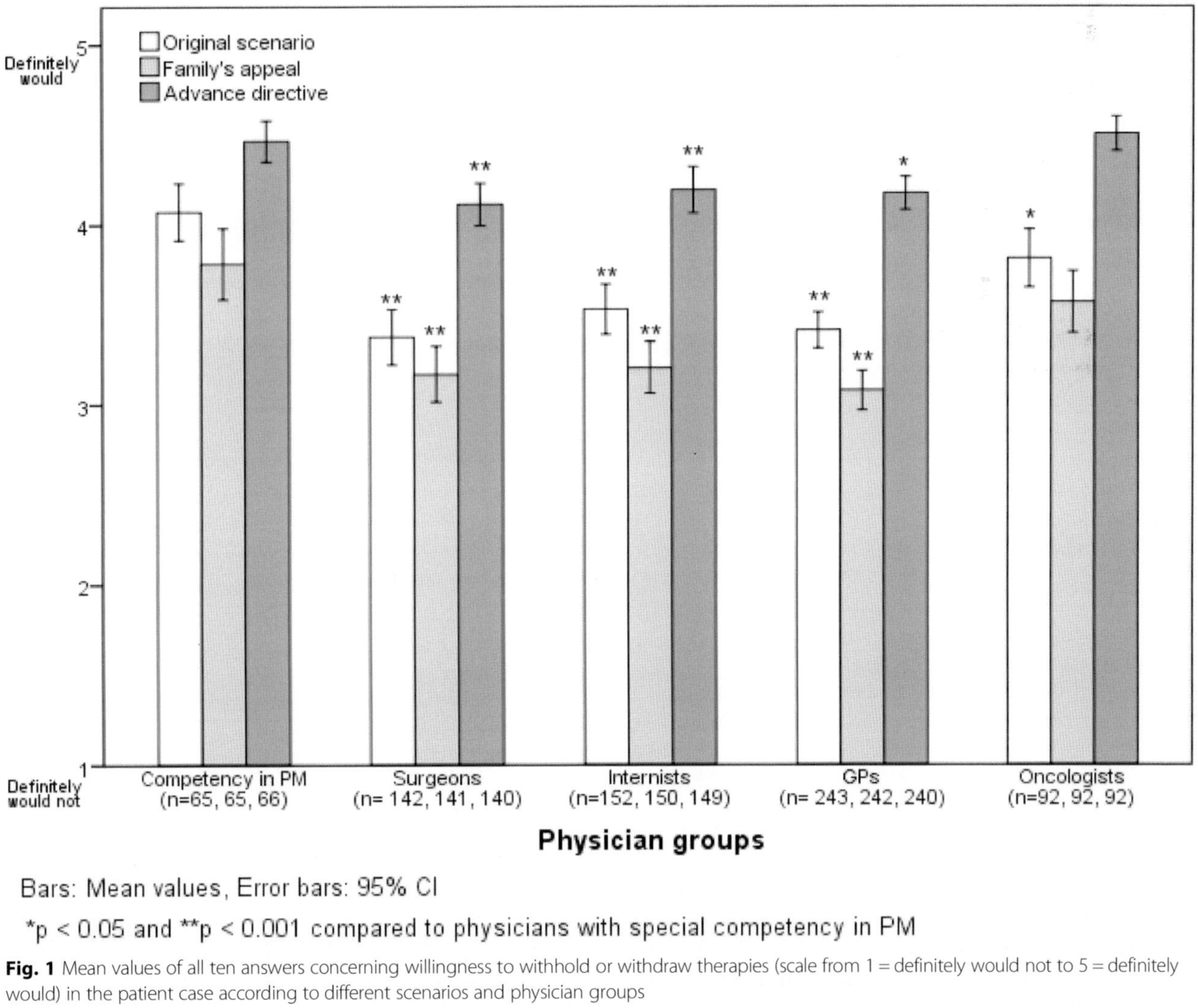

Fig. 1 Mean values of all ten answers concerning willingness to withhold or withdraw therapies (scale from 1 = definitely would not to 5 = definitely would) in the patient case according to different scenarios and physician groups

by using the flexmix package [42] of the statistical program R, version 3.3.0, from the R Foundation for Statistical Computing (R Development Core Team. R: A language and environment for statistical computing. R Foundation for Statistical Computing, Vienna, Austria, 2008, ISBN 3–900,051–07-0, URL). Relative goodness of fit was assessed using Bayesian information Criteria.

Factors (Table 4) affecting the willingness to continue or start therapies (belonging to trajectory groups 3 or 4) compared to withhold or withdraw therapies (belonging to trajectory groups 1 or 2) were examined by univariate and age-adjusted logistic regression models results shown by odds ratios (OR) with 95% confidence intervals (CI). Additionally, a multivariable model, where variables were added simultaneously into the model, was performed for variables with statistical significance under 0.20 in age-adjusted model. Two-sided *p*-values of less than 0.05 were accepted as statistically significant. Data-analyses were performed using IBM SPSS Statistics for Windows, Version 23.0. Armonk, NY: IBM Corp. Released 2014.

Results

Responders

Altogether, 699 valid responses were achieved (response rate 53%). The response rate ranged from 82% among physicians with cPM to 47% among surgeons. Characteristics of the responders are presented in Table 1. A majority of the responders were women, except in the group of surgeons. The median age of the responders was 52 years (interquartile range 43–58), with slight variations between the groups. Most of the GPs worked at out-patient clinics (85%), while the others mainly worked at hospitals (66–87%).

Overall willingness to withhold or withdraw therapies

The mean values of all ten answers according to the three alternatives in the case scenario are shown in Fig. 1. Physicians with cPM were most willing to withhold and withdraw interventions, especially compared to GPs, internists and surgeons. The family's appeal significantly increased the willingness to start or continue life-prolonging therapies in all physician groups, whereas the advance directive decreased it ($p < 0.001$ compared to the original scenario).

Decisions concerning individual treatments

Physicians with cPM were more willing to withdraw and withhold most of the individual interventions, compared to the others (Tables 2 and 3). This difference in decision-making was most striking in withdrawing intravenous hydration, removing nasogastric tube and withholding blood transfusions. In contrast, some decisions (e.g., withdrawing oxygen or antibiotics) varied only slightly between the physicians with cPM and others. Mechanical ventilation was withdrawn by most of the physicians, while supplementary oxygen was frequently continued by all responders.

The daughters' request for "everything to be done" (the family's appeal) increased the willingness to continue or start each life-prolonging treatment, with the only exception the use of oxygen among cPMs. The daughters' request had the largest influence on the decisions concerning intravenous hydration and diagnostic tests (Table 2).

The availability of the advance directive markedly moved decisions towards withdrawing and withholding treatments. Although the differences between responder groups diminished, the physicians with cPM and the oncologists still had the least aggressive approach. Nearly all physicians withdrew mechanical ventilation, discontinued thrombosis prophylaxis and withheld blood transfusion. However, over one third of the physicians without cPM continued intravenous hydration, and supplementary oxygen was frequently continued by all physicians.

Table 1 Characteristics of the participants

	Competency in PM		Surgeons		Internists		GPs		Oncologists		Total	
Number (% of total)	67	(10)	142	(20)	153	(22)	245	(35)	92	(13)	699	(100)
Response rate, %	82		47		51		49		63		53	
Female, n (%)	57	(85)	47	(33)	81	(53)	173	(71)	73	(79)	431	(62)
Median age (IQR)	55	(49–58)	52	(44–59)	53	(46–59)	49	(38–57)	49	(41–56)	52	(43–58)
Age distribution, n (%)												
< 35	0	(0)	4	(3)	4	(3)	42	(17)	2	(2)	52	(7)
35–49	20	(30)	52	(37)	51	(33)	84	(34)	46	(50)	253	(36)
> 49	47	(70)	86	(61)	98	(64)	119	(49)	44	(48)	394	(56)
Years from graduation, median (IQR)[a]	27	(21–32)	26	(17–34)	26	(20–32)	21	(9–31)	22	(14–29)	25	(15–32)

PM, Palliative Medicine, GP, General Practitioner, IQR, Interquartile Range
[a]For nine participants year of graduation was not available

Table 2 Number and proportion (%) of physicians deciding to withdraw a treatment in the patient scenario according to physician groups

Treatment	Scenario	Competency in PM		Surgeons		Internist		GPs		Oncologists		P-value[a]
Antibiotic	Original scenario	41	(65)	72	(51)	78	(51)	128	(53)	45	(54)	0.399
	Family's appeal	33	(50)	55	(39)	55	(36)	89	(37)*	34	(37)	0.353
	Advance directive	58	(87)	116	(83)	122	(82)	204	(84)	82	(89)	0.641
Mechanical ventilation	Original scenario	63	(96)	119	(85)*	135	(89)	195	(81)*	83	(91)	0.008
	Family's appeal	59	(92)	113	(80)*	126	(83)	175	(72)*	76	(84)	0.002
	Advance directive	67	(100)	130	(92)*	147	(98)	228	(94)*	90	(99)	0.011
Intravenous hydration	Original scenario	43	(65)	31	(22)**	39	(26)**	85	(35)**	42	(46)*	< 0.001
	Family's appeal	26	(40)	21	(15)**	19	(13)**	58	(24)*	34	(37)	< 0.001
	Advance directive	58	(88)	64	(46)**	84	(56)**	162	(67)*	75	(82)	< 0.001
Nasogastric tube	Original scenario	62	(95)	85	(60)**	98	(65)**	161	(67)**	63	(69)**	< 0.001
	Family's appeal	60	(92)	76	(54)**	87	(58)**	126	(53)**	64	(70)*	< 0.001
	Advance directive	64	(97)	105	(75)**	126	(84)*	203	(84)*	82	(89)	0.001
Thrombos prophylaxis	Original scenario	55	(85)	108	(76)	105	(69)*	151	(62)*	73	(80)	< 0.001
	Family's appeal	52	(80)	104	(74)	95	(64)*	128	(53)**	67	(73)	< 0.001
	Advance directive	63	(96)	121	(88)	127	(85)*	199	(82)*	86	(94)	0.013
Supplementary oxygen	Original scenario	11	(16)	16	(11)	23	(15)	14	(6)*	11	(12)	0.019
	Family's appeal	12	(18)	14	(10)	13	(9)*	12	(5)	6	(7)*	0.011
	Advance directive	20	(30)	40	(28)	46	(31)	51	(21)	27	(29)	0.189

PM, Palliative Medicine, GP, General Practitioner
[a]Global p-value across all physician groups
*$p < 0.05$ and **$p < 0.001$ pair-wise comparison to physicians with special competency in PM

Trajectory analysis and factors associated with aggressive treatment decisions

When answers were fitted with a trajectory analysis, four differently behaving groups were found (Fig. 2). In the trajectory group 1, responders were consistently willing to withdraw and withhold therapies, and in the trajectory group 2, physicians would probably withdraw and withhold therapies, but their decisions were influenced by the family's appeal and the advance directive. In contrast, responders encompassed in the trajectory group 3 were either uncertain or chose an aggressive approach in about half of their decisions, and they were more influenced by the advance directive, while physicians in the trajectory group 4 were most hesitant to withdraw and withhold therapies.

Table 3 Number and proportion (%) of physicians deciding to withhold an intervention in the patient scenario according to physician groups

Treatment	Scenario	Competency in PM		Surgeons		Internists		GPs		Oncologists		P-value[a]
Blood transfusion	Original scenario	60	(91)	98	(70)*	108	(72)*	185	(76)*	72	(78)*	0.011
	Family's appeal	55	(85)	90	(64)*	85	(56)**	153	(64)*	67	(76)	< 0.001
	Advance directive	66	(99)	132	(94)	136	(91)	227	(94)	90	(98)	0.134
Pleural drainage	Original scenario	43	(65)	59	(42)*	85	(56)	99	(41)**	58	(64)	< 0.001
	Family's appeal	41	(63)	57	(40)*	73	(49)	89	(37)**	51	(56)	< 0.001
	Advance directive	53	(79)	103	(73)	119	(80)	179	(74)	82	(89)	0.030
Chest X-ray	Original scenario	51	(77)	66	(47)**	88	(58)*	119	(60)**	67	(73)	< 0.001
	Family's appeal	44	(67)	61	(43)*	74	(49)*	29	(38)**	59	(65)	< 0.001
	Advance directive	59	(88)	111	(79)	124	(83)	194	(81)	90	(98)*	0.001
Laboratory tests	Original scenario	49	(74)	70	(59)*	87	(57)*	121	(50)*	59	(64)	0.002
	Family's appeal	40	(61)	60	(43)*	67	(45)*	85	(35)**	51	(56)	< 0.001
	Advance directive	58	(87)	115	(81)	119	(78)	190	(78)	88	(96)*	0.006

PM, Palliative Medicine, GP, General Practitioner
[a]Global p-value across all physician groups
*$p < 0.05$ and **$p < 0.001$ pair-wise comparison to physicians with special competency in PM

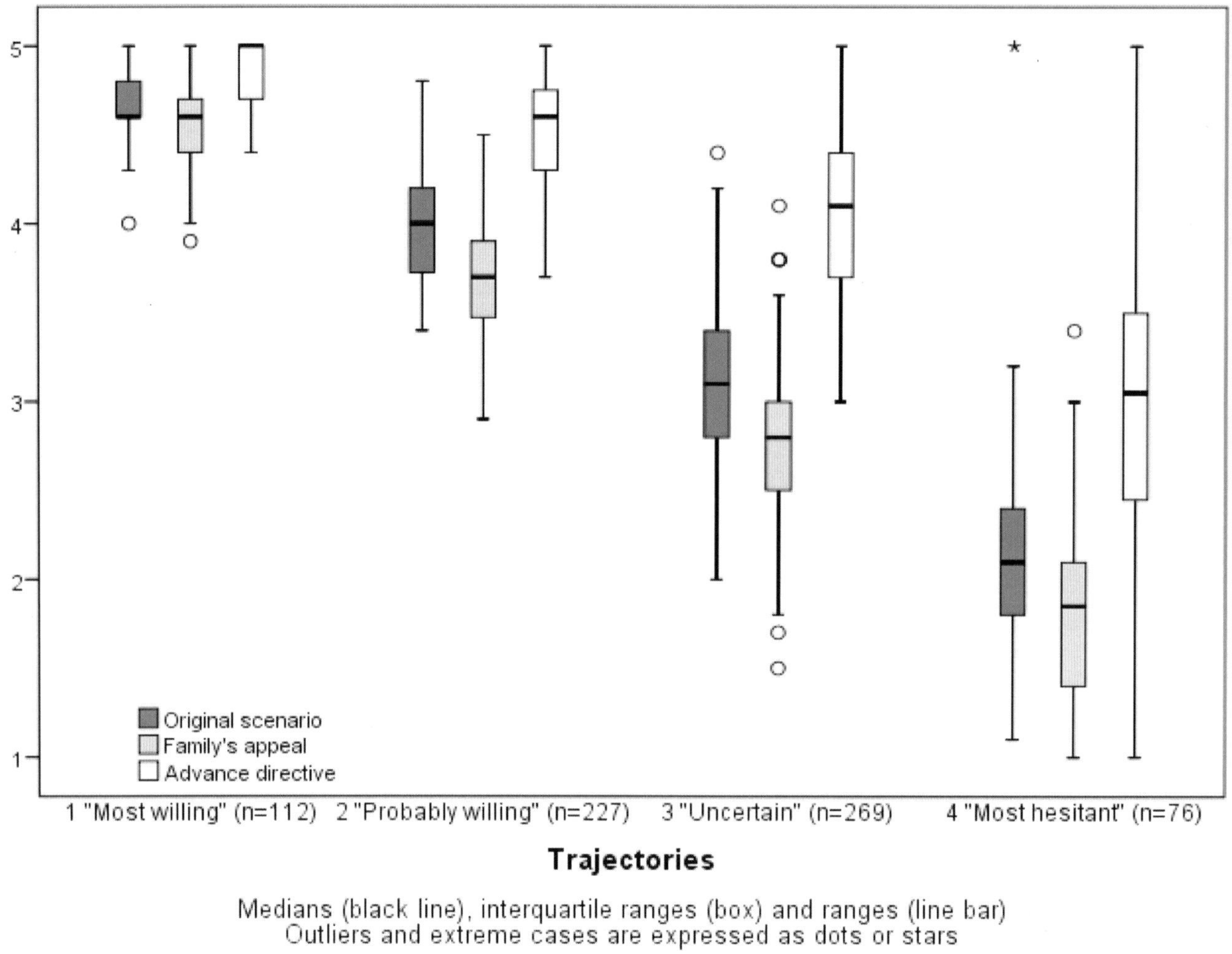

Fig. 2 Distribution of the responses (scale from 1 = definitely would not to 5 = definitely would) in the original scenario, family's appeal and advance directive in the trajectory analysis

Factors associated with the physicians' willingness to continue or start life-prolonging therapies during EOL-care (belonging to trajectory groups 3 or 4) compared to withhold or withdraw therapies (belonging to trajectory groups 1 or 2) are shown in Table 4. By multivariable analysis, younger age and being an internist, surgeon or GP were independent factors behind the decisions not to withhold - or to withdraw – different interventions. In contrast, gender, being in chief-position, having financial responsibility, or a physician's own advance directive and experience in EOL-care among relatives did not have independent influence.

Discussion

We found that physicians with cPM were more willing to withdraw and withhold life-prolonging therapies, especially intravenous hydration and a nasogastric tube, in a patient scenario representing EOL-care. The family's request increased the aggressive approach in all physicians, whereas the availability of an advance directive decreased this. Younger age and being an internist, surgeon or GP without cPM were independent factors for responses reflecting willingness to start or continue life-prolonging treatments in multivariable regression analysis.

In this study, the overall willingness to withhold and withdraw therapies in EOL-care was higher in physicians with cPM, measured by mean values of all the answers and in a multivariable regression analysis, although oncologists and cPMs differed only slightly. We used trajectory analysis to take into account all the scenarios in the given order and found a similar pattern across all four groups. Therefore, the groups starting from a low willingness to withhold or withdraw therapies in the original scenario were finally chosen to be presented in the multivariable analysis. In light of previous studies [43–45], it is understandable that physicians with formal training in PM have good ability to consider and communicate the EOL decisions, probably leading to more decisions to withdraw and

Table 4 Factors associated with the willingness to continue or start life prolonging therapies (belonging to trajectories 3 or 4) compared to withhold or withdraw therapies (belonging to trajectories 1 or 2) in the patient scenario presented by univariate, age-adjusted and multivariable analysis

		Univariate			Age-adjusted			Multivariate		
	n	OR	(95% CI)	p	OR	(95% CI)	p	OR	(95% CI)	p
Age continuous, years	692	**0.96**	**(0.95–0.98)**	< 0.001						
Age				< 0.001						0.002
25–35	52	**4.71**	**(2.35–9.44)**					**3.19**	**(1.54–6.57)**	
35–49	253	**1.49**	**(1.08–2.05)**					**1.46**	**(1.03–2.06)**	
50–67	387	1.00						1.00		
Sex				0.796			0.433			
Female	425	1.04	(0.77–1.41)		0.88	(0.64–1.21)				
Male	267	1.00			1.00					
Chief-position				0.013			0.208			
No	480	**1.51**	**(1.09–2.11)**		1.25	(0.88–1.76)				
Yes	205	1.00			1.00					
Financial responsibility				0.006			0.083			0.183
No	562	**1.75**	**(1.17–2.62)**		*1.44*	*(0.95–2.19)*		1.35	(0.87–2.08)	
Yes	120	1.00			1.00			1.00		
Own advance directive				0.604			0.932			
No	638	1.17	(0.65–2.09)		1.03	(0.57–1.86)				
Yes	49	1.00			1.00					
End-of-life care among relatives				0.066			0.322			
No	336	*1.32*	*(0.98–1.79)*		1.17	(0.86–1.59)				
Yes	352	1.00			1.00					
Physician group				< 0.001			< 0.001			< 0.001
Competency in PM	66	1.00			1.00			1.00		
Oncologists	92	1.63	(0.78–3.40)		1.39	(0.66–2.93)		1.61	(0.75–3.46)	
Internists	150	**3.92**	**(2.00–7.67)**		**3.85**	**(1.96–7.57)**		**4.27**	**(2.13–8.56)**	
Surgeons	142	**4.53**	**(2.30–8.90)**		**4.37**	**(2.21–8.64)**		**4.51**	**(2.25–9.07)**	
GPs	242	**6.27**	**(3.29–12.0)**		**5.34**	**(2.78–10.3)**		**5.60**	**(2.85–11.0)**	

Significant results ($p < 0.05$) bolded and nearly significant ($p < 0.10$) shown by italic font
Age-adjusted significant ($p < 0.05$) or nearly significant ($p < 0.10$) variables included into the multivariate model. Missing values were not analyzed
PM, Palliative Medicine, GP, General Practitioner

withhold treatments. We suggest that this willingness is related to the cPM itself as its influence remained also after multivariate analysis taking into account some important background factors in our study. We have to state, however, that we don't know all the attitudes, which might drive physicians to special education in PM and whether these factors also predispose to withholding and withdrawing life-sustaining treatments.

As our case represented a cancer patient, it is not surprising that responses among physicians with cPM and oncologists were quite similar, although there were differences concerning individual interventions. The relative unwillingness of GPs to make decisions for a palliative approach is a bit concerning, since a vast majority of dying patients in Finland are cared for by GPs. This result was independent of the GPs' younger age. Our results highlight the need for education in PM starting from medical school and continuing throughout specialty training. In addition, palliative care consultations have shown to be beneficial and they should be offered to all specialities to help complex decision-making in EOL-care [6, 46–48].

Younger age was associated with unwillingness to withhold and withdraw therapies in our study. Age seems to be a contradictory factor in decision-making [49]. In some studies, including our own, older age has been associated with more decisions to withhold or withdraw interventions [50, 51], while in others, younger physicians or trainees make less aggressive decisions [52–54]. Younger physicians have less experience in

EOL-care, but on the other hand, PM is currently included in the curriculum of many medical schools, increasing younger colleagues' awareness of the benefits of palliative care. After 1999 two out of the five medical schools in Finland has included an undergraduate curriculum in PM fulfilling the European recommendations [55, 56]. Our results are in line with other studies showing that gender does not influence the decision-making [51, 54]. Some of the other background factors (such as experience in EOL-care with loved ones or a physician's own advance directive) did not influence the decision-making in our study, but are not included in previous studies.

Our results imply, that decisions to withhold or withdraw therapies in a clinical practise is mainly driven by medical education and clinical experience of a physician and preferences of a patient rather than doctor's personal life experience or attitudes.

Advance directive and a healthcare proxy or the family's opinion have been shown to have marked influence on physicians' decision-making [12, 31, 35, 57, 58], but there are no earlier studies about this for palliative care physicians. Our study is in line with previous ones [31, 32], since the family's request for aggressive treatments significantly increased physicians' willingness to continue or start life-prolonging therapies, and advance directive decreased this. This finding was constant through different physician groups including physicians with cPM. Communication and shared decision-making are very important in EOL-care [20, 49–54, 57, 58], but futile therapies should not be used (even if families have requested them), as stated by the Finnish National Supervisory Authority for Welfare and Health [59]. Therefore, this clear influence of family requests on decision-making is controversial and perhaps an issue needing more attention in the education of PM, which should also introduce legal aspects and official recommendations on decision-making. Knowing a patient's own will helps in decision-making [31, 32], and an advance directive naturally moves the decisions towards a palliative approach. However, the content of an advance directive presented here did not describe the patient's will in detail, which is often the case in the real world as well. The understanding of "active treatments" probably influenced the decisions concerning individual therapies in the present study and calls for more detailed advanced care planning and advance directives in clinical practice.

The differences in decision-making between physicians with cPM and others were most striking for nasogastric tube and intravenous hydration. Surgeons, internists and to a lesser extent GPs were unwilling to withdraw hydration, even when an advance directive was found. Artificial nutrition or medically assisted hydration has not been shown to improve survival, quality of life or symptoms in EOL-care, although the evidence about this is scarce [60–64]. There are studies, however, raising concerns about the potential harms, such as increased respiratory secretions, related to hydration during EOL [65]. Although the use of artificial nutrition or intravenous hydration in EOL-care remains controversial, the case scenario in our study represented a dying patient in which these therapies can be considered non-beneficial. The pros and cons of these therapies are included in the formal training in PM, but are probably quite unfamiliar to other physicians.

Supplementary oxygen was the least withdrawn treatment in our study, even among physicians with cPM. This result is in line with reports showing that oxygen is used in more than 70% of patients in EOL-care [66, 67], although the evidence to support this is lacking [68–70]. Perhaps this unwillingness to withdraw oxygen is related to the presumption of its benefit and harmlessness, although it may cause dryness of the mouth and aggravate communication.

In our study antibiotics were withdrawn by about half of the physicians. Use of antibiotics in EOL is controversial, but there is some evidence that antibiotics might relieve symptoms without serious side-effects, which might explain the unwillingness to withdraw them [71, 72]. Internists and GPs were more unwilling to withdraw thrombosis prophylaxis compared to others, probably due to their familiarity with the indications of anticoagulation in the general population. There are no controlled studies to guide when to stop anticoagulation in palliative care, but as our case represented a dying person, withdrawing it can be considered reasonable [73].

The benefits of transfusions in palliative care are experienced briefly and remain controversial [74]. In our study, the physicians with cPM withheld blood transfusions more frequently than others, although the availability of an advance directive increased the willingness to over 90% in all groups.

Pleural drainage can alleviate dyspnoea, but this is an invasive procedure including some risks in EOL-care [75]. Surgeons and GPs were most eager to perform this procedure, which probably reflects their willingness to perform chest X-rays as well. In a Scandinavian study, intensive care physicians withheld laboratory tests [17] more often than all the physicians in our study, which is somewhat surprising. Changing from cure to care might be more complex in a common hospital ward compared to an intensive care unit (ICU), where withdrawing life-supporting treatments commonly leads to relatively rapid patient death.

Limitations

Some limitations of this study need to be acknowledged. Our response rate (53%) is higher than in many of the recent surveys [31, 37, 76], but still sets a limitation.

Although there might be some nonresponse bias, our responders can be considered a representative sample of Finnish physicians providing insight into their decision-making. The distribution of physician groups in the study equals the distribution of different specialities in Finland [39]. Similarly, the high proportion of female respondents in our study is understandable, since 60% of physicians in Finland are women and female dominance is true among all the specialities studied excluding surgeons [39]. Answers to hypothetical scenarios might differ from physicians' decision -making in real life situations. In addition, the scenario forced the responder to give simple "yes" or "no" answer without the possibility for example to discuss with the family to achieve shared decision. Further studies on physicians' decision-making in clinical practice are needed, although this might be difficult to study in large physician groups, as each clinical circumstance is very different. We suggest, however, that the factors behind decision-making remain similar in real life situations and in our hypothetical scenarios. Finally, most of the treatments in our case clearly intend to prolong life (e.g., mechanical ventilation), while some of them may be partly considered as supporting ones (e.g., pleural drainage). Similarly, oxygen or transfusions may be given for symptom relief only or to prolong life, which should be distinguished.

Therefore, "palliative" or "life-prolonging" intent may be questioned in some decisions, but we suggest that the overall tendency to withdraw or withhold therapies in our study reflects reasonable decision-making in EOL-care. The intention itself behind these decisions is an interesting subject for future studies.

Conclusions

Physicians with special education in palliative medicine are more willing to withdraw and withhold life-prolonging therapies in EOL-care. This is especially true concerning decisions on hydration, artificial nutrition and transfusions. Families' request and advance directives have a significant influence on decision-making in all physicians.

Younger age and specialty of a physician are main factors influencing the willingness to start or continue life-prolonging treatments. Therefore, education about decision-making in EOL-care should be mandatory at medical schools and in the training of all the specialities facing dying patients. Palliative care consultations might be needed for complex cases of decision -making in EOL-care.

Abbreviations

cPM: Special competency in palliative medicine; EOL: End-of-life; GP: General health care practitioner; ICU: Intensive care unit; IQR: Interquartile range; PM: Palliative medicine

Funding

This study was funded by the Seppo Nieminen Legacy Fund, the Signe and Ane Gyllenberg foundation, the Finnish Medical Association and the Cancer Society of Pirkanmaa.

Authors' contributions

RP, JL, HH and PLKL designed the study outline and the questionnaire. RP, JL and PLKL collected the data. RP, JL, PLKL and TL analysed the data. RP and TL did the final statistical analysis. All the authors contributed to the writing and reviewing of the manuscript and approved the final manuscript.

Competing interests

The authors declare that they have no competing interests.

Author details

[1]Faculty of Medicine and Life Sciences, University of Tampere, Tampere, Finland. [2]Department of Oncology, Tampere University Hospital, Tampere, Finland. [3]Department of Oncology, Tampere University Hospital, Palliative Care Unit, Teiskontie 35, R-building, 33520 Tampere, Finland. [4]Research and Innovation Center, Tampere University Hospital, Tampere, Finland. [5]Health Sciences, Faculty of Social Sciences, University of Tampere, Tampere, Finland. [6]Rehabilitation Center Apila, Kangasala, Finland.

References

1. Cardona-Morrell M, Kim J, Turner RM, Anstey M, Mitchell IA, Hillman K. Non-beneficial treatments in hospital at the end of life: a systematic review on extent of the problem. Int J Qual Health Care. 2016;28(4):456–69.
2. Zimmermann C, Swami N, Krzyzanowska M, Hannon B, Leighl N, Oza A, Moore M, Rydall A, Rodin G, Tannock I, Donner A, Lo C. Early palliative care for patients with advanced cancer: a cluster-randomised controlled trial. Lancet. 2014;383(9930):1721–30.
3. Temel JS, Greer JA, Muzikansky A, Gallagher ER, Admane S, Jackson VA, Dahlin CM, Blinderman CD, Jacobsen J, Pirl WF, Billings JA, Lynch TJ. Early palliative care for patients with metastatic non-small-cell lung cancer. N Engl J Med. 2010;363(8):733–42.
4. Smith TJ, Temin S, Alesi ER, Abernethy AP, Balboni TA, Basch EM, Ferrell BR, Loscalzo M, Meier DE, Paice JA, Peppercorn JM, Somerfield M, Stovall E, Von Roenn JH. American Society of Clinical Oncology provisional clinical opinion: the integration of palliative care into standard oncology care. J Clin Oncol. 2012;30(8):880–7.
5. Obermeyer Z, Makar M, Abujaber S, Dominici F, Block S, Cutler DM. Association between the Medicare hospice benefit and health care

utilization and costs for patients with poor-prognosis cancer. JAMA. 2014; 312(18):1888–96.
6. Henson L, Gao W, Higginson I, Smith M, Davies J, Ellis-Smith C, Daveson B. Emergency department attendance by patients with cancer in the last month of life: a systematic review and meta-analysis. Lancet. 2015;385(Suppl 1):S41. 6736(15)60356–7
7. Smith S, Brick A, O'Hara S, Normand C. Evidence on the cost and cost-effectiveness of palliative care: a literature review. Palliat Med. 2014; 28(2):130–50.
8. Tan A, Seah A, Chua G, Lim TK, Phua J. Impact of a palliative care initiative on end-of-life care in the general wards: a before-and-after study. Palliat Med. 2014;28(1):34–41.
9. Daher M. Ethical issues in the geriatric patient with advanced cancer 'living to the end'. Ann Oncol. 2013;24(Suppl 7):vii55–8.
10. Hinkka H, Kosunen E, Metsanoja R, Lammi UK, Kellokumpu-Lehtinen P. To resuscitate or not: a dilemma in terminal cancer care. Resuscitation. 2001;49(3):289–97.
11. Hinkka H, Kosunen E, Lammi EK, Metsanoja R, Puustelli A, Kellokumpu-Lehtinen P. Decision making in terminal care: a survey of finnish doctors' treatment decisions in end-of-life scenarios involving a terminal cancer and a terminal dementia patient. Palliat Med. 2002;16(3):195–204.
12. Hinkka H, Kosunen E, Metsanoja R, Lammi UK, Kellokumpu-Lehtinen P. Factors affecting physicians' decisions to forgo life-sustaining treatments in terminal care. J Med Ethics. 2002;28(2):109–14.
13. Ilemona ER. An appraisal of ethical issues in end-of-life care. Niger J Med. 2014;23(4):358–64.
14. Parks SM, Winter L. End of life decision-making for cancer patients. Prim Care. 2009;36(4):811–23. table of contents
15. Reichlin M. On the ethics of withholding and withdrawing medical treatment. Multidiscip Respir Med. 2014;9(1):39-6958-9-39. eCollection 2014
16. White B, Willmott L, Cartwright C, Parker MH, Williams G. Doctors' knowledge of the law on withholding and withdrawing life-sustaining medical treatment. Med J Aust. 2014;201(4):229–32.
17. Hynninen M, Klepstad P, Petersson J, Skram U, Tallgren M. Process of foregoing life-sustaining treatment: a survey among Scandinavian intensivists. Acta Anaesthesiol Scand. 2008;52(8):1081–5.
18. Solomon MZ, O'Donnell L, Jennings B, Guilfoy V, Wolf SM, Nolan K, Jackson R, Koch-Weser D, Donnelley S. Decisions near the end of life: professional views on life-sustaining treatments. Am J Public Health. 1993;83(1):14–23.
19. Vincent JL. Forgoing life support in western European intensive care units: the results of an ethical questionnaire. Crit Care Med. 1999;27(8):1626–33.
20. Levin PD, Sprung CL. Withdrawing and withholding life-sustaining therapies are not the same. Crit Care. 2005;9(3):230–2.
21. Chung GS, Yoon JD, Rasinski KA, Curlin FA. US Physicians' opinions about distinctions between withdrawing and withholding life-sustaining treatment. J Relig Health. 2016;55(5):1596–606.
22. Centeno C, Rodriguez-Nunez A. The contribution of undergraduate palliative care education: does it influence the clinical patient's care? Curr Opin Support Palliat Care. 2015;9(4):375–91.
23. Thoonsen B, Vissers K, Verhagen S, Prins J, Bor H, van Weel C, Groot M, Engels Y. Training general practitioners in early identification and anticipatory palliative care planning: a randomized controlled trial. BMC Fam Pract. 2015;16:126–015. 0342-6
24. Quinn K, Hudson P, Ashby M, Thomas K. "palliative care: the essentials": evaluation of a multidisciplinary education program. J Palliat Med. 2008; 11(8):1122–9.
25. Reville B, Reifsnyder J, McGuire DB, Kaiser K, Santana AJ. Education and referral criteria: impact on oncology referrals to palliative care. J Palliat Med. 2013;16(7):786–9.
26. Hinkka H, Kosunen E, Metsanoja R, Lammi UK, Kellokumpu-Lehtinen P. General practitioners' attitudes and ethical decisions in end-of-life care after a year of interactive internet-based training. J Cancer Educ. 2002;17(1):12–8.
27. McConigley R, Aoun S, Kristjanson L, Colyer S, Deas K, O'Connor M, Harris R, Currow D, Yates P. Implementation and evaluation of an education program to guide palliative care for people with motor neurone disease. Palliat Med. 2012;26(8):994–1000.
28. Wallace CL. Family communication and decision making at the end of life: a literature review. Palliat Support Care. 2015;13(3):815–25.
29. Heyland DK, Allan DE, Rocker G, Dodek P, Pichora D, Gafni A. Canadian researchers at the end-of-life network (CARENET): discussing prognosis with patients and their families near the end of life: impact on satisfaction with end-of-life care. Open Med. 2009;3(2):e101–10.
30. Pardon K, Deschepper R, Stichele RV, Bernheim JL, Mortier F, Bossuyt N, Schallier D, Germonpre P, Galdermans D, Van Kerckhoven W, Deliens L. EOLIC-Consortium: preferences of patients with advanced lung cancer regarding the involvement of family and others in medical decision-making. J Palliat Med. 2010;13(10):1199–203.
31. Escher M, Perneger TV, Rudaz S, Dayer P, Perrier A. Impact of advance directives and a health care proxy on doctors' decisions: a randomized trial. J Pain Symptom Manag. 2014;47(1):1–11.
32. Escher M, Perrier A, Rudaz S, Dayer P, Perneger TV. Doctors' decisions when faced with contradictory patient advance directives and health care proxy opinion: a randomized vignette-based study. J Pain Symptom Manag. 2015;49(3):637–45.
33. Shin DW, Cho J, Kim SY, Chung IJ, Kim SS, Yang HK, Ahn E, Park BR, Seo H, Park JH. Discordance among patient preferences, caregiver preferences, and caregiver predictions of patient preferences regarding disclosure of terminal status and end-of-life choices. Psychooncology. 2015;24(2):212–9.
34. Hong JH, Kwon JH, Kim IK, Ko JH, Kang YJ, Kim HK. Adopting advance directives reinforces patient participation in end-of-life care discussion. Cancer Res Treat. 2016;48(2):753–8.
35. Horn R. "I don't need my patients' opinion to withdraw treatment": patient preferences at the end-of-life and physician attitudes towards advance directives in England and France. Med Health Care Philos. 2014;17(3):425–35.
36. Winter L, Parks SM, Diamond JJ. Ask a different question, get a different answer: why living wills are poor guides to care preferences at the end of life. J Palliat Med. 2010;13(5):567–72.
37. Nakazawa K, Kizawa Y, Maeno T, Takayashiki A, Abe Y, Hamano J, Maeno T. Palliative care physicians' practices and attitudes regarding advance care planning in palliative care units in Japan: a nationwide survey. Am J Hosp Palliat Care. 2014;31(7):699–709.
38. Hinkka H, Kosunen E, Lammi UK, Metsanoja R, Kellokumpu-Lehtinen P. Attitudes to terminal patients' unorthodox therapy: Finnish doctors' responses to a case scenario. Support Care Cancer. 2004;12(2):132–6.
39. The Finnish Medical Association: Phycisians in Finland, Statistics on phycisians and the health care system 2016. [https://www.laakariliitto.fi/site/assets/files/1268/ll16_tilasto2016_net1_170114.pdf] Accessed 27 Dec 2017.
40. The Finnish Medical Association: Special education [https://www.laakariliitto.fi/en/medical-education/] Accessed 15 Mar 2016.
41. Nagin D. Group-based modeling of development. Cambridge: Harvard University Press; 2005.
42. Leisch F. FlexMix: a general framework for finite mixture models and latent class regression in R. J Stat Soft. 2004;11(8):1–8.
43. Ahluwalia SC, Tisnado DM, Walling AM, Dy SM, Asch SM, Ettner SL, Kim B, Pantoja P, Schreibeis-Baum HC, Lorenz KA. Association of early patient-physician care planning discussions and end-of-life care intensity in advanced cancer. J Palliat Med. 2015;18(10):834–41.
44. Brighton LJ, Bristowe K. Communication in palliative care: talking about the end of life, before the end of life. Postgrad Med J. 2016;92(1090):466–70.
45. Chung HO, Oczkowski SJ, Hanvey L, Mbuagbaw L, You JJ. Educational interventions to train healthcare professionals in end-of-life communication: a systematic review and meta-analysis. BMC Med Educ. 2016;16:131–016. 0653-x
46. May P, Normand C, Morrison RS. Economic impact of hospital inpatient palliative care consultation: review of current evidence and directions for future research. J Palliat Med. 2014;17(9):1054–63.
47. Parikh RB, Kirch RA, Smith TJ, Temel JS. Early specialty palliative care--translating data in oncology into practice. N Engl J Med. 2013;369(24):2347–51.
48. Wachterman MW, Pilver C, Smith D, Ersek M, Lipsitz SR, Keating NL. Quality of end-of-life care provided to patients with different serious illnesses. JAMA Intern Med. 2016;176(8):1095–102.
49. Frost DW, Cook DJ, Heyland DK, Fowler RA. Patient and healthcare professional factors influencing end-of-life decision-making during critical illness: a systematic review. Crit Care Med. 2011;39(5):1174–89.
50. Alemayehu E, Molloy DW, Guyatt GH, Singer J, Penington G, Basile J, Eisemann M, Finucane P, McMurdo ME, Powell C. Variability in physicians' decisions on caring for chronically ill elderly patients: an international study. CMAJ. 1991;144(9):1133–8.
51. Garland A, Connors AF. Physicians' influence over decisions to forego life support. J Palliat Med. 2007;10(6):1298–305.

52. Larochelle MR, Rodriguez KL, Arnold RM, Barnato AE. Hospital staff attributions of the causes of physician variation in end-of-life treatment intensity. Palliat Med. 2009;23(5):460–70.
53. Forte DN, Vincent JL, Velasco IT, Park M. Association between education in EOL care and variability in EOL practice: a survey of ICU physicians. Intensive Care Med. 2012;38(3):404–12.
54. Christakis NA, Asch DA. Physician characteristics associated with decisions to withdraw life support. Am J Public Health. 1995;85(3):367–72.
55. Elsner F, Centeno C, Cetto G et al: Recommendations of the European Association for Palliative Care (EAPC) For the Development of Undergraduate Curricula in Palliat Med At European Medical Schools. EAPC 2013. [http://www.eapcnet.eu/LinkClick.aspx?fileticket=S1MI-tulutQ%3d&tabid=1717.] Accessed 02 Jan 2018.
56. Lehto JT, Hakkarainen K, Kellokumpu-Lehtinen PL, Saarto T. Undergraduate curriculum in palliative medicine at Tampere University increases students' knowledge. BMC Palliat Care. 2017;16(1):13. 016-0182-8
57. Esteve A, Jimenez C, Perez R, Gomez JA. Factors related to withholding life-sustaining treatment in hospitalized elders. J Nutr Health Aging. 2009;13(7):644–50.
58. Pautex S, Herrmann FR, Zulian GB. Role of advance directives in palliative care units: a prospective study. Palliat Med. 2008;22(7):835–41.
59. The Finnish National Supervisory Authority for Welfare and Health: Patient's rights. [http://www.valvira.fi/web/en/healthcare/patient_rights] Accessed 09 May 2017.
60. Finucane TE, Christmas C, Travis K. Tube feeding in patients with advanced dementia: a review of the evidence. JAMA. 1999;282(14):1365–70.
61. Good P, Cavenagh J, Mather M, Ravenscroft P. Medically assisted hydration for palliative care patients. Cochrane Database Syst Rev. 2008;2:CD006273. doi(2):CD006273
62. Bruera E, Hui D, Dalal S, Torres-Vigil I, Trumble J, Roosth J, Krauter S, Strickland C, Unger K, Palmer JL, Allo J, Frisbee-Hume S, Tarleton K. Parenteral hydration in patients with advanced cancer: a multicenter, double-blind, placebo-controlled randomized trial. J Clin Oncol. 2013; 31(1):111–8.
63. Goldberg LS, Altman KW. The role of gastrostomy tube placement in advanced dementia with dysphagia: a critical review. Clin Interv Aging. 2014;9:1733–9.
64. Good P, Richard R, Syrmis W, Jenkins-Marsh S, Stephens J. Medically assisted nutrition for adult palliative care patients. Cochrane Database Syst Rev. 2014;4:CD006274. doi(4):CD006274
65. Fritzson A, Tavelin B, Axelsson B. Association between parenteral fluids and symptoms in hospital end-of-life care: an observational study of 280 patients. BMJ Support Palliat Care. 2015;5(2):160–8.
66. Campos-Calderon C, Montoya-Juarez R, Hueso-Montoro C, Hernandez-Lopez E, Ojeda-Virto F, Garcia-Caro MP. Interventions and decision-making at the end of life: the effect of establishing the terminal illness situation. BMC Palliat Care. 2016;15(1):91.
67. Sato K, Miyashita M, Morita T, Tsuneto S, Shima Y. End-of-life medical treatments in the last two weeks of life in palliative care units in Japan, 2005-2006: a Nationwide retrospective cohort survey. J Palliat Med. 2016; 19(11):1188–96.
68. Abernethy AP, McDonald CF, Frith PA, Clark K, Herndon JE 2nd, Marcello J, Young IH, Bull J, Wilcock A, Booth S, Wheeler JL, Tulsky JA, Crockett AJ, Currow DC. Effect of palliative oxygen versus room air in relief of breathlessness in patients with refractory dyspnoea: a double-blind, randomised controlled trial. Lancet. 2010;376(9743):784–93.
69. Campbell ML, Yarandi H, Dove-Medows E. Oxygen is nonbeneficial for most patients who are near death. J Pain Symptom Manag. 2013;45(3):517–23.
70. Uronis HE, Currow DC, McCrory DC, Samsa GP, Abernethy AP. Oxygen for relief of dyspnoea in mildly- or non-hypoxaemic patients with cancer: a systematic review and meta-analysis. Br J Cancer. 2008;98(2):294–9.
71. Helde-Frankling M, Bergqvist J, Bergman P, Bjorkhem-Bergman L. Antibiotic treatment in end-of-life Cancer patients-a retrospective observational study at a palliative Care Center in Sweden. Cancers (Basel). 2016;8(9) https://doi.org/10.3390/cancers8090084.
72. Rosenberg JH, Albrecht JS, Fromme EK, Noble BN, McGregor JC, Comer AC, Furuno JP. Antimicrobial use for symptom management in patients receiving hospice and palliative care: a systematic review. J Palliat Med. 2013;16(12):1568–74.
73. O'Brien CP. Withdrawing medication: managing medical comorbidities near the end of life. Can Fam Physician. 2011;57(3):304–7. e89-92
74. Uceda Torres ME, Rodriguez Rodriguez JN, Sanchez Ramos JL, Alvarado Gomez F. Transfusion in palliative cancer patients: a review of the literature. J Palliat Med. 2014;17(1):88–104.
75. Strasser F, Blum D, Bueche D. Invasive palliative interventions: when are they worth it and when are they not? Cancer J. 2010;16(5):483–7.
76. Cartwright CM, White BP, Willmott L, Williams G, Parker MH. Palliative care and other physicians' knowledge, attitudes and practice relating to the law on withholding/withdrawing life-sustaining treatment: survey results. Palliat Med. 2016;30(2):171–9.

10

Building Bridges, Paediatric Palliative Care in Belgium: A secondary data analysis of annual paediatric liaison team reports from 2010 to 2014

Marie Friedel[1,2*], Bénédicte Brichard[3], Christine Fonteyne[4], Marleen Renard[5], Jean-Paul Misson[6], Els Vandecruys[7], Corinne Tonon[8], Françoise Verfaillie[6], Georgette Hendrijckx[4], Nathalie Andersson[4], Ilse Ruysseveldt[5], Katrien Moens[9], Jean-Marie Degryse[1,10] and Isabelle Aujoulat[1]

Abstract

Background: Although continuity of care in paediatric palliative care (PPC) is considered to be an essential element of quality of care, it's implementation is challenging. In Belgium, five paediatric liaison teams (PLTs) deliver palliative care. A Royal Decree issued in 2010 provides the legal framework that defines the PLTs' missions, as ensuring continuity of curative and palliative care between the hospital and home for children diagnosed with life-limiting conditions. This national study describes how PLTs ensure continuity of care by describing their activities and the characteristics of the children they cared for from 2010 to 2014.

Methods: Thematic analysis of open-ended questions was performed and descriptive statistics of aggregated data issued from annual reports, collected by the Belgian Ministry of Public Health through the Cancer Plan was used. A review panel of PLT members discussed the results and contributed to their interpretation.

Results: Between 2010 and 2014, 3607 children and young adults (0–21 years) were cared for by the 5 Belgian PLTs (mean of 721/per year). Of these children, 50% were diagnosed with an oncological disease, 27% with a neurological or metabolic disease. Four hundred and twenty eight (428) children had died. For 51% of them, death took place at home. PLT activities include coordination; communication; curative and palliative care; education; research and fundraising. Different perceptions of what constitutes a palliative stage, heterogeneity in reporting diagnosis and the current lack of specific valid indicators to report PPC activities were found.

Conclusion: PLTs are offering highly individualised, flexible and integrated care from diagnosis to bereavement in all care settings. Improvements in data registration and implementation of outcome measures are foreseen.

Background

Children with life-limiting or life-threatening conditions require paediatric palliative care (PPC) to various degrees and intensity. The World Health Organization and the European Association of Palliative Care define activities of PPC as "the active total care of the child's body, mind and spirit, (as well as) giving support to the family. It begins at diagnosis, and continues regardless of whether or not a child receives treatment directed at the disease. Health-care providers must evaluate and alleviate a child's physical, psychological and social distress. Effective palliative care requires a broad multidisciplinary approach that includes the family and makes use of available community resources" [1].

A recent cross-sectional analysis conducted in 23 countries revealed that 11 million children warrant a PPC approach, with 8 million of them needing access to specialised PPC services [2].

* Correspondence: marie.friedel@uclouvain.be; marie.friedel@vinci.be
[1]Institute of Health and Society- Institut de recherche Santé et Société (IRSS), Université catholique de Louvain, 30, Clos Chapelle-aux-Champs, Boite 1.30.13, B-1200 Brussels, Belgium
[2]Haute Ecole Vinci, Institut Parnasse-ISEI, 41, Clos Chapelle-aux-Champs, 1200 Brussels, Belgium
Full list of author information is available at the end of the article

Various types of PPC services have developed over the past 20 years in Europe. These can be classified into three main categories: hospital-based; freestanding facilities or home-based services. To date, it is not known which one of these services best ensures continuity of care [3].

Continuity of care is a fundamental part of PPC because of the high number of health professionals the family is in contact with, the various care settings involved (in and out of hospital), and the significant distress experienced by the child and his/her family at different stages (illness, death, bereavement). From the perspectives of families, continuity of care is seen as a "seamless" organisation of care [4] and is a major element of quality palliative care. What remains unclear is how continuity is defined and what are the enablers and barriers to continuity of care in PPC.

Haggerty defines 3 types of continuity: informational continuity, management continuity and relational continuity [5]. Informational continuity involves the delivery of relevant information in a timely manner. Management continuity involves sharing consistent and adaptable goals across care teams and between patients and their carers. Relational continuity refers to a therapeutic relationship with one or more health professionals over time.

Further definitions of continuity of care can be found in the multicomponent model described by Freeman [6, 7] and reported as follows by Parker: "Continuity was defined as the experience of a co-ordinated and smooth progression of care from the service user's perspective (experienced continuity), dependent on services that had: excellent information transfer (continuity of information), effective communication between professionals and services, and with patients (cross-boundary and team continuity), the ability to be flexible and adjust to the needs of the individual over time (flexible continuity), one or more named individual professionals with whom the patient could establish and maintain a therapeutic relationship (relational or personal continuity)" [8].

Saultz calls relational continuity the interpersonal continuity of care [9]. This is characterised by a trusted relationship between care providers and patients. Similarly the concept of continuing bonds is found to be critical in a PPC context, [10] where patients need to be cared for long periods and are in contact with many different health professionals in several care settings. Continuity of care can be achieved through nurse-led care coordination or a nurse case manager offering individualised, family-centred care [11, 12].

Inherent to these definitions and according to international recommendations is that PPC should start at the time of diagnosis of a life-limiting disease [1, 13]. More recently, the World Health Assembly called for governments to integrate PPC within a continuum of care promoting quality of life [14].

Early referral to PPC services is challenging [15]. Cultural barriers and organizational hurdles must be identified and overcome. Whilst there is a lack of descriptions of and comparisons of models in PPC, indicators of continuity of care have been established [11, 16–20].

These include the following characteristics: family-centred; accessible 24 h/day care; coordinated between in-and out-patient settings; delivered by an effectively communicating interdisciplinary team and including the possibility to access respite care and bereavement support.

Context of Paediatric Palliative Care in Belgium

The first paediatric home care service was initiated in 1989 in Gent (Flanders) as a mobile team originating from the Oncology Department of a university hospital with the objective of providing curative care to children suffering from cancer. The aim was to reduce visits to the oncology day hospital. This team accepted the challenge to ensure continuity of care for children requiring palliative care who wished to return home.

The Belgian Act on Palliative Care (2002) protects the rights of all patients to receive comfort care in case of an incurable disease, [21] after disease-oriented therapies have failed.

In Belgium, PPC is offered through 5 specialised paediatric liaison teams (PLTs) affiliated to 5 university hospitals. Two are located in Flanders, 2 in Brussels (capital) and 1 in Wallonia. In 2010 a Royal Decree [22] stated that continuity of care should be available for in- and out-patients with serious illnesses (according to the 4 groups defined by the Royal College of Paediatrics and Child Health in 1997) [23] and categorised into 3 different groups of care: curative care, palliative care and terminal care at end-of-life stage.

Standards for accreditation requirements include the affiliation to a hospital which treats a minimum of 50 new patients < 16 years of age per year suffering from a haemato-oncological or haematological non-oncological illness which requires complex care, such as a stem cell transplantation. Furthermore, the Royal Decree foresees an interdisciplinary team with 4,0 Full-time equivalent (FTE) nurses, 0,5 FTE psycho-social care worker, 0,5 FTE physician and 0,5 FTE administrative assistant. Tandem work is required with the so-called first line, considered a primary health care team including a GP and home care nurses.

The liaison teams were first financed by "Kom op tegen Kanker" (a cancer charity) and by private funding. Since 2006, they have been predominantly funded by the Belgian Federal Government of Health with funds that were initiated by action point 23 of the Cancer Plan [24]. Since 2012 this action point is used to further develop and expand the function of a paediatric liaison team and its accompanied tasks. Financial funding is allocated according to the number of children cared for.

Based on the data collected through annual reports and addressed to the Belgian Federal Government of Health, this study aims to (i) describe the characteristics of children cared for by PLT, (ii) the different activities provided by PLT in order to document how continuity of care is ensured in Belgium. To the best of our knowledge, it is the first publication describing the characteristics of children cared for by the paediatric liaison care teams and the activities they deliver to families, offering important insights on the number and the characteristics of children accessing paediatric palliative care services in Belgium.

Methods

Study design

This study is a secondary analysis of the data provided by the 5 PLTs in the form of their annual reports and data collected by the federal government. Preliminary findings were presented to the PLTs and thereafter enriched by their nuanced interpretation of the results.

Data collection

Aggregated quantitative data and narrative responses to open-ended questions issued from the annual reports 2010–2014 were transmitted to the first author. The data had been extracted from an existing database and is collected by the Cancer Plan then stored at the Belgian Federal Government of Public Health which holds the results of standardised annual PLT activity reports from 2010 to 2014. Annual reports have been mandatory since 2010, the year of the Royal Decree pertaining to the role of PLTs. The head nurse of each PLT completed the annual activity reports and sent them to the Cancer Plan.

The variables required for annual reports are presented in Table 1 and include the number of children cared for, their pathologies, the length of follow-up, as well as the number and places of deaths (hospital or home).

Table 1 Variables for aggregated quantitative data and open-ended questions included in the annual activity reports of the paediatric liaison teams

Age range classification	0–1 Y, > 1–10 Y, 11–20 Y, > 20 Y
Disease classification	Haematology/Oncology
	Neurology/Degenerative
	Genetic/Metabolic
	Cardiovascular
	Gastroenterology
	Nephrology
	Congenital abnormalities
	Immunological
	Respiratory
	Others (Neonatology, Transplantation)
Origin of referral	Origin of referral for new patients (same hospital/other hospital)
Classification of patients	Curative/palliative/end-of-life patients
Number of patients	Total patients followed-up per year
Death	Place of death (home, hospital, other) Total number of deaths Duration of follow-up Frequencies of admission in hospital Mean average duration of admission Number of contacts with families post-death
Objectives and needs	What objectives did you have? Which objectives did you achieve? Which objectives did you partially achieve? Why? What are your needs? Which objective(s) did you not achieve? Why? What are your objectives for next year? Did your team change during this year?
Strengths and weaknesses	What are the strengths of your team? What are the weaknesses of your team?
Needs assessment	What are the requests of the target group? What are the requests of the PLT? What are the requests of services/institutions/hospitals?

Data analysis

Firstly, the characteristics of the children cared for by the five PLT over a five-year period, were summarised, using descriptive statistics.

Secondly, in order to identify and describe the various activities carried out by the PLT as part of their work, responses to the open-ended questions included in the annual reports were analysed by the first author inductively, ie. without any preconceived idea or hypothesis, to identify the themes that would best describe the range of activities undertaken by the PLTs [25].

Finally, the relevance and accuracy of the themes derived from the analysis performed by the first author were discussed with the representatives of the PLTs, as well as the Cancer Plan. The latter was consulted during a formal expert review panel meeting, held on 12th April 2016, which included 4 paediatric liaison nurses (CT,GH,FV,NA); 2 specialist physicians supervising the liaison teams (MR, CF); 1 social worker (IR) acting as a coordinator of a PLT and 2 researchers (IA, MF).

During this meeting, six themes were validated as describing the range of activities undertaken by the PLTs: coordination; communication; care; fundraising; training; quality improvement and research.

Moreover, several challenges encountered by PLT emerged in the annual reports and were discussed during the meeting. Those specific challenges will be presented in the results section.

The results presented hereafter, are therefore the expression of a collaborative approach of data analysis and interpretation, which involved the main stakeholders with the aim to collectively engage in a process of reflecting on past, present and future challenges to improve continuity of care in PPC.

Results

What are the characteristics of the children followed?

Based on the aggregated data from the annual reports for the period 2010–2014, a total of 3607 children in Belgium benefitted from a follow-up of one of the five PLT (average of 721 children per year). Among all the children >followed, the proportion of palliative patients was 25% (n = 910). The mean duration of follow-up was 226 days per child. Of the 3607 children, 47% were > 1 and < 10 of age, 25% were < 1 year, 25% were > 11 and < 20 years and 3% were > 20 years.

Fifty percent suffered from an oncological pathology, 27% from neurological, genetic abnormalities, metabolic or degenerative diseases and 23% consisted of others diseases (including cardiovascular, immunological, gastro-enterological, respiratory, nephrological or perinatal diseases).

Four hundred and twenty eight children (12%) died during the study period. 51% percent of these children died at home, 47% died in hospital and 2% died in respite care services or institutions for disabled children. Each year, more than 40 home deaths were coordinated by PLTs across Belgium.

The characteristics of the children followed from 2010 to 2014 by the PLT are presented in Table 2.

What are the main activities of PLT?

The thematic analysis of the answers given by each PLT to the open questions in the annual activity reports, enriched through discussions with the review panel, resulted in the identification of 6 main types of activities, which are presented hereafter with quotes from the annual reports (AR) or from the review panel meeting (RP).

Coordination

Coordination between home care services, hospital services, schools and respite care services was reported as an important activity. Early referral to a PLT allows the team to build relationships with the families. The referring hospital-based-specialist physician continues to be responsible for the care of the patient until death. Interdisciplinary meetings within hospital units and out-patient services are initiated and coordinated by PLTs.

In order to enhance coordination reports of home-visits and interdisciplinary meetings are stored as electronic records. The phone calls made are recorded in "liaison notebooks" which are kept at the home. These notebooks can be used by the child, family members and caregivers to write down their observations.

Several difficulties in coordination were identified by PLT. These are linked to the absence of a social worker or a permanent coordinator, but also sometimes to the lack of a general practitioner identified by the family, which is a condition to the initiation of PPC home care.

PLTs express "that *the first line is established better in Flanders (northern Flemish speaking-part of Belgium) facilitating therefore the identification of a GP and home care nurses, which seems occasionally, to be a problem in Wallonia (south French-speaking part of Belgium).*" (RP).

One team has created the role of a "coordinator of information", who is based permanently in the hospital to share the information among all health professionals, both for in-hospital and out-patients, and with families. "*This new function represents a valuable support for PLT.*" (RP).

Some PLT developed not only PPC home-based care, but also in-hospital PPC consultations, depending on institutional support and sometimes person-related factors.

> *"It depends on certain individuals in the hospital whether or not your PLT is recognised. This has consequences for early referral. But I must say; now it's better than before. The other in-hospital services know who we are and what we do."* (RP)

Communication

Raising awareness among hospital teams, home care services and general society is achieved through brochures, conferences and fundraising, because PPC is still perceived as being limited to end-of-life care. The term "palliative" frightens the families and may represent an obstacle to accessing palliative care services.

> *"Sometimes the families do not even know that we are the paediatric palliative care team. We are called liaison teams and introduced sometimes as a supportive team by the physicians.(...)The word 'palliative' frightens families.(...) Some families consider us as 'the angel of death', even though we know very well that palliative care is not restricted to end-of life care.(...) Right from the beginning, we should explain clearly, what the term palliative care means and repeat it as often as necessary!"(RP)*

Teams express the urgent need to represent and advocate for PPC through active membership at federal commissions and associations for palliative care.

> *"I have been involved in the Palliative Care Federation*

Table 2 Characteristics of the children followed from 2010 to 2014 by the paediatric liaison teams ($n = 3607$)

Characteristics of children	Number of children (%)	Mean per year/per team (min/max)	Median per year/per team (P25/P75)
Age of children			
0–1 y	885 (25%)		
1–10 y	1689 (47%)		
11–20 y	879 (24%)		
> 20 y	116 (3%)	144 (43–240)	144 (103–196)
	Total of children: 3607 (100%)		
Pathologies			
Haematology/Oncology	1816 (50%)		
Neurology-/Degenerative/Metabolic	989 (27%)		
Other (Neonatology/Gastroenterology/Respiratory)	849 (23%)		
	Total: 3654 (100%)		
Curative/Palliative Patients			
Curative patients	2540 (70%)	102 (1–181)	105 (82–135)
Palliative patients	910 (25%)	36 (10–86)	23 (20–58)
Undefined	157 (5%)		
	Total: 3607 (100%)		
Referral of new patients			
From originating hospital	1848 (51%)		
External hospital	108 (3%)		
Total new patients	2056 (54%)		
	Total: 3607 (100%)		
Length follow-up (children who died)		226 days/child (1–4612 days)	32 days/child (21–201 days)
< 120 days	272 (64%)		
121–240 days	65 (15%)		
241–400 days	31 (7%)		
> 401 days	60 (14%)		
	Total: 428 (100%)		
Location of death			
Hospital	200 (47%)	8 (2–22)	6 (6–10)
Home	221 (51%)	9 (1–22)	9 (3–16)
Others (respite care home, others)	7 (2%)	18 (3–32)	19 (12–26)
	Total: 428 (100%)		

of Flanders as an administrator since 2015 and am also the delegate in the Cell of Federal Assessment of Palliative Care (first meeting in 2015)." (AR)

Care

PLTs provide complex individualised, patient-centred curative and palliative care at home or in hospital settings, when home based care teams are not available or not trained enough. Families can call and receive home visits at any time (available 7 days/24 h). PLTs have observed progressively more complex chronic conditions in children resulting in increasingly higher burdens for the family, who in turn require additional social assistance, financial resources, support for administrative procedures and in-home respite care services.

Coordination for complex procedures such as chemotherapy, blood transfusion, assisted ventilation, feeding through gastrostomy, tracheotomy care, patient controlled analgesia and intravenous sedation, requires constant professional training.

« Liaison teams are small teams where patient care is the priority; the patient population is very diverse often with very complex issues. Delivering care takes time and is very intensive.» (AR)

Care continues even after a child's death. For each family, who wished it, bereavement care was offered via telephone, home visits or letters up to 1 year after the child's death. In 2014, for example 672 contacts were established for 99 families who had lost their children (mean of 7 contacts/family).

Fundraising

Concerns regarding lack of resources were repeatedly expressed by the PLTs. Lack of trained PPC nurses in first-line home care services is also reported. One team states they do not even have an office. For other teams, a full complement of staff members to be able to ensure bereavement care, psychological support for siblings or a supervision of PLT is only possible thanks to private donations.

Monthly, mandatory supervision sessions are offered via an external psychologist. All team members can suggest some themes they want to discuss. Usually, debriefing is provided for challenging clinical situations. The main objectives of these sessions are to promote quality communication, to prevent compassion fatigue and assist team members to process vicarious trauma they may experience.

Lack of adequate governmental financing was repeatedly mentioned as obliging teams in time-consuming activities to find additional private funding to cover the total operating costs of the team. Including a social worker and a coordinator in the team was particularly emphasised.

"Strengthening the team by the presence of a social worker (halftime) would free up time spent on many serious social tasks." (AR)

"A special fundraising was undertaken for the provision of a vehicle." (AR)

"We would like to offer regular bereavement care for siblings, but we lack funding. It's a pity, because siblings are really overlooked." (RP)

"We continue to seek additional help (when lack of personnel) through our own members' networks." (AR)

Training

Continuous training for the team itself regarding pain control, paediatric palliative care, and complex care techniques such as intravenous chemotherapy or blood transfusion is carried out. When a new nurse enters the PLT, a long training period is offered for peer training; integration of care delivery; organisational elements of services; awareness and knowledge of key contacts. Thus acquiring competences in PPC needs time due to the complexity of the interventions provided.

Teams also ensure specific child and family counselling, the education of first line home care services who are not always specialised in paediatrics (for e.g. handling a gastrostomy, patient controlled analgesia pump, insertion of a nasogastric tube) as well as various professionals in hospital settings. Tailored support for schools around issues related to bereavement is also provided. Many PLT members are offering PPC education in nursing schools, faculties of medicine or hospitals.

"We should implement or reinforce training in paediatric palliative care for physicians and nurses of the 1st line." (AR)

Quality improvement and research

Teams are aware of the importance of quality improvement, and are keen to establish workload indicators and patient-reported outcome measures (PROMS). Caring for patients limits the teams' ability to engage in quality improvement and research activities. This was a source of frustration for health professionals.

"These projects are carried out with a minimum of resources and staff and rely heavily on volunteers although our Government imposes these indicators and record keeping. The same sector attaches great importance to the quality indicators and recording because it improves the professionalisation of care and the development of care is factual." (AR)

Protocols on several themes are elaborated in different ways in each PLT. Some create flow-charts to determine feasibility of PPC home care, others create protocols on how to respond to a euthanasia request, should it occur, or how to implement Advanced Care Planning tools.

"Palliative care, but especially early advanced care planning should be implemented in a better and more structurally sound way in paediatric services. Advanced care planning is very important in the care pathways for children with chronic conditions. This would fight therapeutic obstinacy; place care on a different and broader perspective, and allow parents /

families to participate in the implementation of care goals. In paediatric palliative care, advanced care planning is an essential part of the care for children with chronic complex diseases. This still must be implemented." (AR)

What are the specific challenges faced by PLTs?

In addition, during the review panel held in April 2016, the representatives of the 5 PLTs asserted that the workload of their teams was not truly reflected through the data reported in the annual reports. PLT's highlighted 3 difficulties. These involved i) the way of reporting on cases, ii) the criteria to define when a palliative stage starts and iii) when to end a follow-up.

Firstly, with regards to reporting on cases, children followed by the PLTs present, over time, more complex chronic conditions, defined as medical conditions that can last at least 12 months and involve either several different organ systems or one organ system severely enough to require specialty paediatric care and probably a period of hospitalisation in a tertiary care center [26]. The PLTs expressed their difficulty to identify the principal disease of the child and in which category or categories of illness it should be reported.

Secondly, PLTS expressed difficulty in distinguishing patients requiring palliative care: "When curative treatment is no longer an option», «when death approaches", "when the illness isn't curable anymore and will lead to a premature death. But this does not mean that the patient doesn't receive an illness-directed therapy. It has already happened that a patient labelled "palliative" shifted to "curative" because an experimental therapy succeeded. But for patients with neurometabolic illnesses, with a slow disease progression, the patient arrives at a palliative stage later on, when his quality of life deteriorates. It's very different."

This difficulty expressed by PLT to define when palliative care starts and actually stated in the annual reports, is significant and could be explained by the principle role played by PLT in being a seamless service starting at the time of diagnosis and offering a progressive step by step provision of PPC. Further, a distinction between patients receiving palliative versus curative care did not affect service provision. This discussion led to the reflection on whether a formal distinction between those two stages is required.

Finally the review panel expressed difficulty in determining the criteria by which a PLT should decide to end a follow-up. The duration of follow-up for patients can be difficult to determine, particularly when children become more stable and is variable depending on type and severity of disease, and family specific needs.

Discussion

The results obtained in this national study showed that PLTs ensure continuity of care through a number of complex and complementary activities. More specifically, several results demonstrate how continuity of care is ensured, namely the long follow-up period (average of 7 months); starting at the time of diagnosis, often at a curative stage; the high number of home deaths; and the capacity to offer bereavement care to the family. Moreover, the difficulty for PLTs, to distinguish between curative and palliative stages, might indicate that those conceptual distinctions are not relevant to ensure continuity of care, whatever the child's care pathway might be.

While other studies have reported a higher proportion of neurological diseases, [27–29] the large quantity of oncology cases in our study can be explained by several reasons. First of all, this is linked to the historical roots of the PLTs in Belgium that originated in oncology wards. Secondly the accreditation criteria defined by the Royal Decree, focusses on specialised oncology centres. Finally, the origin of funding for this programme, namely the Cancer Plan, likely influences the target population.

Regarding activities of the PLTs, our findings revealed a high number of home deaths, which requires an optimal degree of coordination among home care workers and hospital based professionals. It is commonly assumed that home would be the best place to care for a child at end-of-life, [30] but a study from Bluebond-Langner questions this assumption [31]. According to her, better outcome measures would be to assess the possibility for children and parents to have their preferences taken into account. This is the case for PLTs who offer families not only the possibility to express the location to have their child cared for at end-of-life (at home or at hospital), but also to rapidly adapt the place if preferences change over time.

Continuity of care such as provided by PLTs might be positively influenced through policies. In Belgium, considered among other European countries as offering optimal PPC provision [32], a bill voted in 2016 has enhanced the smooth integration of PPC within the national health system by enlarging the definition of palliative care beyond end-of-life care [21].

This is in line with the results of a systematic review conducted by Knapp et al. on PPC provision worldwide. Of the 43 European countries surveyed, 24 had some services in PPC. Belgium was one of only 5 countries providing the highest level of PPC services (level 4: measure of integration with mainstream services provided) [33].

Nevertheless, Noyes et al. demonstrate several potential barriers to accessing PPC services. Among these, cultural beliefs are highlighted as lowering the use of specialised PPC services [34].

Social acceptance of palliative care might influence optimal early access to specialised palliative care services and therefore continuity of care. One example is the terms used in the team's name, which seems to matter [35]. Fear of the term 'palliative' can be explained by common social representation's associating palliative care with end-of-life care, giving the impression that death is near. It has been reported that families call PPC teams "the angel of death".

Therefore, the term "paediatric liaison teams", instead of PPC teams, adopted by the Federal Government through the Royal Decree [22] seems to be more appropriate and efficacious to ensure acceptability of those services among families. Some solutions around this include for the team better communicating to the family what palliative care is and the use of the term Liaison as an alternative.

PLTs provide humane and professional support to families throughout the journey of a child's illness and death. Quality of relationship is a core element of care, whether for curative or palliative care. Characteristics of this relationship, essential to ensure continuity of care, were found in several theoretical frameworks presented hereafter and linked to the PLT's activities.

Although Harding et al. highlight the lack of an ideal PPC model, [36] the pop-up model [37] suggests a shared care model of palliative care, where primary health services and specialist PPC providers collaborate. This is the case for the Belgian PLTs, considered mostly as a second line service, which aim is to assist and support the primary health care team (GP and home care nurses). The pop-up model underlines the necessity to provide flexible care.

This coordination between specialists and primary health services can be found in community-based PPC such as reported by Kaye et al. [16]. According to Goldhagen et al. this model was even found to improve health-related quality of life and to reduce hospitalisation utilisation and costs [38].

The elements of continuity of care described by Haggerty, [5] can be achieved through nurse-driven care activities, [39–41] which are demonstrated by the PLTs studied here. Moreover, continuity of care can be rooted in the fundamentals of humanistic nursing theories applied to palliative care, [42–44] which are focused on individualised, holistic and family-centred care.

Those components can by summarised in the paradigm of integrated care suggested by Milstein, [45] which advocates the development of professional attitudes of "being with" families throughout the child's disease trajectory, both in curative and palliative stages. This constant presence of the team alongside the family can be seen as a form of companionship, and is an important resource of healing. PLTs report that parents express the valuable presence of teams being there for them "day after day".

This is supported by Weaver et al. [46] and Moonley et al., [47] who strengthen the role of relationships between parents and health care professionals in order to help families to cope with the uncertainty and adversity of their child's illness, leading to mixed, sometimes dichotomous feelings such as joy and sadness, hope and despair as reported by Rallison [48].

Furthermore, Carter introduces the concept of liminality which is an expression used in anthropology. Liminality refers to the intimate parental experience being nowhere, in a place where usual landmarks are becoming evanescent [49]. This can be the case for parents experiencing isolation when caring for their ill child. Through home visits, active listening and coordination of care, PLTs aim to reach parents where they are, in order for them to feel less isolated and help them reconnect to social life.

Several authors [50, 51] have extrapolated the concept of holding developed by the psychoanalyst D.W. Winnicott [52] as the essence of palliative care, arguing the importance of offering a secure and compassionate environment. At the same time paternalistic or judgmental attitudes should be avoided. Such support is essential for families who may be both vulnerable and isolated. Transposing Winnicott's concept of the 'good enough mother' to the 'good enough paediatric liaison team' could offer new perspectives of developing clinical guidelines which best ensure continuity of care.

Following on from the results of and challenges highlighted in our study, several developments of PPC in Belgium are presented hereafter.

Perspectives

Further discussions and workgroups on how to implement valid indicators of activity, identify children's palliative stages, and record diseases according to ICD-10 classification are in preparation among the PLT, the Cancer Plan and several authors of this manuscript. This could improve the quality of reporting, align the data collected to international research [53, 54] and strengthen the legitimacy and sustainability of those specialised paediatric liaison teams.

In conjunction with this, constructive national guidelines on the organisation of PPC are currently being prepared by the Belgian Paediatric Palliative Care Group (BPPC) [55]. Started in 2014, the BPPC assembles about 70 actors of PPC in Belgium from different professional backgrounds. The BPPC aims to elaborate guidelines on 5 themes: pain and symptom control, definition of paediatric palliative care, shared decision-making, organization of care, ethics and end-of life care.

It is presumed that better reporting of activities and developing guidelines might partially improve the quality of PPC. Promoting quality in PPC is a potential area of research [56]. This is in line with the EAPC recommendation on outcome measures in palliative care and quality indicators which are currently restricted to studies on adults [57, 58].

Belgian PLTs express strong interest for implementing tools to identify eligible children for PPC, to explore the individual quality of life of children benefitting from PPC, and to measure the impact of care provided. The relevance and feasibility of using several instruments, such as the Paediatric Palliative Screening Scale (PaPas Scale), [59] the direct weighted Scheduled Evaluation of Individual Quality of Life (SEI-QoL-dw) [60] or the Children's Palliative Outcome Scale (c-POS) was discussed [61] with paediatric liaison teams.

Limitations

To our knowledge, this is the first study describing the paediatric patients followed in Belgium by the specialised PPC teams, called liaison teams. The activities of these teams, including collaborative practice, are summarised to give a national snapshot of activity of PPC over a 5 year period.

However, the main limitation of the study lies in the fact that access to exclusively aggregated data did not permit further statistical analysis. Furthermore, some definitions in relation to curative and palliative care, reporting of patients with more than one diagnosis, and criteria for when follow-up might be concluded may assist in reducing disparities in reporting between different teams.

Conclusion

This secondary data analysis shows that Belgian PLTs ensure continuity of care through personalised, integrated care which starts at the time of diagnosis and continues, after a child's death, through bereavement care. The provision of contact with a PLT in all care settings gives the opportunity to build trusted relationship, which might reduce the important burden of a life-limiting condition on the entire family's life.

Nevertheless, improvements in data collection, development of national guidelines in PPC and implementation of specific outcome measures in routine clinical care are areas that could be further developed and described in future years.

Acknowledgments

We wish to thank Dr. Saskia Van den Bogaert and Mrs. Flore Alix from the Cancer Plan at the Federal government of Public Health for the trust they showed me which was manifested in extraction and delivery of the aggregated data issued from the PLT annual reports; Charline Martens de Noordhout and Tharcisse Nkunzimana for their help in statistics; Shelagh Mc Connell, Jenny Hunt and Claudine Pauwels for their long-lasting moral support; Alison Parnell, Shaheen Shaw, Elizabeth Mc Donald, Mandana Mehta and Hannelore Andries for the proofreading of this article; Pr. Yves Benoît for his courage to initiate the first PPC home care team in Gent; Sonja Develter, for her perseverance to promote PPC in Belgium and Anne-Catherine Dubois for her engagement in developing paediatric respite care.

Funding

This study is part of a PhD which is supported by a grant from the Fonds de Soutien Marguerite-Marie Delacroix and a financial support of the Institut Parnasse-ISEI, Haute Ecole Léonard de Vinci, Brussels, Belgium. The Sister Leontine Foundation supported partially the travel fees in order to make a poster presentation of those results possible, during the 2nd International Children's Palliative Care Network Conference (ICPCN): Paediatric Palliative Care: NOW! in Buenos Aires, Argentinia, May 2016.

Authors' contributions

MF conceived the design of the study together with IA. All data were analysed by MF. IA and JD took part in the analysis of the data. BB, JPM, EV, CT, FV, NA, MR, IR, GH and CF participated to the interpretation of the results. MF, IA and KM reviewed the final manuscript. All authors read and approved the final manuscript.

Author's information

The first author is currently a research assistant and a PhD student at Institute of Health and Society (IRSS) - Université catholique de Louvain, and lecturer at the Nursing school Parnasse-ISEI/Haute Ecole Léonard de Vinci. marie.friedel@uclouvain.be

Competing interests

The authors declare that they have no competing interests.

Author details

[1]Institute of Health and Society- Institut de recherche Santé et Société (IRSS), Université catholique de Louvain, 30, Clos Chapelle-aux-Champs, Boite 1.30.13, B-1200 Brussels, Belgium. [2]Haute Ecole Vinci, Institut Parnasse-ISEI, 41, Clos Chapelle-aux-Champs, 1200 Brussels, Belgium. [3]Cliniques universitaires St-Luc, 10, av Hippocrate, 1200 Brussels, Belgium. [4]Hôpital universitaire des enfants Reine Fabiola, Equipe de liaison pédiatrique, 15, av. JJ Crocq, 1020 Brussels, Belgium. [5]Universitair Ziekenhuis Leuven, Department of Paediatric Hemato-Oncology, Kites-Team (Kinderen In Thuis En Supportieve zorgteam), Herestraat, 49, 3000 Leuven, Belgium. [6]Centre hospitalier régional de la Citadelle, 1, Bd du 12ème de Ligne, 4000 Liège, Belgium. [7]Universitair Ziekenhuis Gent, KOESTER - liaisonequipe Kinderziekenhuis Prinses Elisabeth, C. Heymanslaan, 9000 Ghent, Belgium. [8]Cliniques universitaires st Luc, Interface pédiatrique, 10, av Hippocrate, 1200 Brussels, Belgium. [9]Scientific Institute of Public Health (ISP-WIV), 14, rue J. Wytsman, 1050 Brussels, Belgium. [10]Katholieke Universiteit Leuven, Oude Markt 13, 3000 Leuven, Belgium.

References

1. Abu-Saad Huijer H, Benini F, Craig F, H. Kuttner L, Wood C, Feraris P, Zernikow B. IMPaCCT. Standards for paediatric palliative care in Europe. Eur J Palliat Care 2007; 14:2–7.

2. Connor SR, Downing J, Marston J. Estimating the global need for palliative Care for Children: a cross-sectional analysis. J Pain Symptom Manag. 2017;53(2):171–7. https://doi.org/10.1016/j.jpainsymman.2016.08.020. Epub 2016 Oct 17
3. Gethins M. Pediatric palliative Care in Europe Expands. JNCI. 2012;104(1):10–1.
4. Miller A, Condin C, Mc Kellin W, Shaw N, Klasse A, Sheps S. Continuity of care for children with complex chronic health conditions: parent's perspectives. BMC Health Serv Res. 2009;21(9):242.
5. Haggerty J, Reid R, Freeman G, Starfield B, Adair C, McKendry R. Continuity of care: a multidisciplinary review. BMJ. 2003;327(7425):1219–21.
6. Freeman G, Shepperd S, Robinson I, Ehrich K, Richards S. Continuity of care: report of a scoping exercise for the NCCSDO. London: National coordinating Centre for Service Delivery and Organisation; 2001.
7. Freeman G, Woloshynowych M, Baker R, Boulton M, Guthrie B, Car J, Haggerty J, Tarrant C, et al. Continuity of care 2006: what have we learned since 2000 and what are policy imperatives now? London: National Coordinating Centre for Service Delivery and Organization; 2007.
8. Parker G, Corden A, Heaton J. Experiences of and influences on continuity of care for service users and carers: synthesis of evidence from a research programme. Health Soc Care Community. 2011;19(6):577.
9. Saultz JW. Defining and measuring interpersonal continuity of care. Ann Fam Med. 2003;1(3):134–43.
10. Foster T, Gilmer M. Continuing bonds: a human response within paediatric palliative care. Int J Palliat Nurs. 2008;14(2):85–91.
11. Mastro K, Johnson J, McElvery N, Preuster C. The benefits of a nurse-driven, patient- and family-centered pediatric palliative care program. J Nurs Adm. 2015;45(9):423–8.
12. Johnson S, Giesie P, Ireland A, Rice R, Thomson B. On the scene: developing a nurse care coordinator role at City of hope. Nurs Adm Q. 2016;40(1):39–50.
13. World Health Organization. WHO Definition of Palliative Care for Children. http://www.who.int/cancer/palliative/definition/en/. Accessed 10 Feb 2018.
14. World Health Assembly (WHA), Strengthening of palliative care as a component of integrated treatment within the continuum of care. 134th session EB134.R7. http://apps.who.int/gb/ebwha/pdf_files/EB134/B134_28-en.pdf.
15. Kaye E, Friebert S, Baker J. Early integration of palliative Care for Children with high-risk Cancer and their families. Pediatr Blood Cancer. 2016;63(4):593–7.
16. Kaye E, Rubenstein J, Levine D, Baker J, Dabbs D, Friebert S. Pediatric palliative care in the community. CA Cancer J Clin. 2015;65(4):316–33.
17. Miller E, Levy C, Linebarger J, Klick J, Carter B. Pediatric palliative care : current evidence and evidence gaps. J Pediatr. 2015;166(6):1536–40.
18. Lichtenthal W, Sweeney C, Roberts K, Corner G, Donovan L, Prigerson H, Wiener L. Bereavement follow-up after the death of a child as a standard of care in pediatric oncology. Pediatr Blood Cancer. 2015;62(5):S834–69.
19. Weaver M, Heinze K, Kelly K, Wiener L, Casey R, Bell C, Wolfe J, Garee A, Watson A, Hinds P. Palliative care as standard in pediatric oncology. Pediatr Blood Cancer. 2015;62(5):S829–33.
20. Niswander L, Cromwell P, Chirico J, Gupton A, Korones D. End-of-life care for children enrolled in a community-based pediatric palliative care program. J Palliat Med. 2014;17(5):589–91.
21. Ministry of Justice. Loi du 14 juin 2002 relative aux soins palliatifs in http://www.etaamb.be/fr/loi-du-21-juillet-2016_n2016024163.html. Accessed 10 Feb 2018.
22. Royal Decree of the 15th November 2010 which defines the norms on which the function of the paediatric liaison must respond in order to be accredited in http://www.etaamb.be/fr/arrete-royal-du-15-novembre-2010_n2010024459.html. Accessed 10 Feb 2018.
23. Association for Children with Life Threatening or Terminal conditions and their families (ACT) and the Royal College of Paediatrics and Child Health (RCPCH). A guide to the development of children's palliative care services. UK. 1997.
24. Action 23 of Cancer Plan in https://www.health.belgium.be/sites/default/files/uploads/fields/fpshealth_theme_file/actions.pdf. Accessed 10 Feb 2018.
25. Marks D, Yardley L. Content and thematic analysis, in: research methods for clinical and Health Psychology. London: SAGE; 2004.
26. Feudtner C, Christakis DA, Connell FA. Pediatrics. 2000;106(1):205–9.
27. Palliative care for infants, children and young people. The Facts. EAPC Taskforce for Palliative Care in Children and Maruzza Lefebvre d'Ovidio Onlus Foundation. 2009. In http://www.eapcnet.eu/LinkClick.aspx?fileticket=DeiV2yhtOZA%3D. Accessed 10 Feb 2018.
28. Fraser LK, Miller M, Hain R, Norman P, Aldridge J, McKinney PA, Parslow RC. Rising national prevalence of life-limiting conditions in children in England. Pediatrics. 2012;129(4):e923–9. https://doi.org/10.1542/peds.2011-2846. Epub 2012 Mar 12
29. Fraser LK, Lidstone V, Miller M, Aldridge J, Norman P, McKinney PA, Parslow RC. Patterns of diagnoses among children and young adults with life-limiting conditions: a secondary analysis of a national dataset. Palliat Med. 2014;28(6):513–20. https://doi.org/10.1177/0269216314528743.
30. Kassam A, Skiadaresis J, Alexander S, Wolfe J. Parent and clinician preferences for location of end-of-life care: home, hospital or freestanding hospice? Pediatr Blood Cancer. 2014;61(5):859–64.
31. Bluebond-Langner M, Beecham E, Candy B, Langner R, Jones L. Preferred place of death for children and young people with life-limiting and life-threatening conditions: a systematic review of the literature and recommendations for future inquiry and policy. Pall Med. 2013;27:705–13.
32. Ministry of Justice. Loi du 21 juillet 2016 modifiant la loi du 14 juin 2002 relative aux soins palliatifs en vue d'élargir la définition des soins palliatifs in http://www.etaamb.be/fr/loi-du-21-juillet-2016_n2016024163.html. Accessed 10 Feb 2018.
33. Knapp C, Woodworth L, Wright M, Downing J, Drake R, Fowler-Kerry S, Hain R, Marston J. Pediatric palliative care provision around the world: a systematic review. Pediatr Blood Cancer. 2011;57(3):361–8. https://doi.org/10.1002/pbc.23100.
34. Noyes J, Edwards RT, Hastings RP, Hain R, Totsika V, Bennett V, Hobson L, Davies GR, Humphreys C, Devins M, Spencer LH, Lewis M. Evidence-based planning and costing palliative care services for children: novel multi-method epidemiological and economic exemplar. BMC Palliat Care. 2013;12(1):18. https://doi.org/10.1186/1472-684X-12-18.
35. Maciasz R, Arnold R, Chu E. Does it matter what you call it? A randomized trial of language used to describe palliative care services. Support Care Cancer. 2013;21:3411.
36. Harding R, Albertyn R, Sherr L, Gwyther L. Pediatric palliative care in sub-saharan Africa: a systematic review of the evidence for care models, interventions, and outcomes. J Pain Symptom Manag. 2014;47(3):642–51.
37. Mherekumombe MF, Frost J, Hanson S, Shepherd E, Collins J. Pop up: a new model of paediatric palliative care. J Paediatr Child Health. 2016; https://doi.org/10.1111/jpc.13276.
38. Goldhagen J, Fafard M, Komatz K, Eason T, Livingood WC. Community-based pediatric palliative care for health related quality of life, hospital utilization and costs lessons learned from a pilot study. BMC Palliat Care. 2016;15:73. https://doi.org/10.1186/s12904-016-0138-z.
39. Pontin D, Lewis M. Maintaining the continuity of care in community children's nursing caseloads in a service for children with life-limiting, life-threatening or chronic health conditions : a qualitative analysis. J Clin Nurs. 2009;18(8):1199–206.
40. Johnson S, Giesie P, Ireland A, Rice R, Thomson B. On the scene a nurse care coordinator role at City of hope. Nurs Adm Q. 2016;40(1):39–50.
41. Jankowski J. Professional boundaries issues in pediatric palliative care. Am J Hosp Palliat Care. 2014;31(2):161–5.
42. Wu HL, Volker DL. Humanistic nursing theory: application to hospice and palliative care. J Adv Nurs. 2012;68(2):471–9.
43. Dobrina R, Tenze M, Palese A. An overview of hospice and palliative care nursing models and theories. Int J Palliat Nurs. 2014;20(2):75–81.
44. Magante MC. Developing a care model for hospice and palliative nurses. Int J Palliat Nurs. 2015;21(2):96.
45. Milstein JA. Paradigm of integrative care: healing with curing throughout life, "being with" and "doing to". J Perinatol. 2005;25(9):563–8.
46. Weaver MS, Heinze KE, Bell CJ, Wiener L, Garee AM, Kelly KP, Casey RL, Watson A, Hinds PS. Pediatric Palliative Care Special Interest Group at Children's National Health System. Establishing psychosocial palliative care standards for children and adolescents with cancer and their families: an integrative review. Palliat Med. 2016;30(3):212–23.
47. Mooney-Doyle K, Dos Santos MR, Szylit R, Deatrick JA. Parental expectations of support from healthcare providers during pediatric life-threatening illness: a secondary, qualitative analysis. J Pediatr Nurs. 2017;36:163–72.
48. Rallison LB, Raffin-Bouchal S. Living in the in-between: families caring for a child with a progressive neurodegenerative illness. Qual Health Res. 2013;23(2):194–206.
49. Carter B. Liminality in pediatric palliative care. Am J Hosp Palliat Care. 2017;34(4):297–300.
50. Bioy A, Van Lander A, Mallet D. Belloir M-N (dir.) Soins palliatifs. 9th part. 40th Chapt. Dunod. 2017:265.

51. Duflot C. L'art thérapie en soins palliatifs. Eres. 2016.
52. Winnicott DW, Winnicott on the Child. Cambridge 2002:238.
53. Feudtner C, Feinstein J, Zhong W, Hall M, Dai D. Pediatric complex chronic conditions (CCC) classification system version 2 : updated for ICD-10 and complex medical technology dependence and transplantation. BMC Pediatr. 2014;14:199.
54. Hain R, Devins M, Hastings R, Noyes J. Paediatric palliative care: development and pilot study of a "directory of life-limiting conditions". BMC Palliat Care. 2013;11(12(1)):43.
55. Renard M, Brichard B, Francotte N, Fonteyne C, Misson J-P, Faingnaert M, Mattheeuws K, Ruysseveldt I. Belgian pediatric palliative care: spreading the ideas of pediatric palliative Care in the Different Fields of pediatric medicine. P050 3rd congress on Paediatric palliative care. A global gathering. Rome, 16–19 2016.
56. Kassam A, Skiadaresis J, Habib S, Alexander S, Wolfe J. Moving toward quality palliative cancer care: parent and clinician perspectives on gaps between what matters and what is accessible. J Clin Oncol. 2013;31(7):910–5.
57. Bausewein C, Daveson B, Currow D, Downing J, Deliens L, et al. EAPC white paper on outcome measurement in palliative care: improving practice, attaining outcomes and delivering quality services - recommendations from the European Association for Palliative Care (EAPC) task force on outcome measurement. Palliat Med. 2016;30(1):6–22.
58. Leemans K, Deliens L, Van den Block L, Vander Stichele R, Francke A, Cohen J. Systematic quality monitoring for specialized palliative care services: development of a minimal set of quality indicators for palliative care study (QPAC). Am J Hosp Palliat Care. 2016;
59. Bergstraesser E, Hain R, Pereira J. The development of an instrument that can identify children with palliative care needs: the Paediatric palliative screening scale (PaPaS scale): a qualitative study approach. BMC Palliat Care. 2013;12:20.
60. O'Boyle C, Browne J. Schedule for the Evaluation of Individual Quality of Life. A direct weighting procedure for quality of life domains. Administration Manual. Department of Psychology. Royal College of Surgeons in Ireland, 1995.
61. Harding R. Outcome measures for children: current state of science and views of professional stakeholders. Conference. August 2015. United Kingdom.

Access to palliative care for homeless people: complex lives, complex care

Anke J E de Veer[1*], Barbara Stringer[2], Berno van Meijel[3,4,5,6], Renate Verkaik[1] and Anneke L Francke[1,7,8]

Abstract

Background: People experiencing homelessness often encounter progressive incurable somatic diseases in combination with psychiatric and psychosocial problems, and many need palliative care at the end of their lives. Little is known about how palliative care for this group can be started in good time and provided optimally. The objective of this paper is to give insight into the extent people experiencing homelessness have access to good palliative care.

Methods: Qualitative in-depth interviews were held to reconstruct the cases of 19 people experiencing homelessness in the Netherlands. Eight cases concerned persons being in the palliative phase (using the surprise question) and the other 11 cases concerned persons recently died after a period of ill health due to somatic illness. We used purposive sampling until data saturation was reached. The total number of interviews was 52. All interviews were transcribed verbatim and analysed inductively.

Results: Three key themes were: 'late access', 'capricious trajectory' and 'complex care'. The first key theme refers to the often delayed start of palliative care, because of the difficulties in recognizing the need for palliative care, the ambivalence of people experiencing homelessness about accepting palliative care, and the lack of facilities with specific expertise in palliative care for them. The second key theme refers to the illness trajectory, which is often capricious because of the challenging behaviour of people experiencing homelessness, an unpredictable disease process and a system not being able to accommodate or meet their needs. The third key theme refers to the complexity of their care with regard to pain and symptom control, psychosocial and spiritual aspects, and the social network.

Conclusions: The care for in the palliative phase does not satisfy the core requirements of palliative care since there are bottlenecks regarding timely identification, the social network, and the assessment and management of physical symptoms and psychosocial and spiritual care needs. Education in palliative care of outreach professionals, training staff in shelters in the provision of palliative care, and building a network of palliative care specialists for people experiencing homelessness.

Keywords: Palliative care, People experiencing homelessness, End-of-life care, Psychiatric care, Interviews, Qualitative study

Background

The United Nations states that health facilities, goods and services must be accessible to all, especially the most vulnerable or marginalized sections of the population [1]. This also accounts for palliative care. Palliative care "improves the quality of life of patients and their families facing the problem associated with life-threatening illness, through the prevention and relief of suffering by means of early identification and impeccable assessment and treatment of pain and other problems, physical, psychosocial and spiritual." [2] People working with the homeless, however, often have doubts about whether they have equal access to good palliative care. Palliative care facilities and expertise are often organized with the general population in mind. In the Netherlands, palliative care is preferably provided at home or, for those who need care that cannot be delivered at home, in nursing homes or hospices.

* Correspondence: a.deveer@nivel.nl
[1]Netherlands Institute for Health Services Research (Nivel), P.O. Box 1568, 3500, BN, Utrecht, The Netherlands
Full list of author information is available at the end of the article

However, for people experiencing homelessness good palliative care, preferably 'at home', is not a matter of course. A 'person experiencing homelessness' is someone without permanent housing who may live on the streets, in a shelter, in temporary accommodation, or in some other unstable or non-permanent situation [3]. Based on the number of people known to the Dutch social shelter system, the number of people experiencing homelessness is estimated at 30,000, and this number is thought to be growing [4, 5]. In the Netherlands, ill people experiencing homelessness often stay in special shelters at the end of their lives, which can be seen as their 'home'. Types of shelters, usually organized by the municipality or the Salvation Army, vary across towns. There are temporary shelters for those who are ill or frail, nursing home wards, and shelters offering hospice care.

People experiencing homelessness are a specific target group not only because of their living conditions but also because they have a short life expectancy, their high prevalence of illness and symptom burden, their concerns how their life will end, and the reduced availability of palliative care. In a cohort study in one of the largest cities in the Netherlands, life expectancy at age 30 was 11.0 (95% CI 9.1–12.9) years less for men experiencing homelessness compared to men in the general population and 15.9 (95% CI 10.3–21.5) less for women experiencing homelessness [6]. People experiencing homelessness aged 50 and older were found to have higher rates of age-related conditions (functional impairments, cognitive impairments, falls, urinary incontinence) than the general population aged 20 years older [7]. Those who do not die suddenly, for instance in an accident, by suicide, or from a drug overdose, violence or hypothermia, often need palliative care in the final phase of their life.

Heart diseases, respiratory diseases, diseases of the digestive system and alcohol-related diseases (such as liver problems or cancer) have been cited as major chronic diseases causing death among people experiencing homelessness [8–11]. Complex comorbidity may occur due to the co-occurrence of physical illness, psychiatric conditions (such as depression, psychosis, post-traumatic stress disorder, and schizophrenia) and addictions [7, 12]. When nearing the end of life, people experiencing homelessness suffer a high incidence of symptoms, especially pain, fatigue, and psychological symptoms such as worrying and feeling sad [13].

Previous studies have reported that people experiencing homelessness often have concerns about how their life will end, e.g. about dying anonymously and being undiscovered or unidentified after death [14, 15]. They also frequently worry about the funeral and notification of family members [14]. Older people experiencing homelessness often see a good death as dying peacefully, not suffering, experiencing spiritual connection, and making amends with significant others [16].

These concerns and the diversity and complexity of health problems and needs in different areas of life pose challenges to the access to good palliative care, i.e. people-centred care. Studies indicated that such care is less widely available to people experiencing homelessness [15, 17–22].

Hence the objective of this paper is to give an insight into the extent good palliative care is accessible for people experiencing homelessness in the Netherlands. Answers on this question may give a better understanding of how palliative care for this target group can be improved.

Methods

Design

Qualitative interviews were held with people experiencing homelessness at the end of life, as well as with people who were close to them at the end of life. In this way we tried to collect as much information about a case as possible.

Recruitment and participants

With the surprise question (see below), we purposively recruited people experiencing homelessness, both men and women, in different living circumstances, who were at the end of their lives. We also included cases of persons who were already deceased. The interviewees and deceased cases were selected through contact persons at 13 different shelters, e.g. run by the Salvation Army or municipalities. In the Netherlands, the national healthcare policy is to have no one sleeping rough on the streets, but instead to have them sleep in night-care shelters for the homeless, for instance. Those who do not want to live on the streets anymore have access to sheltered accommodation. There are also special convalescence care shelters for sick people [23]. The shelters involved in our study were in seven cities located in different parts of the Netherlands. This diverse range of settings was selected to take into account the variety of possible palliative care circumstances, since the facilities for people experiencing homelessness can vary between municipalities.

A contact person at each shelter was asked to select cases for our interview study. They were asked to identify persons in the palliative phase with the aid of the surprise question: "Would you be surprised if this person died within the next two years as a result of his/her underlying somatic illness?". If the answer was "No, this would not surprise me", the contact person asked that person whether they would be willing to participate in the study and whether they gave permission to have their name and address passed on to the researcher. The contact person verbally gave information and handed the researchers' information letter plus an informed consent form to the person. After interviewing the person experiencing homelessness, we asked their consent for also interviewing the professionals closest to them, specifically at least one professional who knew their personal circumstances (e.g. a social worker) and one professional who knew their medical circumstances (i.e. physician or nurse). Information of social workers and medical professionals supplemented each other because the nature of their contacts with the person experiencing homelessness was different. After this informed consent, we contacted the professionals for an interview.

In addition, contact persons were asked to identify cases of deceased persons who had died less than 1 year ago after a period of ill health due to a somatic illness. The contact person informed the professionals who had been most closely involved about the research and gave them an information letter with an informed consent form. After obtaining their informed consent, we contacted the professionals for an interview.

We also tried to find a family member or friend to interview (via the person experiencing homelessness or, if deceased, via the professionals). However, about half of the persons in the study cases did not have any contact with family or friends. In the other half of the cases, the relatives refused to participate or professionals were ambivalent asking them.

Participants were provided with a €20 gift voucher, participants who were homeless received €20 in cash.

Data collection

In total 52 individual in-depth interviews were held dealing with 19 cases of people experiencing homelessness: seven interviews with people themselves ($n = 7$), 13 with social workers, 12 with physicians, 16 with registered nurses, three with nurse assistants, and one interview with a sheltered housing facility coordinator.

The interviews were almost always held in the shelter in which the person was living or had lived. The interviews with people experiencing homelessness were conducted by the first author (AdV), where another author (BS) was co-interviewer during the first three interviews. The interviewers were a psychologist (AdV) who worked in a walk-in centre for homeless people, and a mental health nurse specialized in treatment of patients with severe personality disorders (BS). Both are experienced qualitative researchers. BS – with her experience in mental health nursing - trained AdV in how to interact with people from our target group and how to develop trust. After three interviews, each extensively evaluated afterwards, AdV carried out the interviews. The interviews lasted between 20 and 90 min. Open questions were used, encouraging interviewees in their own words to describe the care the person needed and the care they received.

The interviews with the people experiencing homelessness started with a general question concerning their perceived health ("Can you tell me something about your health?"), followed by questions about the care they needed and the care they received. The first question for professionals was: "Can you tell me something about the care you give/gave?" Depending on the answer, questions were asked about the palliative care that was needed and the care provided. A topic list (Table 1) was used to see if the different aspects of palliative care were being addressed. For all groups we used the same topic guide, reminding the interviewer of possible topics to cover and areas to probe. However, during the interview this topic guide was individualized taking into account the specific situation of the interviewee and the findings from previous interviews. The primary focus was on the information the interviewee had and what the interviewee found important to tell. Because people experiencing homelessness and facing the end of their life are very vulnerable in many ways [24] the interviewers continuously paid attention to whether topics could be addressed.

Analysis

Each interview was audiotaped and transcribed verbatim. The analysis was part of a cyclical process of data collection – data analysis – new data collection, ultimately ending in data saturation [25]. Data saturation was obtained after 52 interviews based on 19 cases.

The data were analysed inductively. All transcripts were analysed by the first author (AdV), while each of the other authors analysed at least three transcripts. Initially, codes were generated that remained close to the words of the interviewees. Subsequently, the meaning of clusters of codes was discussed within the research team and key themes

Table 1 Topic list used in the interviews

- The care needed and the care provided (physical, ADL, psychosocial, spiritual, social, symptoms)
- The beginning of the palliative phase
- Proactive care
- Communication with the person experiencing homelessness, wishes of the person
- Autonomy of the person experiencing homelessness
- Family and friends
- Communication and cooperation between professionals
- End-of-life decisions
- After-death care
- Care for other residents
- Care for professionals
- Competencies of professionals

were identified. Transcripts of previous interviews were reanalysed and new interviews analysed, guided by these themes, which in turn were sometimes refined or reformulated during the analysis process. Interim analyses were discussed by several pairs of authors. Differences between the researchers in the analysis and interpretations were discussed until consensus was reached. Thus the coding scheme was jointly refined over time. Finally, the transcripts were coded with the final themes and subthemes, which are also used as the headings and subheadings in the Results section (see below).

Strategies to ensure rigour in our data were purposive sampling aimed to reflect the diversity in the population and multiple interviews per person experiencing homelessness aimed to capture rich, descriptive data. Interviews were analysed by the researchers from early on and after 19 cases and 52 interviews data saturation was reached.

The software program MAXQDA (release 11.0.9b) was used to facilitate the process of data analysis (www.MAXQDA.com). To validate the results, we discussed the central themes that emerged from our analyses in two focus groups with professionals and a representative of the homeless group (11 participants in total).

Results

Characteristics of people experiencing homelessness

Table 2 shows that the cases consisted of 16 men and three women: eight were in the palliative phase and 11 were people who were deceased. Five of the latter group died in the shelter, three in a hospice, two in a nursing home and one in a hospital. The mean age at death was 58. All had a background of homelessness, and most of them also had a history of drugs and/or alcohol abuse.

Three key themes

The interviews revealed three key themes in the provision of palliative care for people experiencing homelessness: late access to palliative care, capricious healthcare trajectories, and the high degree of complexity of the care (Table 3). These key themes were subdivided into eight subthemes. To illustrate the themes, we present the cases of Jane, John, Mitch, Anthony and William (Table 4). John and William were interviewed in the study. Jane, Mitch and Anthony were deceased at the time of the study.

Late access

People experiencing homelessness were found to have late access to palliative care. Three subthemes were factors in this late access: difficulty among professionals in recognizing palliative care needs, the ambivalence felt by them towards searching for and accepting care, and the lack of services specialized in palliative care for people experiencing homelessness.

Table 2 Characteristics of the people experiencing homelessness ($n = 19$)

	n	Percentage
Person is		
- deceased	11	58%
- in palliative phase (1)	8	42%
Sex		
- male	16	84%
- female	3	16%
Age (mean, range)	Total group: 59.8 (45–72)	Deceased: 58.4 (45–70)
Problems preceding palliative phase (multiple categories possible)		
- drug addiction (including alcohol)	17	89%
- psychiatric diagnosis (e.g. schizophrenia)	5	26%
- (mild) intellectual disability	3	16%
- financial problems	1	5%
- illegal resident	2	11%
Expected or actual cause of death (multiple answers possible)		
- cancer	8	42%
- liver cirrhosis	3	16%
- COPD	3	16%
- sepsis	2	11%
- renal failure	2	11%
- cardiovascular disease	2	11%
- diabetes	1	5%

(1) One person initially agreed to participate in an interview but refused when the interviewee arrived. This person gave permission for interviews with his caregivers

Difficulty in recognizing palliative care needs People experiencing homelessness often do not have a recorded medical history due to their often chaotic lifestyles and the paths their lives have taken. Earlier somatic problems were often not documented, which made current signals difficult to interpret. Interpretation was also difficult because people experiencing homelessness mostly had a combination of psychiatric symptoms, addiction

Table 3 Map with the three key themes and eight subthemes characterizing the provision of palliative care in people with a background of homelessness

Late Access	• difficulties in recognizing need
	• ambivalence towards accepting care
	• no palliative care facilities
Capricious trajectory	• challenging behaviour
	• unpredictable disease progression
Complex care	• pain and symptom control
	• psychosocial and spiritual care
	• social network

Table 4 Cases illustrating the results of the analysis

*Jane** was a woman without family or friends, diagnosed with schizophrenia. After a period of homelessness she lived in an assisted living facility. She died of colon cancer in a hospital aged 60. In the final two years of her life she had a small apartment and received assertive community treatment.
John is an illegal resident in the Netherlands aged 52, addicted to alcohol and drugs. Because of his bad health and with the support of a street doctor, he got permission to stay in a shelter. After a hospitalization, he moved to a nursing ward for people experiencing homelessness.
Mitch was a former offender, aged 56, diagnosed with an antisocial personality disorder and long-lasting and severe drugs abuse. He was a drugs dealer and had received several convictions for serious violent crimes. He had been living for some years with his wife in his own apartment and had been receiving assertive community treatment. He died in a hospice of oesophageal cancer.
Anthony was born with a mild intellectual disorder and was addicted to alcohol. Lived in a shelter for people with addiction problems or severe psychiatric problems with somatic complaints. Remarkably, Anthony still had close ties with his family: every day they met each other in his mother's home to play games and drink beer. He died of throat cancer at the age of 53 in a hospice.
William is a friendly man aged 52. He is addicted to alcohol and drugs and his aggression regulation is distorted. He suffers from COPD and is oxygen dependent. He lives in a shelter for people experiencing homelessness with somatic health problems.

* Names are pseudonyms and bear no resemblance of those interviewed

problems, intellectual disabilities and challenging behaviours. A social worker: *"There is not much continuity in my relationships with people experiencing homelessness. They come and go again. This makes it extra difficult to notice changes in health care needs."*

The professionals involved were often social workers who were not trained in recognizing medical problems and potential palliative care needs. As Jane's case illustrates, for most professionals it was difficult to recognize that someone was incurably somatically ill and in need of palliative care (Table 5, E1).

Ambivalence towards accepting care People experiencing homelessness did not readily ask for help, even when they experienced healthcare needs. They had often suffered many losses in the past (e.g. their job, home, family and friends, dreams and hopes, and now their health), suffered from social exclusion, and had learned to solve things themselves. They often had no confidence in professionals due to previous disappointing contacts, feelings of not being treated equally, perceived stigmatization and being disparaged by professionals. Feelings of shame, for instance because of physical neglect or persistence in addiction, were also mentioned as a barrier to seeking help. The maintenance of autonomy and self-control was generally very important for them. From this perspective they did not easily ask for help, nor did they easily accept help, even if they had a strong need for help. Members of an assertive community treatment (ACT) team said that it was difficult to remain in touch with people experiencing homelessness. Despite this difficulty, the ACT team members said that they did not abandon the person (Table 5, E2).

No palliative care facilities In the Netherlands, there are a limited number of nursing-home facilities with specific expertise in palliative care for people experiencing homelessness. However, in most parts of the Netherlands there is insufficient capacity in specialized nursing homes for people experiencing homelessness and so these people depend on mainstream care, for instance in hospitals, nursing homes, hospice facilities or shelters. Just as people experiencing homelessness are ambivalent about accepting care, so mainstream care facilities are also ambivalent about providing care for them, or even reluctant to do so. If a person failed to show up to an appointment in a hospital, for instance, the physician generally did not undertake further initiatives and in the worst-case scenario they just closed the file. Nursing homes and hospices had difficulty with their way of life, especially if they persisted in their addiction. People experiencing homelessness were generally not willing or able to make changes in their way of life, such as refraining from drugs.

At the same time, shelters for people experiencing homelessness were not able to offer palliative care. Social workers were not trained in providing the nursing care, or even the ADL care that is often needed at the end of life. As a social worker put it: *"We always focus on resocialisation, resocialisation, and resocialisation..., whereas another strategy is needed."* Shelters for convalescent care primarily provided ADL care; other nursing care was not available 24/7. Many professionals in shelters thought that palliative care and terminal care were the same, not realizing that many of their clients were in need of palliative care even though they were not in the terminal stage of life. But the professionals in the shelters were very skilled in providing a safe environment and trusting relationships for and with their clients. If the person became sicker, professionals struggled with the dilemma of whether the client could stay or should go to a mainstream palliative care facility (Table 5, E3).

Capricious trajectory

Access to palliative care facilities was often impeded by big fluctuations in care provision. Two subthemes underlie these fluctuations. Firstly, the behaviour of people experiencing homelessness presents a challenge for a

Table 5 Examples (indicated as E1 to E8) illustrating the characteristics of palliative care provision

Subtheme	No.	Quote
Difficulty in recognizing need	E1	Jane's social worker described their search: *"Jane complained about her stomach and intestines... we thought that was part of her psychiatric illness. In retrospect I think these were the first signs of cancer....We arranged admission to a psychiatric hospital... a forced admission because she refused to go voluntarily. If you work in psychiatry, you sometimes focus too much on mental issues, you forget that it may just be something somatic."* In the psychiatric hospital no further medical examinations were done. After discharge from the psychiatric hospital, the social workers noticed that Jane was rapidly losing weight. Because Jane had not visited a GP for years and occasionally made remarks about hospital experiences, the social workers contacted all the hospitals in the region to search for more medical information, but no file on Jane was found. Gradually they realized that Jane was probably very ill. Her social worker: *"If there had been a medical file, we might have spotted signs of digestive problems earlier".*
Ambivalence towards accepting care	E2	A nurse talking about Mitch: *"I persist in motivating him to come to our yearly somatic screening, for instance, but some will never come... Every time, we try to make contact with a person again. We can be very persistent. Even when I see someone on the street or in a shop I talk to him, both during working hours and during my free time."*
No palliative care facilities	E3	A nurse at Anthony's shelter: *"I work in this shelter two days a week, mainly to arrange all kinds of things. ... We can do a lot, that's not the problem. Anthony wants to stay here and, however fragile, some of us sometimes have a little talk with Anthony. But there are different points of views in the team as to how far we can go in offering care for the dying... In this shelter there are no nurses or nurse assistants. But Anthony didn't want to leave and, besides, what nursing home will tolerate his behaviour?"*
Challenging behaviour	E4	The nurse involved with John explained why John had not yet transferred to a nursing home, despite his care needs which they could not meet properly: *"John can't go to the nursing home yet. He won't stick to the rules. He will persist in smoking in his room. In the past someone was refused care in the nursing home because he persisted in smoking, despite warnings. Some nurses didn't dare enter the room because they were afraid of him. Therefor John will only be transferred to the nursing home when this behaviour has faded...so, for the final days of his life."*
Unpredictable disease progression	E5	John's nurse: *"..we thought...this will not last long. But one way or another, he recovered again. He was admitted to hospital and we thought this is the end. But then...suddenly...after two days he returned and was on the streets to take his heroin. As if he rose from the dead ... I'll never forget his will to live."*
Pain and symptom control	E6	A social worker: *"Anthony persisted in smoking. The pain medication made him muzzy. Even when he couldn't leave his bed anymore he still wanted to smoke. Because we were afraid he might fall asleep, some member of staff had to go to his room to let him smoke. But often we don't have enough time to sit there several times a day. Then it is either medication, or smoking..."*
Psychosocial and spiritual care	E7	William, who had to stay in his room because of a lack of mobile oxygen: *"I would like to arrange some things, the funeral, that I have a bit of certainty... It's just a surprise to me now. It is in the surprise package. [Laughing] [I: Did you ask for this?] I don't know. No, well, I've mentioned it here a few times... but yes ... that would be nice. They know I'm very ill ... No one has come to me yet, what do you want when you're dead, what should happen? [I: What do you want] Well, for now I want a mobility scooter ...Now it's still possible, so I can meet some people."*
Social network	E8	Mitch's GP: *"Of course they clearly missed something [tumour] on the CT. If there had been relatives with him, I'm sure the urologist would have said 'Well, gosh, what's up there...?' I'll ask... but yes up to a certain point, of course. It's because you're not so emotionally connected to someone. But I often get this kind of thing, that somebody takes less of a serious look at someone. Right, it shouldn't be that way, but it is."*

continuous, workable relationship with professionals. Secondly, professionals experienced the disease progression as unpredictable.

Behaviour that is challenging for professionals Many of the professionals interviewed, both in facilities for people experiencing homelessness and professionals elsewhere, mentioned that the behaviour of people experiencing homelessness is often challenging and difficult for them to handle. If addicted, they spent a great deal of their time arranging and using alcohol or drugs. Social contacts were mainly based on drugs use. This instrumental behaviour was experienced as often impeding genuine social contacts and communication with professionals. The professionals used a variety of labels when describing frequently occurring difficult behaviours of people experiencing homelessness: aggressive, rejecting, passive, manipulative, norm-breaking and rule-breaking, and an associated loss of decorum (Table 5, E4).

Intellectual and cognitive disabilities, sometimes congenital and sometimes resulting from long-term addiction, further complicated communication and effective interactions. Some had schizophrenia, psychoses or other psychiatric disorders hindering communication. These challenges for professionals threatened the continuity of the care and of the relationship with the professional. Professionals invested a lot of energy in ensuring continuity in medical care by reminding people of their appointments with physicians and accompanying them to the hospital, despite the challenging behaviour they exhibited. The ACT nurse about Mitch's contacts with the medical specialist in the hospital: *"He behaved very pettishly, very badly. He let happen what had to happen, but he was absolutely condescending... He could not accept authority at all."*

Unpredictable disease progression The state of physical health often stabilized or even got better when the sick person moved from living on the streets into a shelter. There, the person not only received somatic care but was also supported in having a regular structure to their day, a day-night rhythm and better food intake, and they received personal attention. The person was also supported in their adherence to the medical treatment. As a consequence, the person's condition could improve more than would have been expected if the sick person had continued in their normal living conditions.

The fact that the temporary improvement was unexpected was also due to a lack of knowledge among professionals, for instance about the course of COPD. If the person had recovered from an exacerbation, many professionals interpreted the improvement as genuine recovery, not realizing that this process of recurring exacerbations characterizes COPD.

Finally, it was also difficult for professionals to get good insight into the disease progression because a person experiencing homelessness often wanted to pick up their usual way of life as quickly as possible. If, after a deterioration, the health status improved slightly, the person often tended to go back to living on the streets. The professionals said people experiencing homelessness had learned to survive from early on in life and did not easily give up. Sometimes their craving for drugs made them leave the shelter or hospital as soon as possible (Table 5, E5). These circumstances made it particularly difficult for professionals to predict the disease progression.

Complex care

The third key theme that prevents people experiencing homelessness from having access to good palliative care is the complexity of this care. In particular the control of pain and other symptoms, the psychosocial and spiritual care, and the care for relatives were perceived as difficult.

Pain and symptom control Many of the professionals interviewed experienced difficulties with pain management and control. Recommendations in general palliative care guidelines or protocols often do not take into account the specific characteristics of persons who use or have used cocaine, methadone, mood stabilizers or antidepressants. People who already use or have used these drugs were found to react differently to the usual doses of pain medication. Some people got suboptimal pain control because professionals believed higher doses might increase the risk of premature death (Table 5, E6).

End-of-life decisions such as palliative sedation also turned out to be different, i.e. the prescribed doses did not have the expected effects due to a long history of drug use. Physicians involved in the health care for residents in shelters sometimes noticed that pharmacists and psychiatrists could not give them appropriate advice either and this made them insecure and reticent about giving higher doses of pain medication than usually recommended. Anaesthesiologists in hospitals were sometimes approached as consultants able to give useful advice in the event of problems with pain control.

In addition to the control of pain, psychological symptoms were also seen as difficult to control. In the case of psychological symptoms such as anxiety and depression, this was often due to the difficulties the people experiencing homelessness had communicating their feelings. 'Self-medication' (the use of alcohol or drugs) made it more difficult to take a satisfactory decision about what should best be prescribed to control the symptoms. A lack of knowledge about what the proper treatment is in the case of long-term use of all kinds of medicines in the past further hindered symptom control.

The interviewees also mentioned dyspnoea as a frequently occurring symptom that was difficult to control. For example, many people experiencing homelessness suffer from COPD and frequently have shortness of breath with regular exacerbations in COPD symptoms. They are very anxious about choking but also experience suboptimal symptom treatment. Smoking when oxygen dependent was sometimes considered as an unacceptably high fire risk in the shelter. The policy then was the suboptimal treatment of low levels of oxygen in the blood.

Psychosocial and spiritual care Except for the shelters run by the Salvation Army, additional psychosocial and spiritual palliative care was not always available in the shelters. Professionals often did not know that psychosocial and spiritual care is also part of palliative care. Some professionals were afraid to talk about dying with the person experiencing homelessness. Others said that they sometimes tried to speak to the person about the fact that they were going to die, but that many people experiencing homelessness avoided having that conversation. The explanation they gave was that talking about the past and meaningful events in their lives could bring back memories that were too painful. Just 'being there' for the sick person was seen as the most important thing, trying to grab an opportunity to talk about it. They tried to indulge the person with attention, comfort, good food, sweets and kindness. Psychosocial and spiritual care was sometimes particularly difficult at the end of life when the person was too ill to leave the room and spend time in a common room. Professionals in shelters said that they usually did not have enough time to go to the person's room to talk with that person, other than bringing them meals and offering physical care. Therefore most of the time the person was all alone in their room (Table 5, E7).

Social network The social network of people experiencing homelessness often only consisted of other people experiencing homelessness with whom they used to drink or use drugs. If someone got sick, these contacts usually faded. Family ties were mostly broken due to painful events in the past. As William told about his relationship with his sister: *"I have neglected her entire life. I only called her when I was in jail. Then I ordered her to buy a game computer...that kind of things."* It usually cost a lot of time to find an address and restore family ties. Renewed relationships were often painful and fragile, and needed continuous supervision so that the relationship did not break again. In most cases there were no family or friends available who could help the person experiencing homelessness to discuss complaints with medical specialists and to increase the chance of receiving good palliative care (Table 5, E8). The lack of a social network also increased the chance of dying without the presence of the immediate family or other relatives.

Discussion

The main aim of this paper was to give insight into whether people experiencing homelessness in the Netherlands have access to good palliative care. We must conclude that there are some serious barriers that make good palliative care for this target group particularly challenging. These barriers can be clustered into three key themes: 'late access', 'capricious trajectory' and 'complex care'.

The first theme refers to the often limited use of palliative care because of the difficulties in recognizing the need for palliative care, the ambivalence people experiencing homelessness towards accepting palliative care, and the lack of facilities with specific expertise in palliative care for the homeless.

The difficulties in recognizing a need for palliative care in this target group as identified in our study might be related to the phenomenon of diagnostic overshadowing, which is often seen in the care for people with a mental illness [26]. The person's physical symptoms are misattributed to their mental illness, which leads to a worse physical condition.

Ambivalence towards accepting care also increases the chance of worse care. We found that this ambivalence was related to perceptions that people experiencing homelessness often have of being stigmatized. Other research shows that these perceptions are based on frequent actual prejudice and stigmatizing attitudes in services [27, 28]. The ambivalence seems to result from an interplay between the person experiencing homelessness and the social and health care services. This phenomenon in the system is also described as 'care paralysis', referring to the inability to help clients with multiple and complex problems by social services and care facilities [29]. Care avoidance and care paralysis can be considered as reinforcing and recalling each other. Late access to palliative care also relates to our finding that mainstream care facilities in the Netherlands often lack expertise in care for people experiencing homelessness while shelters often lack expertise and facilities regarding palliative care. An international review of studies showed that in other countries comparable challenges lie in providing good palliative care in for the target group both in hostels for people experiencing homelessness and in mainstream healthcare systems [30].

The second theme refers to the illness trajectory, which is often capricious because of the challenging behaviour of people and the unpredictable disease process. The illness trajectories of people experiencing homelessness were often found to be difficult to predict for a number of reasons, not least because care in a shelter, after having lived on the streets, might temporarily improve health. This phenomenon makes it more difficult to arrive at a proper estimation of the evolving healthcare needs of the person in question. Previous research [31] showing significant improvements in health status after a person enters the shelter system, confirms these observations. The capricious illness trajectories were also described in other research as a barrier for palliative care discussions [32].

In addition, we found that maintenance of autonomy and self-control was generally very important for the target group, which often resulted in an avoidance of care, non-cooperative behaviour and subsequently late access to palliative care. Professionals might face a dilemma in how to support the person experiencing homelessness in maintaining their autonomy: whether no further insistence to accept care or to continue to discuss the situation and the need for care with them. No further insistence respects their wish to avoid care, but ongoing discussion of the person's situation and needs provides an opportunity for advance care planning and puts the person in control of the future situation. Although the effectiveness of existing advance care planning interventions, such as completing advance directives, has not yet been fully proven for the population of people experiencing homelessness [33], planning may help the person maintain autonomy and self-control. Further research should be done on how this dilemma can best be handled. Care providers who establish contact and win trust employ 'non-judgemental appreciation'. They show empathy, accept what is and try to connect with the client and their world [28, 34].

The third major theme identified in our study refers to the complexity of pain and symptom control, psychosocial and spiritual care, and the lack of involvement of relatives. People experiencing homelessness frequently have complex care needs, and multiple problems and symptoms that are difficult to recognize and interpret. For instance, persons who are homeless often haven psychiatric disorders, such as schizophrenia. One of the characteristics of people with schizophrenia is that they often express lower intensity of pain when compared to other people [35]. Besides, pain people experiencing homelessness is often difficult to identify and control because of drug abuse. In addition, it is often difficult to control dyspnoea because many of these people want to carry on smoking, giving a risk of fire when oxygen is used. This may cause undertreatment.

The care is also complex because of difficulties to involve relatives. Whereas in the general population relatives are often directly involved in palliative care, in the homeless population the family is often absent, also at the end of life. Supporting individuals experiencing homelessness in restoring family bonds is an exceptionally challenging task for professionals. The absence of family is also illustrated by the fact that we were not able to involve immediate family or other relatives, either because they had their own problems or because they did not want to resurrect the past. The lack of a social network and the ambivalence felt by professionals about contacting the immediate family or other relatives are also found in other research among people experiencing homelessness [14, 15, 36].

In addition, we found that providing good psychosocial and spiritual care is often difficult. Professionals sometimes did not know that this kind of care is also part of palliative care, were afraid of talking about dying, or did not have enough time for it. People experiencing homelessness also often avoid such conservations. Our study however also showed that some wanted to talk to someone else about psychosocial and spiritual issues, such as reflecting about their life and the near future. This is in accordance with studies showing that people experiencing homelessness do worry about the end of life [11–13]. Respect for the person is a precondition for developing trust and improving the engagement with them, which is needed for tailored psychosocial and spiritual care [36].

Strengths and limitations

A strength of this study is the multi-perspective approach: the cases of 19 people experiencing homelessness in need of palliative care were described incorporating information of all the people most closely involved. A second strength is that we selected a variety of cases of people experiencing homelessness, receiving care from a variety of services. This variety contributed to the validity of the results.

A limitation is that no immediate family members or other relatives were interviewed. Family members refused, mainly because the memories were too painful and/or they wanted to close the book on this. Often, there were no contact details for family members. Underlying processes and how to deal with them are worthwhile studying.

Practice implications

Late access to palliative care, a capricious illness trajectory and the complexity of care have consequences for professionals involved in the care for people experiencing homelessness at the end of life.

Based on the results we recommend the following for timely, good palliative care for the homeless:

- Informing outreach professionals, such as street workers, about palliative care. They can play an important role they can play in signalling, documenting and reporting whenever they suspect that someone is seriously ill. People experiencing homelessness themselves or those who were formerly experiencing homelessness can easily make contact with other people experiencing homelessness. They may also have a role in signalling a need for palliative care.
- Training staff in shelters in palliative care and the ways palliative care can be organized is a first step towards improving palliative care for people experiencing homelessness living in shelters. Staff in mainstream palliative care facilities (nursing homes, hospices) can be trained and supported to deal with clients with challenging behaviour and the special needs they may have (e.g. regarding addiction, pain and symptom control, and involvement of family and friends).
- Building a network of palliative care specialists for people experiencing homelessness, who can advise professionals in mainstream facilities, e.g. regarding the complexities of pain and symptom management in this target group. This can stimulate growth of the body of knowledge about palliative care for people who are homeless.

There is some evidence that interventions aimed at advance care planning, documenting wishes, and better cooperation may be a potentially effective ways to encounter the concerns and needs of homeless people in the final phase of their life [14, 17, 33]. However, further research is needed on the effectiveness of these interventions.

Conclusion

According to the definition of the World Health Organization [2], palliative care is "an approach that improves the quality of life of homeless individuals and their families facing the problem associated with life-threatening illness, through the prevention and relief of suffering by means of early identification and impeccable assessment and treatment of pain and other problems, physical, psychosocial and spiritual." This study shows that people experiencing homelessness have less access to this care. The absence of a medical record, the lack of palliative care expertise and ambivalence of people who are homeless to ask for and accept care make timely identification of a need for palliative care difficult. Complex social relationships and no or fragile family bonds make involvement of the social network challenging. Assessment and treatment of pain and other problems is complicated by in particular the ambivalence towards accepting care, challenging behaviour, and (former) use of alcohol or drugs. We conclude that the palliative care currently provided to the people experiencing homelessness does not meet the core requirements of palliative care due to bottlenecks regarding timely identification, care for the social network, and the assessment and management of physical symptoms and psychosocial and spiritual care needs.

Abbreviations

ACT: assertive community treatment; ADL: Activities of Daily Living; CI: Confidence Interval; COPD: Chronic Obstructive Pulmonary Disease; FNO: Fonds Nuts Ohra; RCOAK: Roomsch Catholijk Oude Armen Kantoor; WHO: World Health Organization

Acknowledgements

We are grateful to the persons who were experiencing homelessness and all professionals for participating in the study.

Funding

The study was funded by FNO and RCOAK.

Authors' contributions

RV, AF and BvM wrote the research proposal and contributed to the design of the study. AdV and BS conducted the interviews. All authors were involved in the analysis and interpretation of data and the critical revision of the paper. All authors read and approved the final manuscript.

Competing interests

The authors declare that they have no competing interests with respect to the research, authorship, and/or publication of this article.

Author details

[1]Netherlands Institute for Health Services Research (Nivel), P.O. Box 1568, 3500, BN, Utrecht, The Netherlands. [2]Center for Consultation and Expertise, Gouda, The Netherlands. [3]Inholland University of Applied Sciences, Amsterdam, The Netherlands. [4]University Medical Center, VU, Department of Psychiatry, Amsterdam Public Health Research Institute, Amsterdam, The Netherlands. [5]Parnassia Psychiatric Institute, The Hague, The Netherlands. [6]GGZ-VS, Academy for Masters in Advanced Nursing Practice, Amsterdam, The Netherlands. [7]University Medical Center, VU, Department of Public and Occupational Health, Amsterdam Public Health Research Institute, Amsterdam, The Netherlands. [8]Expertise Center for Palliative care, Amsterdam, The Netherlands.

References

1. UN. CESCR General Comment No. 14: The Right to the Highest Attainable Standard of Health (Art. 12). Adopted at the Twenty-second Session of the Committee on Economic, social and cultural rights, on 11 August 2000 (Contained in Document E/C.12/2000/4).
2. World Health Organization. WHO definition of palliative care. 2002. http://www.who.int/cancer/palliative/definition/en/ (accessed date 8 August 2017).
3. National Health Care for the Homeless Council. Official definition of homelessness. https://www.nhchc.org/faq/official-definition-homelessness/. Accessed on March 21, 2018.
4. Van Straaten B. On the way up? Exploring homelessness and stable housing among homeless people in the Netherlands. IVO Addiction Research Institute Available from: http://hdl.handle.net/1765/93459. Accessed June 6, 2017.
5. CBS Statline. Daklozen; persoonskenmerken. 2017. Available from: http://statline.cbs.nl/Statweb/publication/?VW=T&DM=SLNL&PA=80799ned&D1=a&D2=a&D3=a&HD=150303-1405&HDR=T,G2&STB=G1. Accessed June 6, 2017.
6. NusselderWJ SMT, Krol L, Slockers CT, CWN L, van Beeck EF. Mortality and life expectancy in homeless men and women in Rotterdam: 2001–2010. PLoS One. 2013;8(10):e73979.
7. Fazel S, Geddes JR, Kushel M. The health of homeless people in high-income countries: descriptive epidemiology, health consequences, and clinical and policy recommendations. Lancet. 2014;384:1529–40.
8. Aldridge RW, Story A, Hwang SW, Nordentoft M, Luchenski SA, Hartwell G, Tweed EJ, Lewer D, Katikireddi SV, Hayward AC. Morbidity and mortality in homeless individuals, prisoners, sex workers, and individuals with substance use disorders in high-income countries: a systematic review and meta-analysis. Lancet. 2018;391:241–50.
9. Baggett TP, Hwang SW, O'Connell JJ, Porneala BC, Stringfellow EJ, Orav EJ, Singer DE, Rigotti NA. Mortality among homeless adults in Boston: shifts in causes of death over a 15-year period. JAMA Intern Med. 2013;173(3):189–95.
10. Stenius-Ayoade A, Haaramo P, Kautiainen H, Gissler M, Wahlbeck K, Eriksson JG. Mortality and causes of death among homeless in Finland: a 10-year follow-up study. J Epidemiol Community Health. 2017;0:868–75. https://doi.org/10.1136/jech-2017-209166.
11. Vuillermoz C, Aouba A, Grout L, Vandentorren S, Tassin F, Moreno-Betancur M, Jougla E, Rey G. Mortality among homeless people in France, 2008-10. Eur J Pub Health. 2016;26(6):1028–33.
12. Podymow T, Turnbull J, Coyle D. Shelter-based palliative care for the homeless terminally ill. Palliat Med. 2006;20(2):81–6.
13. Tobey MT, Manasson J, Decarlo K, Ciraldo-Marynuk K. Homeless individuals approaching the end of life. J Pain Symptom Manag. 2017;53(4):738–44.
14. Hubbell SA. Advance care planning with individuals experiencing homelessness: literature review and recommendations for public health practice. Public Health Nurs. 2017;34(5):72–478.
15. Song J, Bartels DM, Ratner ER, Alderton L, Hudson B, Ahluwalia JS. Dying on the streets: homeless persons' concerns and desires about end of life care. J Gen Intern Med. 2007;22(4):435–41.
16. Ko E, Kwak J, Nelson-Becker H. What constitutes a good and bad death?: perspectives of homeless older adults. Death Studies. 2015;39(7):422–32.
17. Klop HT, de Veer AJE, van Dongen SI, Francke AL, Rietjens JAC, Onwuteaka-Philipsen BD. Palliative care for homeless people: a systematic review of the concerns, care needs and preferences, and the barriers and facilitators for providing palliative care. BMC Palliative Care. 2018;17(67). https://doi.org/10.1186/s12904-018-0320-6.
18. Krakowsky Y, Gofine M, Brown P, Danziger J, Knowles H. Increasing access-a qualitative study of homelessness and palliative Care in a Major Urban Center. American Journal of Hospice and Palliative Medicine. 2013;30(3):268–70.
19. McNeil R, Guirguis-Younger M. Illicit drug use as a challenge to the delivery of end-of-life care services to homeless persons: perceptions of health and social services professionals. Palliat Med. 2012;26(4):350–9.
20. Mac Williams J, Bramwell M, Brown S, O'Connor M. Reaching out to ray: delivering palliative care services to a homeless person in Melbourne, Australia. Int J Palliat Nurs. 2014;20(2):83–8.
21. Webb WA. When dying at home is not an option: exploration of hostel staff views on palliative care for homeless people. Int J Palliat Nurs. 2015;21(5):236–44.
22. Shulman C, Hudson BF, Low J, Hewett N, Daley J, Kennedy P, et al. End-of-life care for homeless: a qualitative analysis exploring the challenges to access and provision of palliative care. Palliat Med. 2018;22(1):36–45.

23. Van Laere I, de Wit M, Klazinga N. Shelter-based convalescence for homeless adults in Amsterdam: a descriptive study. BMC Health Serv Res. 2009;9(208). https://doi.org/10.1186/1472-6963-9-208.
24. Koffman J, Morgan M, Edmonds P, Speck P, Higginson IJ. Vulnerability in palliative care research: findings from a qualitative study of black Caribbean and white British patients with advanced cancer. J Med Ethics. 2009;35:440–4.
25. Guest G, Bunce A, Johnson L. How many interviews are enough? An experiment with data saturation and variability. Field Methods. 2006;18(1):59–82.
26. Jones S, Howard L, Thornicroft G. 'Diagnostic overshadowing': worse physical health care for people with mental illness. Acta Psychiatr Scand. 2008;118(3):169–254.
27. Canavan R, Barry MM, Matanov A, Barros H, Gabor E, Greacen T, et al. Service provision and barriers to care for homeless people with mental health problems across 14 European capital cities. BMC Health Serv Res. 2012;12:122.
28. Klop HT, Evenblij K, Gootjes JRG, de AJE V, Onwuteaka-Philipsen BD. Care avoidance among homeless people and access to care: an interview study among spiritual caregivers, street pastors, homeless outreach workers and formerly homeless people. BMC Public Health. 2018;18(1):1095. https://doi.org/10.1186/s12889-018-5989-1.
29. Schout G, de Jong G, Zeelen J. Beyond care avoidance and care paralysis: theorizing public mental health care. Sociology. 2011;45(4):665–81.
30. Hudson BF, Flemming K, Shulman C, Candy B. Challenges to access and provision of palliative care for people who are homeless: a systematic review of qualitative research. BMC Palliative Care. 2016;15:96.
31. Schanzer B, Boanerges Dominguez MPH, Shrout PE, Caton CLM. Homelessness, health status, and health care use. Am J Public Health. 2005;97(3):464–9.
32. Hudson BF, Shulman C, Low J, Hewett N, Daley J, Davis S, Brophy N, Howard D, Vivat B, Kennedy P, Stone P. Challenges to discussing palliative care with people experiencing homelessness: a qualitative study. BMJ Open. 2018;7:e017502. https://doi.org/10.1136/bmjopen-2017-017502.
33. Sumalinog R, Harrington K, Dosani N, Hwang SW. Advance care planning, palliative care and end-of-life care interventions for homeless people: a systematic review. Palliat Med. 2017;31(2):109–19.
34. Schout G, de Jong G, Zeelen J. Establishing contact and gaining trust: an exploratory study of care avoidance. J Adv Nurs. 2010;66(2):324–33.
35. Engels G, Francke AL, van Meijel B, Douma JG, de Kam H, Wesselink W, Houtjes W, Scherder EJA. Clinical pain in schizofrenia: a systematic review. Journal of pain. 2014;15(5):457–67.
36. Moore G, Manias E, Gerdtz MF. Complex health service needs for people who are homeless. Aust Health Rev. 2011;35:480–5.

12

Experiences and challenges of home care nurses and general practitioners in home-based palliative care

Britt Viola Danielsen[1*], Anne Marit Sand[1], Jan Henrik Rosland[2,3] and Oddvar Førland[4,5]

Abstract

Background: Norway has one of the lowest home death rates in Europe. However, it is the health authorities´ ambition to increase this by facilitating palliative care at home. The aim of this study was to achieve more insight, through home care nurses and general practitioners, of conditions that facilitate or hamper more time at home and more home deaths for patients with terminal disease and short life expectancy.

Methods: We used a qualitative research design with four focus groups with a total of 19 participants, of either home care nurses or general practitioners, using semi-structured question guides. The data were processed by systematic text condensation and encompassed thematic analysis of meaning and content of data across cases, which included four steps of analysis.

Results: Three main themes were identified: 1) The importance of a good start for the patient and family with five sub-themes, 2) 'Passing the baton' – the importance of collaboration across the health system with four sub-themes, and 3) Avoiding new hospitalization by establishing collaboration and competence within primary health care with four sub-themes.

Conclusions: This study demonstrates that optimum palliative care at home depends on close collaboration and dialogue between the patient, family, home care nurses and general practitioner. It suggests the need for safer discharge routines and planning when hospitals transfer patients with terminal disease to their homes. A good start for the patient and family, where the initial interdisciplinary collaboration meeting takes place in the patient's home, is crucial for a good result. The general practitioners' perception of their 'disconnection' during hospitalization and prior to discharge has the potential to reduce patient safety. The family seems to be fundamental in gaining more time at home for the patient and supporting the patient to eventually die at home. Home-based palliative care demands experience and competence as well as regular supportive mentoring.

Keywords: Palliative home care, Home care nurse, General practitioner, Home deaths, Qualitative study

Background

Norway has one of the lowest home death rates in Europe. Only 13% of deaths in Norway took place at home in 2016, while 50% died in a nursing home and 30% in a hospital [1]. In Norway, there is, so far, no trend towards an increasing proportion of home deaths, even though the health care authorities have tried to facilitate palliative care services in the home [2, 3]. In some countries, this trend has been reversed in recent decades, particularly in the United States, Canada and the United Kingdom [4–7], with greater proportions of people dying at home.

Dying at home surrounded by family members is considered by some to be the 'gold standard' for a good death [8–10]. Several systematic literature reviews found that most of those with terminal disease and short life expectancy wanted to stay in their homes as long as possible, and eventually die at home [11–13]. One systematic review from 2015 emphasized that many studies highlighted patients´ preferences to be cared for at home

* Correspondence: Britt.Viola.Danielsen@hvl.no
[1]Department of Health and Caring Sciences, Faculty of Health and Social Sciences, Western Norway University of Applied Sciences, P.O. Box 7030, N-5020 Bergen, Norway
Full list of author information is available at the end of the article

as long as possible or to be able to die at home. However, for some patients, dying at home may be difficult to achieve due to an absence of family caregivers [14]. Another systematic review from 2015 concluded that caution should be taken when assuming that most patients prefer to die at home, because studies often excluded the views of those who did not express a preference or who were not asked [15]. Despite this, it is important that health care services support those preferring to stay at home in the last part of their lives [16]. According to Norwegian health authorities, increased time at home can often be a more realistic objective for home-based palliative care than home death, as it says something about the extent to which the patient's desire to live the last time at home is fulfilled [17].

In Norway, research undertaken in a large municipality concluded that a multidisciplinary approach, which involved family physicians and community nurses with support from a multidisciplinary specialist palliative care consultant team, increased the proportion of home deaths and led to fewer people being admitted to nursing homes [18]. In a systematic review, Murray et al. [11] concluded that factors related to the disease, the degree of social support from relatives, the quality and availability of healthcare services and programs, and the patient's preference were the most important factors for determining the place of end-of-life care. This is in line with Gomes and Higginson [19], who found the place of death to be an interplay of factors such as type of disease and disability, sociodemographic characteristics, patients' preferences, health care services, social support from the family, and macrosocial factors such as historical trends. A systematic review and meta-analysis of determinants of home and nursing home deaths from 2016 concluded that early referral to palliative care and the presence of a multidisciplinary home-based palliative care team increase the likelihood of a patient dying in their preferred location [8]. These studies identify the interplay between the patient, family, health care services, general practitioners (GPs) and home care nurses to be critical factors.

To further explore these aspects, interviewing health care personnel could be a method to achieve more precise insight and understanding. We found only a few qualitative studies of experiences with home-based palliative care that included both GPs and home care nurses. In an evaluation study from England, specialist palliative care nurses, district nurses and GPs stressed three elements of importance for keeping patients at home at the end of their life: firstly, an accompanied transfer home element, which could be arranged quickly; secondly, trained hospice aides at home to care and support patients and their families; and thirdly, a crisis intervention team that included a specialist palliative care physician [20]. Focus groups with district nurses and community specialist palliative care nurses in England identified poor co-ordination and discharge planning, difficulty in arranging necessary equipment and services and inadequate out-of-hours medical provision as barriers to dying at home for patients with cancer with a short life expectancy [21].

The aim of the current study was to achieve more insight, through home care nurses and GPs, of conditions that facilitate or hamper more time at home and more home deaths for patients with terminal disease and short life expectancy.

Methods

Study context

Norway has a national tax-funded, universal, public, long-term care service aimed at securing each patient's basic medical and social needs, free of charge or with a small user fee. The service is primarily carried out at a local level in the municipalities through GP cooperatives, home care services, nursing homes and sheltered houses. The home care service is part of the municipality health care service, and includes home care nursing and practical assistance based on each patient's needs [22].

Each Norwegian citizen has a right to have his or her own family doctor, a GP. To be a patient on a GP list is free of charge, and if you need to see the doctor, you have to pay a limited fee, the balance being paid by the state. The GP collaborates with the home care nursing services in the municipality. Home care nursing is a municipal, public service, whereas GPs are self-employed and organised in GP cooperatives. The GP identifies medical needs, gives prescriptions and carries out home visits if considered necessary [23].

Inpatient care is mainly provided by the hospital trusts owned by Regional Health Authorities and founded by the state. The largest hospitals have multidisciplinary palliative care teams providing care and sometimes ambulatory services to patients with the most complex needs in hospital departments and municipalities nearby [23]. Since the late 1980s, there has been a policy of replacing relatively expensive inpatient care with less-costly outpatient care and bringing care closer to patients' homes. This policy has been strengthened by the Coordination Reform implemented in 2012 [24].

According to this policy, the provision of care in Norway has been shifting from institutional care towards more home-based care. The home care nurses play a fundamental role, including palliative care in the home. Home-based care can be provided as a 24-h service, giving health and care services at patients' homes several times during both the day and night. Palliative care for patients staying at home is provided via collaboration between next of kin, home care nurses and GPs, and is sometimes assisted by a hospital-based specialist palliative care team [23, 25]. The GPs often have a history of providing health care for the palliative care patient and the family over many years and are often involved in the early stages of diagnosis, thereby providing some continuity of oversight. In our sample, they generally had one to two palliative care patients in home care each year for whom they had medical responsibility. Medical doctors are the only health professionals in Norway who can prescribe medicines, as nurse practitioners have not yet been introduced.

Study design, participants and sampling populations

Our study had a qualitative approach with a phenomenological dimension. The use of focus groups is a qualitative research method, which is suitable for gaining rich descriptions of the participants' experiences and in-depth knowledge about complex phenomena [26]. We conducted focus groups separately for home care nurses, nursing assistants and GPs, using a semi-structured guide for the research questions. The question guides were thoroughly discussed and refined in the research group in advance. Its main objective was to stimulate the sharing of experiences concerning factors that facilitate or hamper more home time and home deaths for patients with terminal disease and short life expectancy.

Four focus groups were conducted in an urban area of Norway: one with home care nurses, one with home care nurses and home care nursing assistants together, and two with GPs. Each focus group lasted from 80 to 100 min. The two focus groups with home care personnel took place in June and October 2015, whereas the two with GPs took place in May and June 2016. Local nursing managers recruited the nurse participants. The intention was to recruit GPs via the Local Medical Officer; however, this did not eventuate. We had to recruit them via the telephone: 17 GPs were contacted and eight agreed to participate. In total, 19 health professionals participated in the focus groups. Each focus group consisted of 4 to 6 participants. The GPs were recruited from different districts, whereas the nurses and nursing assistants were from one home care district.

The nurses were all experienced. On average, they had 24 years in clinical practice and 17 years in home care nursing. The age varied from 41 to 63 years, with an average of 52 years. Only three of them worked full-time, the rest worked part-time in positions, which varied from 54 to 80% of a full-time load. All Registered Nurses had further education and relevant competencies in home care nursing, palliative care, elderly care and health promotion (See Table 1). The home care nurses had recently attended a course in palliative care in their district. The collaboration with the patient's GP was the responsibility of the home care nurses. The nurse assistants contributed to the primary care of the patients and assisted in contacting the next of kin.

The GPs were all experienced doctors with an average of 24 years in professional practice. Their ages varied from 35 to 65 years, with an average of 56 years. All, except the youngest GP, were specialists in General Practice medicine (See Table 2).

Data collection

The four focus groups were conducted by two of the researchers. In the first focus group with the GPs, written notes were taken. These were subsequently used as the basis for the next focus group with the GPs. The other three focus groups were audiotaped and transcribed.

Data analysis

The data were processed by systematic text condensation before analysis according to Malterud [27], which is

Table 1 Participant characteristics – Home care nurses and nursing assistants

Profession	Age	Full-time / part-time?	Years of working experience as nurse / nurse assistant	Further education
RN Nurse 1	40–50	Part-time	20–25	Elderly and Aging
RN Nurse 2	40–50	Part-time	25–30	Home Care Nursing
RN Nurse 3	50–60	Part-time	35–40	Science in Nursing
RN Nurse 4	50–60	Full-time	10–15	Palliative Care Nursing
RN Nurse 5	50–60	Part-time	10–15	Palliative Care Nursing
RN Nurse 6	50–60	Part-time	25–30	Health promotion and Health prevention
RN Nurse 7	40–50	Full-time	15–20	Cancer Nursing
Nurse assistant 1	50–60	Full-time	10–15	None
Nurse assistant 2	50–60	Full-time	15–20	Dementia Care
Nurse assistant 3	60–70	Part-time	20–25	None
Nurse assistant 4	50–60	Part-time	25–30	Dementia Care

Table 2 Participant characteristics – General Practitioners

Profession	Age	Full-time / part-time	Years of working experience as GP	Specialist competencies
GP 1	30–40	Full-time	1–5	·Under specialisation
GP 2	40–50	Full-time	10–15	GP
GP 3	60–70	Full-time	25–30	GP
GP 4	60–70	Full-time	30–35	GP, Social Medicine
GP 5	60–70	Full-time	30–35	GP
GP 6	50–60	Full-time	25–30	GP
GP 7	60–70	Part-time	25–30	GP
GP 8	60–70	Part-time	30–35	GP

a modification of Giorgi's phenomenological analysis. Systematic text condensation encompasses thematic analysis of meaning and content of data across cases. It includes four steps of analysis: 1) *Total impression – from chaos to themes* - establishing a general impression of all the data from the focus groups with an open mind, looking for preliminary themes related to the participants´ experiences with palliative care in the home; 2) *Identifying and sorting meaning units – from themes to codes* – identifying and arranging meaning units by reviewing the text line by line, followed by coding of the meaning units related to the themes which emerged in the first step (A meaning unit is a text fragment including some information about the research question and may be coded under numerous code labels); 3) *Condensation – from code to meaning* – requiring systematic abstraction of meaning units within each of the code groups identified in the second step of the analysis. The empirical data are reduced to a decontextualized selection of meaning units sorted as thematic code groups. The coded units of meaning are condensed and organized into groups according to their code, sorting them into subgroups; and 4) *Synthesizing – from condensation to description and concepts* – reconceptualising the data by putting the pieces together. By synthesizing the contents of the condensed data, the description and concepts develop as an analytical text supported by citations, which can illustrate the research theme or finding.

Approvals and ethical considerations

Ethics approval was received according to Norwegian research law and regulations. Each participant received written information about the research project in advance and provided informed consent before the focus groups were conducted. The research project was approved by the Data Protection Authority within the Norwegian Centre for Research Data (NSD) (Reg. no. 45256). The participants were informed both in writing and orally about confidentiality and anonymity of the data, and that at any stage they could withdraw from the study without any consequences.

Results

In the current study, we identified the experiences of home care nurses and GPs of the conditions that facilitate or hamper more time at home and more home deaths for patients with terminal disease and short life expectancy. The results from the data analysis are divided into three different themes with 13 sub-themes altogether:

1. *The importance of a good start for the patient and family*
    a. Establishing trust and safety for the patient and family
    b. The important first days at home after discharge from hospital
    c. Establishing collaboration between the home care nurses and the GP
    d. Establishing safety for the patient and family by ensuring availability of the GP
    e. The GP's initial consultation in the patient's home
2. *"Passing the baton" – the importance of collaboration across the health system*
    a. Lack of collaboration with the hospital in the transfer of patients
    b. Good support from the hospital Palliative Care Centre
    c. The GP's disconnection during hospitalization with consequences for the patient and family
    d. A vulnerable gap in preparing the transfer of patients from the hospital
3. *Avoiding new hospitalization by establishing collaboration and competence within primary health care.*

a. Dialogue and interdependence between the GP and home care services
b. Competence, experience and counselling
c. Preparing for the end of the terminal stage for the patient and family – to be ahead
d. Tolerance, acceptance and flexibility within home care personnel

The themes and their sub-themes are defined below, with supporting data drawn verbatim (translated into English) from the focus groups and presented in italics.

The importance of a good start for the patient and family

The home care nurses experienced that most of their patients in palliative care were transferred from hospital. However, some patients were already in home-based care with whom they had already established a close relationship, as well as with the family.

Establishing trust and safety for the patient and family

The nurses emphasized the importance of achieving a close and trusting collaboration with the patient and next of kin. They described how they prioritised these patients when establishing palliative care in the patient's home. A primary group for the patient and family was established among the nurses in order to create more continuity and increase patient safety. The nurses underlined the importance of good collaboration from the very first day with the next of kin who had a key role in the success of home palliation. Empathy for, and time to listen to, the patient and family were considered essential. For reassurance, they gave the patient and next of kin the telephone number of the group and assured them of their availability 24/7.

> *"It all depends on the next of kin for this to work. We cannot do the job unless the family is safe. Without the family, it is very difficult to succeed with palliative care at home."* (Nurse)

The important first days at home after discharge from hospital

The home care nurses stressed the importance of the initial palliative care planning in the patient's home following discharge from hospital in gaining the confidence of, and establishing the necessary safety for, the patient and the family. They emphasized good collaboration with the hospital as a critical factor to prepare for and obtain a good start. Consequently, they found it important to collect adequate information on the patient in advance in order to be prepared with the requisite medicines and medical equipment for the patient, such as a hospital bed, pain relief pump, professional displacement equipment, etc. This was considered important to maintain pain control, comfort, and quality care for the patient at home.

> *"It is so important to have a good start. There are no practical things that paralyze more than lack of medications, displacement equipment, etc. (...) For if the start is chaos, then this chaos can easily continue. "* (Nurse)

In general, the home care services selected an experienced nurse for the first meeting with the patient and next of kin in the patient's home in order to gain confidence and ensure safety. To make sure that everything was properly set up, the first meeting often lasted one hour to fulfil the two key requirements: safety and trust. However, as they had many patients in the district to care for, there were not always adequate resources.

> *"We need to get some extra time from the management on the first days. It's a wish, but we do not always get it."* (Nurse)

The family was often a great help in collecting medicines from the pharmacy or carrying out other practical errands. In recent years, all prescriptions in Norway have become electronic which has improved the daily administration of medications. Despite this, it sometimes takes several days to get the medicines from the pharmacist because they are not available locally.

Establishing collaboration between home care nurses and the GP

It was essential for the nurses to establish collaboration with the patient's GP as soon as possible. They preferred to arrange a meeting at home with the patient, family, GP and nurse together. The GPs involved in the focus groups gave their cell phone number to the home care nurse when the life expectancy of the patient was short. The nurses often experienced good collaboration with the GPs, especially GPs from the local district whom they knew, and with whom they had regular contact. In their view, the GP's involvement was fundamental for success.

> *(...) "When the GP is not doing his or her job, it is simply not acceptable. We cannot take on their responsibility."* (Nurse)

Establishing safety for the patient and family by ensuring availability of the GP

The GPs involved in the focus groups found it natural to give their cell phone number to the patient and family when there was short life expectancy for patients. The

GPs said that they did not experience any misuse. According to the nurses, access to the GP's cell phone made the patient and family feel safer and more confident. They believed that this strengthened the family's ability to cope with the challenges of having to care for a very sick family member and avoid hospitalization. For these patients, the GPs set few limits with regard to working hours and medical support.

> *"Once I had to take an emergency visit on Christmas Eve, where it was necessary to spend time at home in a family with a terminally ill patient who had a lot of pain and unrest. With conversation and drug titration, we managed to get the pain under control. (...) I could not let this occur during perhaps their last night at home together."* (GP)

However, the GPs often sought agreement from the family that they would not call at night between 11 p.m. and 7 a.m. Home visits were made when needed, often in the afternoon after their office work had finished.

The GPs initial consultation in the patient's home

Sometimes the GPs planned home visits together with the home care nurses in the initial phase. They found this useful with regard to responsibilities and further planning.

> *"As a GP, you totally depend on good collaboration with home care nurses. (...) It works best when home care nurses are confident in their role and take clear responsibility."* (GP)

The GPs who participated in the focus groups all favoured home visits. They mentioned that the difficult life and death topic was easier to address there. When life expectancy was short and little time was left, they also experienced that it was far more efficient to visit patients at home.

> *"We become much closer to the patient at home where we can go into the kitchen and perhaps drink a cup of coffee together."* (GP)

"Passing the baton" – the importance of collaboration across the health system

The health care system in Norway is divided into specialized and primary health care which means that the medical responsibility of the hospital doctors and the GPs is separated. When the patient is hospitalized, the GP generally is not involved in medical treatment.

Lack of collaboration with the hospital in the transfer of patients

The home care nurses described how the hospital often promised more on behalf of the home care services than was realistic to achieve, which could often lead to unrealistic expectations from the patient and family. The nurses experienced that short hospital stays were the main focus of the hospital. In Norway, the principal policy is to have as few hospital beds as possible, based on calculations and historical data for optimum use. Early discharge is therefore stressed, putting pressure on doctors to make it possible to receive new patients. There is also a regulation which states that as soon as a hospital doctor declares that medical treatment is completed, the municipality has to take over the care of the patient. Otherwise, the municipality has to pay daily fines. According to the nurses, this often resulted in palliative care patients being discharged too early and being unprepared or with false expectations about what was possible for the home care nursing services to facilitate.

> *"The hospital said that we (the home care nursing team) could be there all the time if needed. They give patients and next of kin unrealistic expectations. (...) We cannot be there 24 hours a day."* (Nurse)

The GPs were concerned with the hospital's responsibility and urged them to "pass the baton" to make discharge of the patient safer. They referred to the formal collaboration agreements between hospital and community care.

> *"Friday is a very bad day for discharging palliative care patients (...) It is their responsibility, and it is the hospital's responsibility to make sure; it's about passing the baton to the next doctor in a proper way."* (GP)

The GPs experienced lack of contact when the palliative care patient was ready for discharge. They described the management in the municipality home care services being contacted by the hospital, but there was no protocol for contacting and establishing collaboration with the GP. Instead, what they did receive was an electronic medical report shortly after a hospital discharge, sometimes the next day.

Good support from the Hospital Palliative Care Centre

According to the GPs, the Palliative Care Centre was the only department in the hospital that worked together with the GPs as a team. The Palliative Care Centre contacted the GP as part of the routine procedure prior to the patient's transfer, in order to establish the necessary collaboration. In general, the

GP's home visits needed to be planned up front, due to their already full schedule with other patients.

The home care nurses had good experiences and collaboration with the Palliative Care Centre, especially with their multidisciplinary ambulatory team. The nurses' experience was that this team could compensate in cases where the GP was not sufficiently involved and sometimes they worked as professional support for both the GP and the home care nurse team.

> *"The patient came home Friday and died the following Tuesday. He got urinary retention due to cancer prostate. I tried to insert a urinary catheter, but I did not succeed. The patient was in terrible pain. The GP came, but he failed too. He called the Palliative Ambulatory Team (...) and a doctor and a nurse came to the patient's home. With a special urinary catheter, they succeeded. The patient calmed down and died just an hour or two afterwards in his own bed at home surrounded by his family".* (Nurse)

The GPs' disconnection during hospitalization with consequences for the patient and family

The GPs said that when one of their patients was hospitalized, they were rarely contacted by the hospital physicians about the patient's medical situation or invited to discuss the medical treatment. They described their situation as being 'disconnected' from the medical treatment, and they urged establishing two-way communication with the hospital physicians, which they thought would benefit the patient and next of kin and increase patient safety.

The GPs often experienced having an important translator and liaison role between the patient and the hospital during medical treatment. The patients met many physicians and health professionals during their hospital stay, and the patients often found it confusing to understand the treatment initiated, etc. In the GPs' view, it could be difficult for the patient to provide informed consent. The nurses reported similar experiences; they needed to explain the treatment, etc. in understandable terms. The GPs underlined that they generally knew their patients very well, and believed they played a central role in patient care.

> *"Patients are in a phase where they are desperate; they meet so many new doctors. It allows me as a GP to become much more important for the patient in the hospital phase."* (GP)

The GPs urged the hospital to build closer collaboration with the GPs in their routines for the benefit of palliative care patients. In their opinion, both medical and ethical dilemmas could have been solved for the better. Their experience was that the hospital did not even consider the GP's knowledge of the patients. The GPs expressed that "overtreatment" and "cowboy medicine" could be reduced by involving them through the medical treatment process.

> *"(...) I have known the patient for more than 30 years. Now she is 87 years old, suffering and multimorbid. (...) They start new treatment without even considering consulting me."* (GP)

A vulnerable gap in preparing transfer of patients from hospital

The home care nurses described the procedures and experiences when a palliative care patient was discharged. The hospital contacted the local management in the Home Services of the appropriate district within the municipality. The management then communicated with the local district's home care nurses who organized the service for the patient. They worked in different offices some miles away. The home care nurses rarely had direct contact with the hospital ward that was responsible for the discharge of the patient, despite this previously having been the practice. Instead, they received electronic information through the management. The nurses worried about patient safety, as they had often experienced that vital information was overlooked or lost during those steps.

Avoiding new hospitalization by establishing collaboration and competence within primary health care

Collaboration, competence-building and flexibility *within* primary health care was emphasized by both the home-based nurses and the GPs.

Dialogue and interdependence between the GP and home care services

Sometimes the nurses struggled to get the GP involved in palliative care. It was a matter of the GP's priorities as well as confidence in the nurses´ clinical judgement of the patient. The patient's condition could deteriorate quite suddenly, and therefore it was of great importance that the nurses and GP established regular contact and confidence in each other and consequently were able to collaborate closely. If this did not occur, the risk of hospitalization increased.

> *"If you don't have a GP who is there for the palliative care patient, it's hard to get the job done properly. Sadly, it often ends with death in the hospital. We are simply not able to manage it at home, because it's not safe when the GP does not participate."* (Nurse)

The communication between home-based nurses and GPs had improved by introducing a system of electronic messages. The nurses could write messages, which the GP could respond to during the day. Both home care nurses and GPs underlined that electronic communication with dialogue messages was a great improvement and increased the availability of both parties for the benefit of the patients.

Competence, experience and counselling

The GP often discovered that many home care nurses had expertise in palliative care with far more experience than they had with these patients. The GPs thought they should be more aware of this aspect in the collaboration.

> *"My experience is that home care nurses are doing well in palliative care and are very familiar with handling pain relief pumps, far better than myself."* (GP)

The GPs appreciated the dedication and engagement of the nurses to do their best for the patients and their next of kin. However, they did expect home care nurses to come forward and express clearly their expectations in the collaboration. The GPs experienced that when the home care nurse was uncertain, it required more of them. They wanted the nurses to have the confidence to come forward and express what they needed from the GP.

On the other hand, the GPs acknowledged that home care nurses had challenging work, and that it was important to have somebody to discuss complex and ethical matters. The GPs said they had little training in palliative care medicine. They highlighted the courses in palliative care medicine organised in collaboration with the Palliative Care Centre and the hospital. If possible, they preferred to have courses together with home-based nurses in their local districts.

The home care service had nurses with special competencies in palliative care in their team. The nurses emphasized the importance of clinical expertise and advanced experience in interpersonal and technical situations to create the necessary safety for palliative care patients and their families. They stressed that this was not an area for novices. The nurses who participated in the focus groups had many years of experience but expressed the need for increasing their competencies by gaining new knowledge. Relevant courses and meetings with professional thematic content and discussions were highly appreciated.

The nurses expressed a need for regular counselling. Intense working periods with palliative care patients could be quite exhausting and stressful both physically and mentally. Sharing experiences happened randomly when the nurses had time or felt it was necessary. However, they called for leaders to take greater responsibility for coordinating systematic mentoring and counselling for the nurses.

Preparing for the end of the terminal stage for the patient and family – to be ahead

Both nurses and doctors were aware of the vulnerability of the patient and family when the patient's situation deteriorated. The nurses tried to be prepared for what was coming and to create a good environment for the patient in close collaboration with the family. At the final terminal stage, home care registered nurses, and not the nurse assistants, took care of the patient and family as they experienced that their competences were needed at all times. They wanted to create predictability for the patient and family and to practise flexibility according to the patient's and family's needs and wishes. Both GPs and nurses were readily available on the telephone.

> *"The daughter of a dying mother could never forget how thankful she was when the nurses acted flexibly and said: "We will come back later, when you and your mother have finished your breakfast." (...) Then you realize that such small things become so important to them."* (Nurse)

The nurses were concerned about the families who had promised their loved ones that they could die at home, as the situation could change very quickly, and the patient's situation could become unbearable. In those situations, they experienced that the hospital could be a better alternative for the patient and family and they needed to support them in that decision.

The nurses made great efforts to have the necessary medication available in time for relieving the most common symptoms in the terminal stage. It was important for the nurses that the GP prescribed the medication in a timely manner, as the patient's situation could change very quickly. Without the requisite medicines, it often ended with hospitalization for the patient. A medical box, similar to that used in an English model, with the four most important medicines for symptom relief in the terminal stage (the 'just-in-case box'), was introduced at the Palliative Care Centre and the Centre for Competence in Palliation consisting of Morphine, Midazolam, Haloperidol and Glycopyrron [2, 28]. The medical box was prescribed from the GP or Hospital Palliative Care Centre, which made it possible for home care nurses to control patient's symptoms in the last terminal stage and avoid hospitalization.

Tolerance, acceptance and flexibility within home care personnel

The home care nurses had been a team for many years with little turnover and they highlighted the importance of good collaboration within their own group. They helped each other out, shared experiences and supported each other, which was essential to keep up the enthusiasm and pleasure in the work. Competence, clinical experience, palliative care experience, maturity, situation recognition and acceptance of each other's different skills were highlighted.

They seemed to handle new technical equipment and procedures with great competence to ensure patient safety. They expressed having a good and supportive atmosphere and an ability to speak openly with each other.

> *"We certainly have the will to help each other. (...) There is mutual understanding that those who work with palliative care patients and dying patients, they need time.* So, *we help each other."* (Nurse)

The home care nurses practised flexibility in the shift roster when it came to situations where they needed more time in the palliative care patient's home. They could not always get hold of an extra nurse. They relieved each other of different additional tasks and assignments during the day to make it possible for the nurses involved to handle the situation without having to think about every task that awaited them. They had a kind of "silent agreement". The flexibility made it easier for them to cope with challenging situations, which could occur quite suddenly.

> *"I went overtime and started with morphine, satisfied since we had "saved the situation" (...) Then you cannot leave your job. You simply must stay at work an extra couple of hours."* (Nurse)

Discussion

Several studies have shown connections between individual, collaborative and organizational aspects of the palliative care services and the rates of home deaths [11, 19]. Early referral from hospital to home-based care and multidisciplinary palliative home care teams are essential findings [8]. In our study, we wanted to achieve more insight, through home care nurses and GPs, of conditions that that facilitate or hamper more time at home and more home deaths for patients with terminal disease and short life expectancy.

The importance of a good start

The nurses underlined that it was essential to establish close collaboration with the patient and family early as well as emotional support for the family who took on such a great responsibility. The primary group contributed to more continuity and safety stressing the importance of not leaving the professional responsibility of palliative care to the family. This is in line with other studies which have identified the significance of close and personal collaboration and contact with the family in palliative home-based care [29, 30].

The nurses emphasized that the collaboration meeting between the patient, next of kin, GP and home care nurse ought to take place as soon at the patient arrives home. This is essential to secure a good start. This meeting needs a fixed agenda. It must be clarified if the patient really wants to stay at home as long as possible and even die there. The capacity and support from the next of kin is vital. Moreover, the initial preparation dialogue should focus on what kind of complexity they can endure at home [31].

Furthermore, it must be clarified as to what kind of medical complications might make the patient's family think it would be better for the patient to be in hospital. They need to be reassured that their decision can be changed. The dialogue needs to focus on both their current worries, as well as the challenges ahead.

It is important that the nurse has the necessary experience and skill to participate in these meetings [32]. To succeed with a good start, a very competent home care nurse must be present at the first meeting. The main purpose is to create an atmosphere of trust and to reduce anxiety. The home care nurses must give priority to the family and be sure there is enough time to do so. Trust from both the patient and the next of kin is the goal. The nurses in our study stressed that if home-based palliative care started in chaos, the chaos was likely to continue, and they expressed that they would never leave the family unless the family knew who and where to call 24/7.

Our study underlines the importance of creating safety at home for the patient and family by ensuring good planning in advance, together with the hospital, when the patient is still hospitalized. That includes medications and medical equipment necessary for pain control, and other relief for the patient at home. Such practical aspects of discharge planning and coordination were also emphasized by O'Brien & Jack [21] as pivotal. Other studies have found that advance care planning with respect to the place of death reduced the time in hospital in the patient's last year [33] and that patients who had issued directives in advance received care that was strongly associated with their preferences [34]. The participants in our study stressed the importance of establishing a collaboration between the patient's GP and home care nurses. GP home visits create openings for closer collaboration with the patient and family as well as the opportunity to talk about the life and death topic [31]. Another study indicated that GP home visits in palliative care had an important impact on the patient staying and dying at home [35].

Passing the baton between the hospital and home-based palliative care

In Norway, the health care services are regulated by different laws and authorities that can present challenges to collaboration. The specialist palliative care services in the hospitals are administered by one of the four Regional Health Authorities. Home care nurses and self-employed GPs in the primary health care sector are administered by the 428 local municipalities.

Our findings revealed challenges with the continuity of palliative care between the hospitals and the primary health care sector. The GPs were rarely contacted prior to the patient's discharge from hospital, despite having in-depth knowledge of the patient. They did not feel that their knowledge was acknowledged by the hospital doctors concerning further treatment plans for the patient. The GPs were left with a sense of being disconnected from the medical treatment. They were concerned about patient safety and urged the hospital physicians to establish two-way communication. Instead, the GPs received a final medical report. Although the municipal home care services were contacted by the hospital prior to the patient's discharge, either by phone or via a written report, the nurses expressed that the planning and preparation by the hospital was often inadequate.

One problem is that information between the hospital and those responsible for palliative care in the primary health care sector generally goes to the municipality's health care service management rather than directly to the GP or primary home care nurse. Even when given the expectation, participants could not always trust that prescriptions, medicines etc. were in order. The most difficult transfer day in the week was Friday, due to the difficulties of adequate supply of medicines during the weekend, as vital information was often missing upfront. Normally, the patient's GP was not available in the weekends. Our findings emphasize the need for safer discharge routines when hospitals transfer palliative care patients to their homes. Electronic two-way communication between hospital doctors and GPs would increase patient safety.

Sometimes there seemed to be a huge difference between what patients and families had been promised at the hospital and the reality of what home care nurses were able to provide. This caused insecurity and a drop in confidence in the patient and next of kin. According to the home care nurses and the GPs, the hospital should pass the baton in a proper and safe way that is better than that seen in current practice.

The palliative care patients are in vulnerable situations that require special arrangements and a dependence on continuous exchange of knowledge, information and decisions. Several earlier studies have emphasized the importance of early referral and knowledge exchange between the hospital and those delivering palliative care in the primary health care context [36–38]. Earlier involvement and knowledge exchange allows relationships to be built and trust to be developed in the care and treatment planning processes between the collaborators. Such contact promotes safety for the patients and prevents crises from occurring. Some studies have found that the next of kin has a key role [11, 19, 32]. Our findings indicate that without a family member to take responsibility, it is almost impossible to achieve good palliative care at home.

Avoiding hospitalization by establishing safety and competence

In order to avoid hospitalization in the terminal stage of life, our research shows that dialogue and interdependence between nurses and GPs is crucial and prevents unnecessary hospitalization. The nurses appreciated good collaboration with GPs. If the GP does not take an active part, the patient and family is left in a more vulnerable situation. Although the Palliative Care Centre at the hospital is available in some areas, it is necessary to team up with a GP in order to succeed in the delivery of good palliative care.

The health professionals' competence and experience in palliative care are essential. Our study revealed the need for courses in palliative care that include a focus on collaboration across all palliative care providers. This is in line with Smith and Porock [36] who found that training and educational interventions were of crucial importance to improve knowledge and practical competence in palliative care in the community. Both GPs and nurses in this study reported the need to work together, "shoulder to shoulder", and they appeared dedicated to their palliative care work. According to Levine et al. [39] and O'Mahony et al. [40], palliative care work required the health professionals involved to take care of each other.

However, the nurses reported that the GPs did not always trust their clinical judgement. The patient's condition could alter quickly and consequently they needed to be prepared; for instance, in the choice of medication or subcutaneous administration instead of tablets if swallowing problems should occur. Difficulties in establishing collaboration with the GP may be due to GPs' uncertainty caused by their lack of experience with palliative care patients. However, further research into this aspect is needed.

Some GPs emphasized that nurses should be more outspoken in communicating their understanding of the patients´ needs. Instead of expressing despair, they urged nurses to be more assertive and express clearly what they expected from the GP. This feature may be an aspect of health professional hierarchy where nurses have often felt oppressed by doctors [41].

The nurses and GPs in our study stressed the importance of close collaboration with, and emotional support for, the patient and family and the need for flexibility and availability especially in the last part of the terminal stage, which is in accordance with other research in the field [29, 30, 42]. Even if they were dedicated to palliative care, they experienced that the family was fundamental in achieving more time at home for the patient and eventually the chance for the patient to die at home. The use of the medical box for symptom relief was essential and avoided some unnecessary hospitalizations. Instead, they managed to control the symptoms and the patient could die peacefully at home [28].

On the other hand, the nurses reported that patient's condition could worsen very quickly, and the family was not always capable of handling the situation, as it could become unbearable. They found it important to support the family members to change their minds even if they had promised their loved one to die at home. Supporting the family to balance between their needs, wishes and resources has been found to be critical in home-based palliative care [29, 42]. The dying patient and family need reassurance from trusted professionals with experience in palliative care [43].

This study highlights the need for flexibility in shift plans and working lists as well as understanding within the nursing group. The nurses knew each other well and could rely on each other's competencies. When the nurses realized that the death of a patient was imminent, they practiced flexibility in the shift plan. They had a kind of "silent agreement" to handle some of the tasks of the nurses involved so that they could stay longer with their patient. Without this flexibility, these patients would often be sent to the hospital or emergency unit.

The nurses missed being mentored and having the opportunity to talk about difficult situations and ethical dilemmas in an organised way. Working with palliative care patients and their families is demanding in many ways. It is well known that exhaustion and stress is a huge concern for palliative care health professionals [40, 44]. Supportive mentoring on a regular basis could reduce and prevent distress [39].

Methodological considerations

Gaining perspectives from both home care nurses and GPs could be considered a strength. Our participants were particularly experienced and quite dedicated, which might reduce their representativeness. Our study focused on the professionals working with palliative care in primary health care, not professionals working in hospitals. Hence, there is a limitation as the voice of doctors and nurses in hospitals has not been heard regarding the transfer of the palliative care patient from hospital. Because of our context, the findings are probably more relevant to cities, rather than rural areas. However, it was not the aim of the study to investigate this issue in different geographical contexts. Further research into this aspect could be useful.

Conclusion

This study demonstrates that optimum palliative care at home depends on close collaboration and dialogue between the patient, family, home care nurses and general practitioner. Our findings emphasize the need for safer discharge and planning procedures when hospitals transfer palliative care patients to their homes. A good start is crucial for a good result. The initial collaboration meeting at home between the patient, next of kin, general practitioner, and home care nurse requires a fixed agenda. An interesting and thought-provoking finding was that the general practitioner was rarely contacted during their patient's hospitalization and prior to discharge despite having in-depth knowledge of their patient's medical history, which if sought, could benefit the patient and the next of kin. This 'disconnection' with the patient's general practitioner might reduce patient safety. Both general practitioners and home care nurses appeared to be dedicated to their palliative care work. They emphasized the need to work together, "shoulder to shoulder". However, they experienced that the family was fundamental in gaining more time at home for the patient and creating the chance for the patient to eventually die at home. Our study emphasizes that home-based palliative care demands experience and competence as well as regular supportive mentoring.

Abbreviations

GP: General practitioner; NSD: Norwegian Centre for Research Data; RN: Registered nurse

Acknowledgements

We wish to extend our profound gratitude to the nurses and GPs who participated in this study and shared their experiences. We also extend our gratitude to the local nursing managers who recruited the nurse participants.

Data analysis and interpretation

The focus groups were audiotaped and transcribed by AMS and BVD, both performed the main analysis. The data were also analyzed separately by JHR and OF to strengthen the results. All authors then compared the themes and synthesized them into meaningful core themes and sub-themes.

Authors' contributions

BVD: Participated in the concept and design of the study, the data collection, analysis and interpretation of the data, and was the main author responsible for drafting and editing the manuscript. AMS: Participated in the concept and design of the study, took principal responsibility for the data collection, and participated in analysis and interpretation of the data, and the drafting and editing of the manuscript. JHR: Participated in the concept and design of the study, the data collection, analysis and interpretation of the data, and drafting and editing of the manuscript. OF: Participated in the concept and design of the study, the analysis and interpretation of the data, and the drafting of the manuscript, and assumed the key role in the final editing of the manuscript. All authors read and approved the final manuscript.

Competing interests

The authors declare that they have no competing interests.

Author details

[1]Department of Health and Caring Sciences, Faculty of Health and Social Sciences, Western Norway University of Applied Sciences, P.O. Box 7030, N-5020 Bergen, Norway. [2]Department of Clinical Medicine, University of Bergen, Bergen, Norway. [3]Sunniva Centre for Palliative Care, Haraldsplass Deaconess Hospital Bergen, Bergen, Norway. [4]Centre for Care Research - Western Norway, Western Norway University of Applied Sciences, Bergen, Norway. [5]Faculty of Health Studies, VID Specialized University, Bergen, Norway.

References

1. Norwegian Institute of Public Health. Table D3 - Deaths by place of death. In: Norwegian Cause of Death Registry. 2016. [Available from: http://statistikkbank.fhi.no/dar/.
2. Norwegian Directorate of Health. In norwegian: Rapport om tilbudet til personer med behov for lindrende behandling og omsorg mot livets slutt: å skape liv til dagene. Oslo: The Norwegian Directorate of Health; 2015.
3. Norwegian Ministry of Health and Care Services. Future Care. Report to the Storting (White Paper) 29 (2012–2013). Oslo: Ministry of Health and Care Services.
4. Higginson IJ, Sarmento VP, Calanzani N, Benalia H, Gomes B. Dying at home--is it better: a narrative appraisal of the state of the science. Palliat Med. 2013;27(10):918–24.
5. Teno JM, Gozalo PL, Bynum JP, Leland NE, Miller SC, Morden NE, et al. Change in end-of-life care for Medicare beneficiaries: site of death, place of care, and health care transitions in 2000, 2005, and 2009. JAMA. 2013;309(5):470–7.
6. Wilson DM, Truman CD, Thomas R, Fainsinger R, Kovacs-Burns K, Froggatt K, et al. The rapidly changing location of death in Canada, 1994–2004. Soc Sci Med. 2009;68(10):1752–8.
7. Gomes B, Calanzani N, Higginson IJ. Reversal of the British trends in place of death: Time series analysis 2004–2010. Palliative Medicine. 2012;26(2):102–7.
8. Costa V, Earle CC, Esplen MJ, Fowler R, Goldman R, Grossman D, et al. The determinants of home and nursing home death: a systematic review and meta-analysis. BMC Palliat Care. 2016;15(1):8.
9. Kastbom L, Milberg A, Karlsson M. A good death from the perspective of palliative cancer patients. Support Care Cancer. 2016:1–7.
10. Billingham MJ, Billingham S-J. Congruence between preferred and actual place of death according to the presence of malignant or non-malignant disease: a systematic review and meta-analysis. BMJ Support Palliat Care. 2013;3(2):144.
11. Murray MA, Fiset V, Young S, Kryworuchko J. Where the dying live: a systematic review of determinants of place of end-of-life Cancer care. Oncol Nurs Forum. 2009;36(1):69.
12. Gomes B, Calanzani N, Gysels M, Hall S, Higginson IJ. Heterogeneity and changes in preferences for dying at home: a systematic review. BMC Palliat Care. 2013;12(1):7.
13. Higginson IJ, Sen-Gupta GJ. Place of care in advanced cancer: a qualitative systematic literature review of patient preferences. J Palliat Med. 2000;3(3):287–300.
14. Sandsdalen T, Hov R, Hoye S, Rystedt I, Wilde-Larsson B. Patients' preferences in palliative care: a systematic mixed studies review. Palliat Med. 2015;29(5):399–419.
15. Hoare S, Morris ZS, Kelly MP, Kuhn I, Barclay S. Do patients want to die at home? A systematic review of the UK literature, focused on missing preferences for place of death. PLoS One. 2015;10(11):e0142723.
16. World Health Organization. Palliative care for older people: better practices. Denmark. In: Copenhagen: WHO regional office for Europe; 2011.
17. Ministry of Health and Care Services. In norwegian: På liv og død: palliasjon til alvorlig syke og døende. NOU 2017:16. Official Norwegian Reports (NOUs).
18. Jordhoy MS, Fayers P, Saltnes T, Ahlner-Elmqvist M, Jannert M, Kaasa S. A palliative-care intervention and death at home: a cluster randomised trial. Lancet (London, England). 2000;356(9233):888–93.
19. Gomes B, Higginson I. Factors influencing death at home in terminally ill patients with cancer: systematic review. BMJ. 2006;332(7540):515–8.
20. Jack BA, Baldry CR, Groves KE, Whelan A, Sephton J, Gaunt K. Supporting home care for the dying: an evaluation of healthcare professionals' perspectives of an individually tailored hospice at home service. J Clin Nurs. 2013;22(19–20):2778–86.
21. O'Brien M, Jack B. Barriers to dying at home: the impact of poor co-ordination of community service provision for patients with cancer. Health Soc Care Community. 2010;18(4):337–45.
22. Christensen K, Wærness K. Long-term care services in Norway. A historical sociological perpective. In: Christensen K, Pilling D, editors. The Routledge handbook of social care work around the world. Abingdon, Oxon: Routledge; 2018. p. 15–28.
23. Ringard Å, Sagan A, Saunes IS, Lindahl AK, World Health O. Norway: health system review. Copenhagen: World Health Organization on behalf of the European Observatory on Health Systems and Policies; 2013.
24. Ministry of Health and Care Services. The Coordination Reform. Proper treatment – at the right place and right time (White Paper no.47, 2008–2009). In: Ministry of Health and Care Services, editor 2009.
25. Norwegian Ministry of Health and Care Services. The Norwegian Government's plan for the care services field for 2015–2020. Oslo: Norwegian Ministry of Health and Care Services; 2015. Available from: https://www.regjeringen.no/contentassets/af2a24858c8340edaf78a77e2fbe9cb7/careplan2020_eng.pdf.
26. Krueger RA, Casey MA. Focus groups: a practical guide for applied research. 5th ed. Los Angeles: Sage; 2015.
27. Malterud K. Systematic text condensation: a strategy for qualitative analysis. Scand J Public Health. 2012;40(8):795–805.
28. Wilson E, Morbey H, Brown J, Payne S, Seale C, Seymour J. Administering anticipatory medications in end-of-life care: a qualitative study of nursing practice in the community and in nursing homes. Palliat Med. 2015;29(1):60–70.
29. Neergaard MA, Olesen F, Jensen AB, Sondergaard J. Palliative care for cancer patients in a primary health care setting: bereaved relatives' experience, a qualitative group interview study. BMC Palliat Care. 2008;7(1).
30. Sørhus Skeie G, Landmark BT, Grov EK. Ansvarlig og avhengig - Pårørendes erfaringer med forestående død i hjemmet. In English: responsible and dependent - relatives' experience with expected death at home. Klinisk Sygepleje. 2016;43(02):87–100.
31. Friis P, Forde R. Advance care planning discussions with geriatric patients. Tidsskr Nor Laegeforen. 2015;135(3):233–5.

32. Hunstad I, Svindseth MF. Challenges in home-based palliative care in Norway: a qualitative study of spouses' experiences. Int J Palliat Nurs. 2011; 17(7):398–404.
33. Abel J, Pring A, Rich A, Malik T, Verne J. The impact of advance care planning of place of death, a hospice retrospective cohort study. BMJ Support Palliat Care. 2013;3(2):168–73.
34. Silveira MJ, Kim SY, Langa KM. Advance directives and outcomes of surrogate decision making before death. N Engl J Med. 2010;362(13):1211–8.
35. Aabom B, Kragstrup J, Vondeling H, Bakketeig LS, Stovring H. Does persistent involvement by the GP improve palliative care at home for end-stage cancer patients? Palliat Med. 2006;20(5):507–12.
36. Smith R, Porock D. Caring for people dying at home: a research study into the needs of community nurses. Int J Palliat Nurs. 2009;15(12)
37. Austin L, Luker K, Caress A, Hallett C. Palliative care: community nurses' perceptions of quality. Quality Health Care. 2000;9(3):151–8.
38. Luker KA, Austin L, Caress A, Hallett CE. The importance of 'knowing the patient': community nurses' constructions of quality in providing palliative care. J Adv Nurs. 2000;31(4):775–82.
39. Levine S, O'Mahony S, Baron A, Ansari A, Deamant C, Frader J, et al. Training the workforce: description of a longitudinal interdisciplinary education and mentoring program in palliative care. J Pain Symptom Manag. 2017;53(4):728–37.
40. O'Mahony S, Gerhart JI, Grosse J, Abrams I, Levy MM. Posttraumatic stress symptoms in palliative care professionals seeking mindfulness training: prevalence and vulnerability. Palliat Med. 2016;30(2):189–92.
41. Roberts SJ, Demarco R, Griffin M. The effect of oppressed group behaviours on the culture of the nursing workplace: a review of the evidence and interventions for change. J Nurs Manag. 2009;17(3):288–93.
42. Proot IM, Abu-Saad HH, Crebolder HFJM, Goldsteen M, Luker KA, Widdershoven GAM. Vulnerability of family caregivers in terminal palliative care at home; balancing between burden and capacity. Scand J Caring Sci. 2003;17(2):113–21.
43. Wye L, Lasseter G, Percival J, Duncan L, Simmonds B, Purdy S. What works in 'real life' to facilitate home deaths and fewer hospital admissions for those at end of life?: results from a realist evaluation of new palliative care services in two English counties. BMC Palliat Care. 2014;13(1):37.
44. Kamal AH, Bull JH, Wolf SP, Swetz KM, Shanafelt TD, Ast K, et al. Prevalence and predictors of burnout among hospice and palliative care clinicians in the U.S. J Pain Symptom Manag. 2016;51(4):690–6.

Feasibility, acceptability and adaption of dignity therapy: a mixed methods study achieving 360° feedback

Sandra Stephanie Mai[1], Swantje Goebel[1], Elisabeth Jentschke[2], Birgitt van Oorschot[2], Karl-Heinz Renner[3] and Martin Weber[1*]

Abstract

Background: Dignity Therapy (DT) is a short-term intervention to reduce psychological suffering in end-of-life care. Its strength lies in evidenced-based development and investigation. The aim of the present study is to investigate the feasibility of DT at German palliative care units (PCU), as well as the acceptability and adaption of a German version of the DT question protocol (DTQP).

Method: A clinical multicentre mixed methods study, whereby patients and relatives provided quantitative (feedback questionnaires) and qualitative (cognitive interviews) data on the DT intervention. Before using the DTQP on patients, healthcare professionals (HCP) were invited to participate in cognitive interviews to provide input on DT. Therefore 360° feedback was achieved. Finally, the conducted DT interviews were examined.
The study took place at two German PCUs (Mainz and Würzburg). Participating HCPs were physicians, psychologists, nurses and chaplains. Patients admitted to the PCUs were eligible to participate if they had a terminal illness and a life expectancy ranging from 2 weeks to 12 months.
Results: Out of 410 admitted patients, 72 were eligible and 30 (7.3% of all patients and 41.7% of eligible patients) participated. On average, 9 questions from the DTQP were used per DT interview. Subsequent cognitive interviews with patients produced four main categories of feedback (on the title, the question protocol, wording, and the questions actually asked). Finally, of the 30 participants, 19 completed the feedback questionnaire, as did 26 relatives. Of those, 18 patients and 24 relatives evaluated DT as helpful.

Conclusions: DT is feasible for German PCUs. Our research yielded a validated German translation of the DTQP following EORTC guidelines and findings were reported according to the COREQ checklist for qualitative design.
Trial registration.
The study was registered retrospectively on the 22nd of December 2017 at the German Clinical Trials Register (DRKS00013627).

Keywords: Dignity therapy, Palliative care, Qualitative research, Translation

Background

Depression, anxiety, hopelessness and loss of meaning and purpose are central symptoms of the demoralization and psychological distress faced by patients in palliative care [1]. These burdens are associated with loss of dignity [2, 3]. In a systematic review, Monforte-Royo concludes that the loss of dignity and its influence on hopelessness and loss of meaning may result in a wish for hastened death [4]. An updated systematic review added that "loss of self" and the "lived experience of a timeline towards dying and death" were common features of a patient's wish to hasten death [5]. These findings indicate that patients need appropriate supportive care to address psychological symptoms and ensure quality of life in their final days. An evidence-based intervention to care for the terminally ill on a psychosocial and spiritual basis is Dignity Therapy (DT) [6]. DT was first described in 2005 by

* Correspondence: martin.weber@unimedizin-mainz.de
[1]Interdisciplinary Palliative Care Unit, III. Department of Medicine, University Medical Center of the Johannes Gutenberg University of Mainz, Mainz, Germany
Full list of author information is available at the end of the article

Harvey Max Chochinov, based on his findings on dignity in the terminally ill and the dignity model [3]. The dignity model provides three major dignity categories (illness-related concerns, dignity-conserving repertoire, social dignity inventory) and several themes (e.g., dignity-conserving perspectives and dignity-conserving practices) evoked from patients' explanations of their understanding of dignity. The basis of DT is a semi-structured question protocol (Table 1).

During an audio-recorded interview session the therapist guides the patient through these questions to enhance the dignity-conserving perspectives. Most importantly the framework of questions is intended to be flexible with a varying number of questions actually used in order to suit the individual patient ([7], p. 185). The transcript of the interview session is edited and read out to the patient; if necessary, further editing can be performed. The transcript is then finalized to create a permanent generativity document which can be shared with loved ones [7]. Research on the feasibility and efficacy of DT has been published for six countries [8]. Although findings regarding its efficacy have been contradictory in recent randomized controlled trials [8, 9], helpfulness and meaningfulness are proven benefits for patients and relatives, and DT is regarded as feasible in different clinical settings, healthcare systems and cultures. These findings were an encouraging starting point to evaluate the implementation of DT in palliative care units (PCU) in Germany.

Table 1 The Dignity Therapy Question Protocol

(1)* Tell me a little about your life history; particularly the parts that you either remember most or think are the most important. (2) When did you feel most alive?
(3) Are there specific things that you would want your family to know about you, (4) and are there particular things you would want them to remember?
(5) What are the most important roles you have played in life (family roles, vocational roles, community-service roles, etc.)? (6) Why were they important to you, and what do you think you accomplished in those roles?
(7) What are your most important accomplishments, and what do you feel most proud of?
(8) Are there particular things that you feel still need to be said to your loved ones (9) or things that you would want to take the time to say once again?
(10) What are your hopes and dreams for your loved ones?
(11) What have you learned about life that you would want to pass along to others? (12) What advice or words of guidance would you wish to pass along to your (son, daughter, husband, wife, parents, other[s])?
(13) Are there words or perhaps even instructions that you would like to offer your family to help prepare them for the future?
(14) In creating this permanent record, are there other things that you would like included?

*Numbering is only to ensure traceability of methodology and results for the reader

Although DT has already been used in Germany to a limited extent, the Dignity Therapy Question Protocol (DTQP) to date lacks a scientifically verified translation into German. Various unproven translations of the question framework have been used up to this point. What is more, the feasibility and acceptability of DT in Germany have not been examined before. And yet these issues are fundamental to enable further comparable research and the implementation of DT in Germany. The purpose of this research was therefore to conduct a mixed methods study at two German PCUs, in Mainz (M) and Würzburg (W). Similar to the implementation of DT in Denmark [10], the aims of our study were (1) to translate the DTQP and if necessary adapt the question framework, and (2) to test the feasibility and acceptability of DT in an inpatient setting.

Methods

The clinical multicentre study comprises quantitative and qualitative research at two PCUs in the university hospitals of M and W. After their actual DT interview, patients participated in semi-structured cognitive interviews to report their experience of the process through free narratives. Narratives are the most appropriate form of research to report experiences. Patients also completed a feedback questionnaire (quantitative and free text comments) to gather further information on their estimation of DT. Once the patient DT process was complete, relatives were also asked to evaluate DT by completing a feedback questionnaire similar to that of the patients. To achieve 360° feedback, healthcare professionals (HCP) from different disciplines within palliative care were interviewed in expert focus groups. This method allowed critical discussion of the different aspects arising from DT. The information detailed below follows this timeline and complies with the consolidated criteria for reporting qualitative research (COREQ) [11].

Translation of the dignity therapy question protocol (DTQP)

In accordance with the EORTC Translation Procedure [12], two English and two German native speakers conducted forward-backward translations of the DTQP. These translations were discussed at round tables by physicians and psychologists experienced in palliative care and, where necessary, checked back with H.M. Chochinov to obtain a pilot version.

HCP evaluation of the DTQP German translation

In June and July 2015, two experienced researchers (S.S. M., qualified psychologist, and PhD S.G., sociologist) conducted focus groups with HCPs in meeting rooms at the university hospitals of M and W; the meetings lasted 60 and 70 min respectively. Both researchers were clinical and scientific colleagues of the participants from M; however, prior to study commencement, they were not acquainted with the HCP participants from W. Participating HCPs were all highly experienced in palliative care and were purposively recruited by e-mail. The number of participants represents the multi-professionalism of palliative care teams, consisting of five HCPs in M (psychologist, chaplain, nurse and two physicians) and seven HCPs in W (two chaplains, two nurses and three physicians). All participants were informed of the aim to achieve a German translation of the DTQP and they all gave written informed consent to participate. Each participant was attributed an ID to anonymize the qualitative data. As none of the 12 HCPs had previously conducted DT, their statements can be regarded as unbiased. Following a comprehensive interview guideline (developed by S.G. according to Willis' recommendations on cognitive interviewing [13], Additional file 1), the HCPs were requested to express spontaneous associations regarding the title of the intervention, the wording of the DT questions, and the adaption of DT to the German cultural context. As well as visually summarizing and recording the participants' statements on flip charts during the sessions, audio recordings were also made. S.S.M. and S.G. then transcribed and analysed the qualitative data based on the principles of qualitative content analysis as described by Kuckartz [14]. This method enables the elaboration of core messages from the interview transcriptions, by using inductive and deductive approaches in a systematic manner. Only parts of the interviews pertaining to the research questions have been considered, numbered, and arranged within an Excel sheet. Analysis units from the first interview transcript were paraphrased and generalized, and redundancies were identified, and inductively subsumed into main categories and subcategories. This resulting code structure was used to analyse the second interview deductively, and new codes were added inductively to the code structure, as needed. Typical phrases were identified. In the first instance both researchers coded independently. To achieve interrater reliability, categories were discussed and any coding conflicts were resolved. This process was repeated until the final structure of categories was formed and all relevant parts of the text were coded appropriately. The research group reviewed the results to ensure inter-subjectivity and coherence within the code structure. The results constituted the first step in the linguistic and cultural adaption of the DTQP.

Patient evaluation of the DT intervention and the DTQP

Leaning on the experiences and data of the Danish DT feasibility study [10], we decided to include 30 patients from two PCUs in our study. Each patient admitted to the PCUs in M and W was attributed an ID and was screened for eligibility. Inclusion criteria were: having a terminal illness with a clinically estimated life expectancy of up to 12 months; age ≥ 18 years; ability to give informed consent; possibility to nominate a relative for the feedback questionnaire; and appropriate German language skills. Exclusion criteria were: having cognitive impairments or an estimated life expectancy below 2 weeks, especially where the dying process had begun. After giving written informed consent, patients participated in the audio-recorded DT interview led by DT therapists (M: psychologist and male nurse; W: psychologist) trained by H.M. Chochinov. All steps of the DT protocol were fulfilled (interview session, transcribing, editing, reading out to the patients, finalizing the document and taking it to the recipient). Detailed information about the duration of the DT interview and DT intervention was logged. Furthermore each question asked during the DT interview was counted, repetitions were listed, and rewording as well as patients' noteworthy reactions were noted.

After the DT interview using the DTQP, the participants took part in semi-structured cognitive interviews with their therapists to report their experience of the implementation of the DT interview (the interview guideline was produced by S.S.M. and S.G. according to Willis' recommendations on cognitive interviewing [13], Additional file 2). All sessions took place in the patients' single rooms at the PCUs. The cognitive interviews were recorded, transcribed and analysed by S.S.M. and S.G. using qualitative content analysis [14] as described above. The basic coding tree results from the major themes of the cognitive interview. The resulting data constituted the second step in the adaption of the DTQP.

Patient and relative feedback questionnaires

After delivery of the finalized generativity document, patients and relatives (as nominated by the patients and after having given informed consent) were asked to complete the DT Patient Feedback Questionnaire [15] and the DT Family Feedback Questionnaire [16] respectively. Both questionnaires previously had been translated into German by forward-backward translation (Additional file 3 and Additional file 4). They combine quantitative items (5-point Likert scale; 1 = strongly disagree, 5 = strongly agree) and free text comments.

All data were analysed descriptively with SPSS 22.0 and Microsoft Excel®.

Results

The following results are presented in order of the described methodology and timeline.

HCP views on the DTQP

Besides general remarks on the interpretation of the word 'dignity,' which some HCPs viewed in a religious way and others in a more philosophical way, we observed five main categories of comments on DT and the DTQP: (1) negative aspects of DT; (2) positive aspects of DT; (3) Dignity Therapist; (4) conducting DT; and (5) the DTQP (Table 2). There were no comments on financing DT. Among the focus group conclusions was the opinion that the PCU is an appropriate setting for DT, as the patients have single rooms. HCPs also agreed that DT could be an essential part of the interdisciplinary care for patients if it is conducted with compassion: "If DT is conducted with heart, it could be an essential part of care and it becomes effective through this [compassion] and may be guided less by the questions that are asked but by the issue that lies on the patient's heart" (M5). One HCP compared DT to the concept of 'holding spaces': "You give space for life issues, experiences and suffering, and this is dignifying and a valuable encounter" (W1).

Participant characteristics and DT intervention data

A total of 410 patients were admitted to the PCUs in M (215 patients between June 2015 and October 2015) and W (195 patients between June 2015 and April 2016). Of these, 72 patients (17%) (M: 54; W: 18) met the inclusion criteria, and 30 of them (M: 19; W: 11) participated (7.3% of all patients and 41.7% of eligible patients). Participants' inpatient stay ranged from 5 days to 98 days (median = 16 days). The mean age was 63 years (range: 38–88); 20 participants were female; the median Eastern Cooperative Oncology Group performance status

Table 2 Themes, frequencies and example quotations of HCP views on the *DTQP* (M1/W1 = chaplain; M4 = psychologist; M3/M5/W0/W3/W6 = physician; M2/W5 = nurse)

Main Category	Themes	Frequency M / W	Example Quotation (ID)
Negative aspects of DT	Complex for patients and therapists	2 / 1	The time-consuming process is a disadvantage. (M4); Do we need such a sophisticated concept or don't you hit on it yourself when getting a serious diagnosis? (W0)
	Psychological burden could arise	3 / 5	Negative memories could arise and create psychological burden. (M3); DT could have side effects if unconscious aspects arise. (W6)
	Patients fear negative consequences if they decline DT	3 / -	Some patients tell me they're afraid of being treated less well if they decline something, e.g. students' teaching courses. (M1)
	The name of the intervention is inappropriate	2 / 5	You can't say DT. This seems inappropriate. (M1); Therapy [in the name of the intervention] is something that people don't want to have, because they had enough therapy during their illness. (W5)
	Application of DT is limited	- / 5	DT is only appropriate for patients with the ability to communicate verbally, be self-reflective and discuss value-based issues. (W3)
Positive aspects of DT	DT encourages self-reflection	6 / 4	It triggers self-reflection, which is an advantage. (M5); DT is a process to realize what is important in my life, what is personally valuable for me. (W1)
	Generating a legacy	3 / -	The form (written words) creates the possibility to pass something on to your relatives that you couldn't verbalize. (M2)
	DT creates space for a dignifying encounter	3 / 4	DT is about caring for the person. (M1); The concept of the dignifying attitude we find in DT is a good thing. (W3)
Dignity Therapist	Challenges for the therapist posed by DT	4 / 6	The therapist must be very sensitive to decide which statement is meant for the document. (M5); You need to know how to handle negative issues when uncovering negative affect. (W0)
	Consequences for the therapist after DT	2 / -	The interviewer may take on some of the patient's distress. (M4)
Conducting DT	Application site / setting	1 / 5	The thousands of people in nursing homes or wards other than palliative care units should also be able to receive DT. (M1); The questions are great. I even used them during a dialogue about anamnesis. (W6)
DT Question Protocol	(Question) phrasing	11 / 8	Some questions sound awkward. (M1); Subjunctive phrases are irritating. (W2)
	Open-ended questions are stimulating	6 / 3	The first question is a good opening as it is an open-ended question. (M3); For me, open-ended questions are important … they can be heart-opening. (W1)
	Focus on generating legacy	1 / 2	The advantage is to receive a treasure of life experience, e.g., question 11. (M3); [As a participant] I'd wish to know that it doesn't have to be a permanent record for the next generation. (W6)
	Focus on accomplishments	2 / 6	Asking for accomplishments and roles is risky when interviewing a patient who is depressed. (M4); To name something as an accomplishment as an observer from the outside, that is social dignity. (W4)
	Application by DT Therapists	6 / 6	I understood that the therapist uses some but not all of the DT questions. (M1); The effect of the questions depends on asking these questions with a warm, calm and empathic tone. (W6)

(ECOG) was 3 with a 40% Palliative Performance Scale (PPS) rating. Table 3 provides further information on the participants' characteristics.

The main exclusion criteria were: a life expectancy below two weeks (196 patients; 58%), followed by cognitive impairments (74 patients; 22%). A further 10% of eligible patients could not be included due to organizational barriers.

The median time-span of the whole DT process – from introducing it to the patient to returning the generativity document – was 15 days (mean: 24; range: 6–131). During this time, there were four contact sessions between patient and therapist on average. The mean time expenditure for therapists was 7 h (SD: 1.6; range: 4.27–10.38), comprising time to interview, edit, read out to the patient, make final editorial changes and return the finalized document to the recipient (note that this excludes time taken to transcribe the audio recording; this task was conducted by student assistants). The mean time expenditure for the patients was 2.15 h (SD: 0.5; range: 1.25–3.5). The mean time required for the DT interview was 48 min (SD: 19; range: 20–81). Once finalized, 19 of the generativity documents were given to the patients solely (to be handed out to the relatives by themselves or after their death), 3 documents were given to patients and relatives together, and 8 were received directly by relatives.

On average, nine questions were used per interview. Q1 ("Tell me a little about your life history; particularly the parts that you either remember most or think are the most important") was always asked; the least asked question was Q6 ("Why were [these roles] so important to you and what do you think you accomplished within those roles?"). Q2 ("When did you feel most alive?") was asked in 24 out of 30 interviews. In one interview, to match the language used by the patient, the wording changed from "alive" to "bloody good" (M 129). In 17 out of 23 interviews, Q3 ("Are there specific things that you would want your family to know about you?") was responded to with comments like, "I don't have any secrets", "I think they know everything", or "I don't hide anything". Q7 ("What are your most important accomplishments, and what do you feel most proud of?") was used 26 times. We found that Q8 ("Are there particular things that you feel still need to be said to your loved ones?") was sometimes personalized, e.g. "to your son" (5/16). Q10 ("What are your hopes and dreams for your loved ones?") was used 27 times and reworded 17 times (from "dreams" to "wishes"). Similarly, Q12 ("What advice or words of guidance would

Table 3 Study participant (patients and relatives) characteristics

Patients (*N* = 30)				
Age in years		Mean: 63	SD: 9.9	Range: 38–88
Gender	Female: 20 (67%)		Male: 10 (33%)	
ECOG at admission	Median: 3	Mean: 2.77	SD: 0.73	Range: 1–4
PPS at admission	Median: 40	Mean: 45	SD: 12.8	Range: 30–80
Period of time in months *(years)* between first diagnosis and first DT interview		Mean: 33 *(2.76)*	SD: 39.29 *(3.28)*	Range: 1–163 *(0.06–13.62)*
Main diagnosis	Gastrointestinal cancers:		10 (33.3%)	
	Gynaecological cancers:		8 (26.7%)	
	Lung cancers:		5 (16.7%)	
	Urology cancers:		4 (13.3%)	
	Neurological diseases		2 (6.7%)	
	Dermatological cancers:		1 (3.3%)	
Length of inpatient stay in days	Median: 15.5	Mean: 22.5	SD: 18.0	Range: 5–98
Relatives (N = 30)				
Age in years (2 missings)		Mean: 54	SD: 12.83	Range: 24–74
Gender	Female: 14 (46.7%)		Male: 16 (53.3%)	
Relationship to patient	Spouse:		17 (56.7%)	
	Child:		6 (20%)	
	Sibling:		3 (10%)	
	Parent:		2 (6.7%)	
	Other:		2 (6.7%)	
Duration of relationship in years (5 missings))		Mean: 35.48	SD: 17.31	Range: 8–71

Table 4 Themes, frequencies and example quotations of patient views on the DTQP ($N = 29$)

Main Category	Themes	Frequency M / W	Example Quotation (ID)
Title of the intervention (Dignity Therapy ➔ Würdezentrierte Therapie)	The title conveys dignity until the end	1 / -	The title conveys that my entire existence is dignified and I am taken seriously as long as I am alive. I want to be appreciated. (M 136)
	Dignity conveys respect	6 / 1	Dignity means to accept the person and respect him or her as he or she is. (M 163)
	Dignity is an attitude	4 / -	Dignity evokes the idea of appreciating your own life story. (M 128)
	Therapy is irritating	4 / -	Therapy is an action and I don't see how this goes together with dignity. (M 202)
	Therapy conveys help	11 / 2	Therapy conveys a helpful technique to solve a problem. (M 43)
	The title is not informative	8 / 2	First I couldn't understand anything with the title. I had no idea what kind of technique this therapy could be. (M 43)
	The title is suitable	8 / 5	The title is suitable for this intervention as it means to reflect about what was important in your life. (W 23)
Dignity Therapy Question Protocol	Everything is addressed	3 / 2	The questions cover everything like a comprehensive frame. (M 99)
	Open questions provoke reflection	4 / 1	The questions force you to think back and reminisce about what you have gone through. (W 54)
	The DTQP is coherent	5 / 7	I think it was coherent and every question fits; it combines theoretical and practical aspects. (M 117)
	The questions in the DTQP make sense	6 / 1	The questions are all emotional, some make you cry, some make you laugh about something, but it's always liberating. (W 23)
	The DTQP contains duplications	3 / 2	Question no. 8 and no. 9 are similar. (W 007)
	Some questions are difficult	5 / 2	It's difficult to respond to questions that are partly very personal – but it works. (M 83)
	There are no upsetting questions	5 / -	The questions were alright. None of them was disruptive. (M 92)
Wording of individual questions	There are no disruptive words	3 / -	There were no specific words that were upsetting. (M 21)
	Question 5: Change "Remit" (*Aufgabenbereiche*) to "Roles" (*Rollen*)	1 / -	I think it would be better to ask for roles instead of remits. (M 43)
	Question 2: The word "alive" (*lebendig*) is moving	3 / -	I like the word 'alive' because it encompasses everything and is different from being happy or cheerful. (M 57)
	Question 8, 9, 10: Relatives mentioned should be personalized	- / 1	For me, I would replace relatives with children. (W 007)
	Question 7: "Accomplishments" (*Leistungen*) and "Pride" (*Stolz*) are connoted positively	2 / -	Pride and accomplishments belong to us by nature; it's something positive. (M 129)
	Question 7: "Pride" (*Stolz*) is connoted negatively	2 / -	The word "pride" is too strong and should be replaced with contentment. (M 136)
	Question 12: "Advice" (*Rat*) should be replaced	- / 1	The word 'advice' is disruptive because I think everyone lives his or her own life. (W 23)
Set of questions actually asked during DT interview	The photo metaphor is well received	1 /	The question regarding memories as if looking through a photo album is nice. (M 43)
	All questions elicited a response	3 / -	Any question asked was okay, so that it [the interview] was genuine. (M 83)
	Questions concerning loved ones are emotionally evocative	3 / 1	It is important to talk about the emotional things although they trigger sadness. (W 23)

Table 4 Themes, frequencies and example quotations of patient views on the DTQP (*N* = 29) *(Continued)*

Main Category	Themes	Frequency M / W	Example Quotation (ID)
	Additional questions arise situational	3 / -	The DTQP provides the questions to give me an idea of what the interview is about – additional questions come up as we go along. (M 129)
	The interview atmosphere contributes to a successful DT interview	3 / -	The Therapist was very good; I don't think I have opened up that much with many people. (M 136)

you wish to pass along to your ...?") was used in 11 interviews and reworded (skipping 'words of guidance') without prior agreement between the interviewers.

Patient views on the DTQP and the DT intervention

Out of 30 patients, 29 subsequently took part in cognitive interviews to share their views on the DTQP (mean duration: 10 min; SD: 6; range: 2–30). We identified four main categories of feedback: on the title; the DTQP; the wording of individual questions; and the set of questions actually asked during the DT interview (Table 4). In addition, patients gave the following positive remarks and ideas regarding DT: the questions could lead to more openness in talking about cancer; DT preserves pride; DT should be widely offered; DT should be conducted in the presence of relatives; DT is only successful if it is a helpful encounter. More sceptical comments related to the effectiveness or usefulness of DT or to the fear of psychological challenges arising. One patient suggested adding the following question: "What has been your mission in your life?" (M 43). Regarding Q5, she recommended changing "remits" into "roles" (M 43); this was the de facto wording in 8 out of 23 interviews. For comparative purposes, Q7 ("What are your most important accomplishments, and what do you feel most proud of?") was of particular interest: Danish colleagues found that using the word "proud" was not feasible for the Danish culture [10 Pride was only discussed as negative respectively positive by 2 patients each. Case M 136 illustrates this issue. Within the cognitive interview the patient stated that "pride is too strong" and that "it should be replaced with contentment". Yet, during the DT interview she had easily answered that question by recounting what she had achieved on her own after getting divorced. The

Table 5 Patient feedback questionnaires on DT

Item	*N*	strongly agreed or agreed (*n* / %)	disagreed or strongly disagreed (*n* / %)	neither agreed or disagreed (*n* / %)	Selected Comments (ID)
I have found Dignity Therapy to be helpful to me.	19	18 / 94.7	–	1 / 5.3	It was helpful, because warm memories became present; it gave me a feeling of stability. (M 43)
I have found Dignity Therapy to be satisfactory.	19	18 / 94.7	1 / 5.3	–	It was far more than satisfactory. DT is a gift. It was more than I expected. (M 43)
Dignity Therapy made me feel that my life currently is more meaningful.	19	14 / 73.7	2 / 10.5	3 / 15.8	Life had the same meaning before [DT]. (M 43)
Dignity Therapy has given me a heightened sense of purpose.	19	13 / 68.4	2 / 10.5	4 / 21.1	I see that what I did wasn't that wrong after all. (M 47)
Dignity Therapy has given me a heightened sense of dignity.	19	14 / 73.7	3 / 15.8	2 / 10.5	I feel accepted the way I am. (W 42)
Dignity Therapy has lessened my sense of suffering.	19	11 / 57.9	3 / 15.8	5 / 15.8	DT has enhanced issues that help cope with the situation. (M 43) Cancer stays cancer and death is unstoppable. (M 83)
Dignity Therapy has increased my will to live.	19	13 / 68.4	6 / 31.6	–	My way of thinking has changed. (M 83)
I believe Dignity Therapy has or will be of help to my family.	19	14 / 73.7	2 / 10.5	3 / 15.8	I hope that my family's cohesion is strengthened [by DT]. (M 21)
I believe my participation in Dignity Therapy could change the way my family sees or appreciates me.	19	11 / 57.9	4 / 21.1	4 / 21.1	The appreciation of my family will not be affected by the therapy. (M 128)
I believe my participation in Dignity Therapy could change the way my healthcare providers see or appreciate me.	19	8 / 42.1	4 / 21.1	7 / 36.8	I think that healthcare providers won't base their appreciation for a patient on his/her participation in DT. (M 128)
In general, I have been satisfied with my psychosocial care.	19	19 / 100	–	–	I always received help and was never ever let down. (W 42)

interview atmosphere was clearly not negatively affected by the word "proud"; in contrast it seemed to offer her the opportunity to be proud of herself.

Of the 30 patients who took part in the DT interview, 19 returned feedback questionnaires. In all, 18 patients evaluated DT as helpful ("It was helpful, because DT gave me a feeling of stability" [M 43]) or satisfactory ("It was far more than satisfactory. DT is a gift. It was more than I expected" [M 43]); 14 patients agreed that DT heightened their sense of dignity ("I feel accepted the way I am" [W 42]). All patients were satisfied with their psychosocial care. Statistics and selected comments for all items are presented in Table 5.

Family member feedback questionnaires on the DT intervention

Out of 30 nominated relatives, 26 provided feedback and 23 of these evaluated DT as helpful for their loved ones ("To reminisce has brought up many smiles and shown how beautiful his life was and how precious life is." [M N99]); 20 relatives agreed that DT was as important as any other aspect of care ("To talk about former times reduced spiritual pain." [W N23]). Further, 24 relatives would recommend DT to other patients and families ("All terminally ill should receive help in this wonderful way." [M N128]). Statistics and selected comments for all items are presented in Table 6.

Establishment of the final consensus version

The collected data led to the establishment of a consensus version, discussed by a DT expert group (S.S.M., S. G., E.J., and Jan Gramm and Jochen Spang). Slight changes to the intermediate translated version of the DTQP were made for Q3, Q4, Q5, Q8, Q9, Q10 and Q12. As "proud" was not a sensitive issue for HCPs or patients, Q7 remained. The final German version of the DTQP is provided as Additional file 5.

Discussion

This is the first report evaluating DT in Germany. DT is a feasible intervention for PCUs in Germany and has demonstrated high levels of acceptability among patients, relatives and HCPs. The German DTQP has now been proved ready for the implementation of DT in Germany; it also provides a starting point for further research. Our methodological procedure included independent double forward-backward translation, discussions with HCPs, cognitive interviews with patients on their experience of the DT interview and

Table 6 Family member feedback questionnaires on DT

Item	*N*	strongly agreed or agreed (*n* / %)	disagreed or strongly disagreed (*n* / %)	neither agreed or disagreed (*n* / %)	Selected Comments (ID)
I believe Dignity Therapy was helpful to my loved family member.	26	23 / 88.5	–	3 / 11.5	To reminisce has brought up many smiles and shown how beautiful his life was and how precious life is. (M N99)
I believe Dignity Therapy helped to give my family member a heightened sense of purpose or meaning in his life.	26	16 / 61.5	–	10 / 38.5	One week after, my father changed his decision to hasten death and decided to fight again. (M N21)
I believe Dignity Therapy helped to increase my family member's sense of dignity.	26	16 / 61.5	1 / 3.8	9 / 34.6	To "work" within an interview was an accomplishment for her that she made because her testimonies were important. (M N136)
I believe Dignity Therapy helped prepare my family member for death.	26	17 / 65.4	–	9 / 34.6	In doing [DT] my beloved wife could reminisce about various situations or moments while she was dealing with her own death. (M N68)
I believe Dignity Therapy was as important a component of my family member's care as any other aspect of their care, including pain management.	26	20 / 76.9	1 / 3.8	5 / 19.2	To talk about former times reduced spiritual pain. (W N23) Intensive care and pain management make suffering and pain bearable for the patient. (M N128)
I believe Dignity Therapy helped reduce my family member's suffering.	26	14 / 53.8	1 / 3.8	11 / 42.3	Not really reducing the suffering – but in a way bringing comfort. (M N43)
Dignity Therapy helps me during my time of grief.	25	13 / 52.0	1 / 4.0	11 / 44.0	To hold something in your hand does you some good. (W N86)
Dignity Therapy will continue to be a source of comfort for my family and me.	25	16 / 64.0	3 / 12.0	6 / 24.0	It will because it is a kind of 'love-legacy' of my godmother. (M N136)
I would recommend Dignity Therapy to other patients or family members who are dealing with a terminal illness.	26	24 / 92.4	1 / 3.8	1 / 3.8	All terminally ill should receive help in this wonderful way. (M N128)

the set of questions they were asked, and finally, general feedback on DT as an intervention from both patients and their family members. By providing the cognitive interview guidelines (Additional file 1 & Additional file 2), we want to contribute to further research projects on the implementation of DT in different international linguistic and cultural settings. The aspects of acceptability (for HCPs) and helpfulness and meaningfulness (for patients and relatives) were supported within this sample, although this result is limited by a small sample, mainly of patients suffering from cancer. Overall, 30 out of 72 (41.7%) eligible patients participated. For the aspect of feasibility, our results are encouraging compared to a two-year Danish study on DT that included 80 out of 389 eligible patients (23.5%) [17], as well as to a study by Hall [18], where 45 out of 188 (24%) patients responded. However, in a Portuguese study by Julião et al. only 4 of 92 patients declined to participate [9]. As we found within the cognitive interviews, DT is an intervention that is most successful through a respectful relationship between the therapist and the patient; it has to be taken into account that the effectiveness of the intervention might be influenced by the interviewing therapist. The need for further research into the efficacy of DT from the viewpoint of different HCPs and in diverse settings is described at length by Fitchett [8]. The mechanism of action of DT on psychological and spiritual needs is also largely unexplored. Wang et al. have identified a lack of randomized controlled trials on life review interventions in general and especially for DT [19]. So far, only a Portuguese study found significant reductions in psychological distress by DT [9].

Conclusions

In summary, DT appears as a feasible and promising intervention in Germany – as well as in numerous other countries – for patients approaching the end of life. Further research on the mechanism of action and suitable methods to elucidate its effects on patients and relatives is highly warranted. Finally, there is also a need to further evaluate sources of funding for DT, as well as the impact of an extensive implementation.

Additional files

Additional file 1: Interview guide for HCP focus groups. (DOCX 39 kb)
Additional file 2: Interview guide for patient cognitive interviews. (DOC 80 kb)
Additional file 3: DT Patient feedback questionnaire. (DOC 99 kb)
Additional file 4: DT Family feedback questionnaire. (DOC 95 kb)
Additional file 5: German version of the Dignity Therapy Question Protocol. (DOC 24 kb)

Abbreviations

COREQ: Consolidated criteria for reporting qualitative research; DT: Dignity Therapy; DTQP: Dignity Therapy Question Protocol; EORTC: European Organisation for Research and Treatment of Cancer; HCP: Healthcare professionals; M: Mainz; PCU: Palliative care unit; W: Würzburg

Acknowledgements

We thank all patients and relatives for participating in this study and giving us insight into their lives. We thank Harvey Max Chochinov for inspiring us with Dignity in Care and training in Dignity Therapy. His invaluable support was most helpful and appreciated. Thank you to Joerg Hildebrandt, who interviewed several patients for this study in Mainz. Thank you to Jan Gramm and Jochen Spang, who participated in the EORTC translation process of the DTQP. Data used in this study will be published in an MD thesis (Sandra Stephanie Mai, University Hospital Mainz, Germany). Parts of the data were presented as a Poster Abstract (P01-382) at the 15th World Congress of the European Association for Palliative Care. More information on DT in Germany is available at www.patientenwuerde.de/.

Funding

This study received no specific grant from any funding agency in the public, commercial or non-profit sectors.

Authors' contributions

SSM developed the study design, conducted the interviews with HCPs and patients, analysed the qualitative and quantitative data, and drafted the manuscript. SG developed the cognitive interview guidelines, conducted the interviews with HCPs, organized the study conduction in Mainz and analysed the qualitative data. EJ organized the study conduction in Würzburg and conducted the interviews with patients in Würzburg. BvO contributed to the study organization in Würzburg. K-HR contributed to the study design. MW took part in the development of the study design and critically reviewed the manuscript. All authors provided critical comments on drafts of the manuscript and approved the final version.

Competing interests

The authors declare that they have no competing interests.

Author details

[1]Interdisciplinary Palliative Care Unit, III. Department of Medicine, University Medical Center of the Johannes Gutenberg University of Mainz, Mainz, Germany. [2]Interdisciplinary Center for Palliative Medicine, University Hospital Würzburg, Würzburg, Germany. [3]Department of Psychology, Bundeswehr University Munich, Neubiberg, Germany.

References

1. Block SD. Psychological issues in end-of-life care. J Palliat Med. 2006;9:751–72.
2. Vehling S, Mehnert A. Symptom burden, loss of dignity, and demoralization in patients with cancer: a mediation model. Psychooncology. 2014;23:283–90.
3. Chochinov HM, Hack T, McClement S, Kristjanson L, Harlos M. Dignity in the terminally ill: a developing empirical model. Soc Sci Med. 2002;54:433–43.
4. Monforte-Royo C, Villavicencio-Chavez C, Tomas-Sabado J, Mahtani-Chugani V, Balaguer A. What lies behind the wish to hasten death? A systematic review and meta-ethnography from the perspective of patients. PLoS One. 2012;7:e37117.
5. Rodriguez-Prat A, Balaguer A, Booth A, Monforte-Royo C. Understanding patients' experiences of the wish to hasten death: an updated and expanded systematic review and meta-ethnography. BMJ Open. 2017;7:e016659.

6. Chochinov HM, Hack T, Hassard T, Kristjanson LJ, McClement S, Harlos M. Dignity therapy: a novel psychotherapeutic intervention for patients near the end of life. J Clin Oncol. 2005;23:5520–5.
7. Chochinov HM. Dignity therapy: final words for final days: Oxford University Press; 2012.
8. Fitchett G, Emanuel L, Handzo G, Boyken L, Wilkie DJ. Care of the human spirit and the role of dignity therapy: a systematic review of dignity therapy research. BMC Palliat Care. 2015;14:8.
9. Julião M, Oliveira F, Nunes B, Carneiro AV, Barbosa A. Effect of dignity therapy on end-of-life psychological distress in terminally ill Portuguese patients: a randomized controlled trial. Palliat Support Care. 2017:1–10.
10. Houmann LJ, Rydahl-Hansen S, Chochinov HM, Kristjanson LJ, Groenvold M. Testing the feasibility of the dignity therapy interview: adaptation for the Danish culture. BMC Palliat Care. 2010;9:21.
11. Tong A, Sainsbury P, Craig J. Consolidated criteria for reporting qualitative research (COREQ): a 32-item checklist for interviews and focus groups. Int J Qual Health Care. 2007;19:349–57.
12. Dewolf L, Koller M, Velikova G, Johnson C, Scott N, Bottomley A. EORTC quality of life group translation procedure. 3rd ed. Brussels: EORTC Quality of Life Group Publication; 2009.
13. Cognitive Interviewing WGB, Tool A. For improving questionnaire design. London: SAGE Publications; 2005.
14. Kuckartz U. Qualitative text analysis: a guide to methods, practice and using software. London: Sage Publications; 2014.
15. Chochinov HM, Kristjanson LJ, Breitbart W, et al. Effect of dignity therapy on distress and end-of-life experience in terminally ill patients: a randomised controlled trial. Lancet Oncol. 2011;12:753–62.
16. McClement S, Chochinov HM, Hack T, Hassard T, Kristjanson LJ, Harlos M. Dignity therapy: family member perspectives. J Palliat Med. 2007 Oct;10(5): 1076–82.
17. Houmann LJ, Chochinov HM, Kristjanson LJ, Petersen MA, Groenvold M. A prospective evaluation of dignity therapy in advanced cancer patients admitted to palliative care. Palliat Med. 2014;28:448–58.
18. Hall S, Goddard C, Opio D, Speck PW, Martin P, Higginson IJ. A novel approach to enhancing hope in patients with advanced cancer: a randomised phase II trial of dignity therapy. BMJ Support Palliat Care. 2011; 1:315–21.
19. Wang CW, Chow AY, Chan CL. The effects of life review interventions on spiritual well-being, psychological distress, and quality of life in patients with terminal or advanced cancer: a systematic review and meta-analysis of randomized controlled trials. Palliat Med. 2017; doi:10/1177/0269216317705101

14

Palliative care for patients with cancer: do patients receive the care they consider important?

Marianne Heins[1*], Jolien Hofstede[1], Mieke Rijken[1], Joke Korevaar[1], Gé Donker[1] and Anneke Francke[1,2,3]

Abstract

Background: In many countries, GPs and home care nurses are involved in care for patients with advanced cancer. Given the varied and complex needs of these patients, providing satisfactory care is a major challenge for them. We therefore aimed to study which aspects of care patients, GPs and home care nurses consider important and whether patients receive these aspects.

Methods: Seventy-two Dutch patients with advanced cancer, 87 GPs and 26 home care nurses rated the importance of support when experiencing symptoms, respect for patients' autonomy and information provision. Patients also rated whether they received these aspects. Questionnaires were based on the CQ index palliative care.

Results: Almost all patients rated information provision and respect for their autonomy as important. The majority also rated support when suffering from specific symptoms as important, especially support when in pain. In general, patients received the care they considered important. However, 49% of those who considered it important to receive support when suffering from fatigue and 23% of those who wanted to receive information on the expected course of their illness did not receive this or only did so sometimes.

Conclusion: For most patients with advanced cancer, the palliative care that they receive matches what they consider important. Support for patients experiencing fatigue may need more attention. When symptoms are difficult to control, GPs and nurses may still provide emotional support and practical advice. Furthermore, we recommend that GPs discuss patients' need for information about the expected course of their illness.

Keywords: Palliative care, Primary health care, Home care services, Neoplasms, Quality of care

Background

Although survival in patients with cancer has increased markedly in the past few decades, more than a third of patients with cancer still die within 5 years of the diagnosis [1–4]. This is often preceded by a period of months, sometimes years, in which patients receive palliative care. When cure or life prolongation is the main goal, care for patients with cancer is mostly provided by hospital professionals. At the end of life, when the main goal of care is improvement in the quality of life rather than cure or life prolongation, most patients prefer to remain at home [5]. In countries with a strong primary care system, general practitioners (GPs) and home care nurses are often closely involved in the care for patients with advanced cancer [6–12]. The involvement of GPs and home care nurses has several benefits: patients are more likely to die in their preferred place [13, 14] and they are less likely to have emergency department visits [15]. At the same time, the care needs of patients with advanced cancer are complex. Patients often suffer from a combination of complex symptoms, such as pain, fatigue, dyspnoea, anxiety and depression [16]. Given the varied and complex needs of these patients, providing satisfactory care and support in managing these symptoms is a major challenge for the GPs and home care professionals involved.

Besides providing support when a patient suffers from physical or psychological symptoms, GPs and home care

* Correspondence: m.heins@nivel.nl
[1]Netherlands Institute for Health Services Research (NIVEL), P.O Box 1568, 3500 BN Utrecht, The Netherlands
Full list of author information is available at the end of the article

professionals may also find it challenging to ensure good information provision and respect for the patient's autonomy. Patients' preferences are patient-specific and may change over time, and patients may eventually experience problems expressing their wishes. The medical and scientific community is increasingly aware of the importance of respecting patients' autonomy and of satisfactory information provision. This is implemented through the concept of advance care planning: the process of discussing in good time and recording patient preferences concerning the goals of palliative care, and of subsequently planning this care [17]. Advance care planning poses challenges for healthcare providers, such as GPs and home care nurses, in ensuring proper information provision and respecting the autonomy of patients [17].

In addition, studies of the quality of palliative care indicate that symptoms are not always managed properly [18–22], and that information provision and respecting the patient's autonomy could be improved [21, 22]. However, in these studies information was often collected from relatives rather than directly from patients themselves, while other studies did not focus specifically on patients with advanced cancer. Given this lack of knowledge about the specific preferences and experiences of patients with advanced cancer, more insight is needed into their opinions about these subjects in order to optimise these aspects of palliative care. Also, given the important role of GPs and home care nurses in palliative care, it could be helpful to have insight into the extent to which their perspective on respecting autonomy and information provision match with that of their patients with advanced cancer. We therefore formulated the following research questions for this study:

1. What aspects of care do patients with advanced cancer consider important regarding support when experiencing specific symptoms, respect for autonomy and the provision of information?
2. Do the perspectives of patients regarding respect for autonomy and information provision match with what GPs and home care nurses consider important?
3. Does the care that advanced cancer patients actually receive match with what they consider important regarding care for physical and psychosocial well-being, respect for autonomy, and information?

Methods

Study design

We applied a stepwise approach. First we recruited GPs, who then selected patients with advanced cancer in their practice according to the selection criteria provided by the researchers and invited them to participate in the study. Patients who gave informed consent to participate in the study and were receiving home care were asked to invite one of their home care nurses (registered nurses or certified nurse assistants) to participate.

Participants

We randomly selected 3000 GPs from the national GP registry, which holds the addresses of all the GPs in the Netherlands. They were sent an information letter and reply form. In the information letter they were asked whether they were willing to recruit one or more of their advanced cancer patients and – if so – whether they were also willing to complete a questionnaire about these patients. GPs who replied that they were willing to participate were sent a written questionnaire for themselves or, if they preferred, a link to the online version of the questionnaire. Besides, these GPs were sent information letters and questionnaires on paper for their patients and home care nurses. The GPs were asked to recruit patients and hand the information letters and questionnaires to patients with a diagnosis of cancer with a poor prognosis (i.e. the GP would not be surprised if the patient were to die within a year). Patients in the terminal phase or those who were mentally or cognitively unable to fill in a questionnaire in Dutch had to be excluded. There was no restriction on the number of patients that GPs could recruit.

In the information package that the patient received from the GP (which included an information letter and questionnaires), the patient was also asked to pass an information letter and questionnaire on to one of their home care nursing staff if they were receiving home care.

Measures

For data collection among patients, we used the following sections from the Consumer Quality Index ('CQ Index') Palliative care [21]: 'Care for physical and psychosocial well-being (with items on support when a patient had specific symptoms)' 'Respect for autonomy' and 'Information'.

The CQ Index Palliative Care is a valid and reliable instrument [23] that contains questions about how important certain care aspects are for patients or relatives (importance items) and corresponding questions about actual care experiences (experience items). For the importance items, patients are asked to rate the importance of items on a four-point Likert-scale, ranging from 'not important' to 'very important'. For the experience items, patients are asked to rate their experience on a four-point Likert-scale, ranging from 'no/never' to 'always'. For the questions about support when experiencing specific symptoms, the option 'not applicable' could be chosen if a patient had not experienced a symptom. The original CQ Index Palliative Care asks about care given by care professionals in general, while we asked specifically about care received from a GP or home care nurse.

In the questionnaires for the GPs and home care nurses, we rephrased the questions to reflect the perspective of the GP or home care nurse. For instance, 'Are you involved in decisions about your care?' (which was an item in the section on 'Information provision') was changed to 'Do you involve patients in decisions about their care?' Not all of the questions we asked patients were applicable to GPs and home care nurses. For instance, we did not ask the GPs and nurses whether they gave patients contradictory information or a clear explanation, as we expect that GPs and home care nurses will try to give consistent and understandable information. We also did not include questions about support when a patient suffers from a specific symptom, as patients may receive this support from another health professional.

Table 1 Background characteristics of patients

Background characteristic	Patients ($n = 72$)
Age (yrs.)	70.5 (8.9)
Sex	
Male (%)	35 (49%)
Female (%)	37 (51%)
Cancer site	
Lung	21 (29%)
Colorectal	15 (21%)
Breast	11 (15%)
Prostate	6 (8%)
Pancreatic	4 (5%)
Time after diagnosis	
< 6 months	18 (25%)
6 months – 1 year	13 (18%)
1–2 years	16 (22%)
2–5 years	19 (26%)
> 5 years	6 (8%)
Home care	
No	32 (44%)
Personal care	30 (42%)
Medical care	20 (28%)
Housekeeping	14 (19%)
Missing	1 (1%)

Statistical analyses

Descriptive statistics - frequencies and percentages or means (with 95% confidence intervals), depending on the type of variable - were computed for the background characteristics and importance scores. In the analyses of the experience scores, we excluded patients who rated an aspect as 'not important'. Analyses were performed using Stata/SE 14.2.

Results

Participants

A total of 87 GPs participated in the study. They were predominantly male (57%) and had on average 19 years of experience as a GP. 60% had received some form of palliative care education, mostly special courses.

Between June 2015 and January 2016, we recruited 72 patients through the participating GPs. Half of the patients were male and their mean age was 70. Most were diagnosed with lung or colorectal cancer. The time since diagnosis ranged from less than 6 months to over 5 years (Table 1).

We recruited 26 home care nurses via the participating patients. The nurses were predominantly female (85%). They had on average 11 years of experience as a home care nurse and almost all (88%) had received some form of palliative care education.

What aspects of care do patients consider important?

The majority of the patients considered support when experiencing specific symptoms as important or very important, although some patients rated items as not important (9–15%) (Fig. 1). Mean importance scores were between 2.7 and 2.9 on a four-point scale (Table 2). An exception was 'support when in pain' and 'support when experiencing shortness of breath', which hardly any patients rated as not important (0 and 4%, respectively) (Fig. 1).

Almost all patients rated items related to 'respect for autonomy' or 'information provision' as important or very important, ranging from 89% for receiving information about the expected course of the disease to 99% for being involved in decisions about care (Fig. 2). Mean importance scores ranged from 3.4 to 3.6 on a scale of 1 (not important) to 4 (very important).

What do GPs and home care nurses consider important, and does this match with patients' opinions?

Almost all GPs rated aspects of 'respect for autonomy' and 'information provision' as important or very important (96–98%). They considered these aspects even more important than patients themselves (Table 2). Almost all home care nurses considered the items 'involving patients in decisions' and 'assigning a contact person' as very important (96 and 88%, respectively). None of the GPs or home care nurses rated an aspect as not important (Fig. 2).

Do patients receive the care they consider important?

Some patients who considered receiving support when experiencing a certain symptom to be at least somewhat

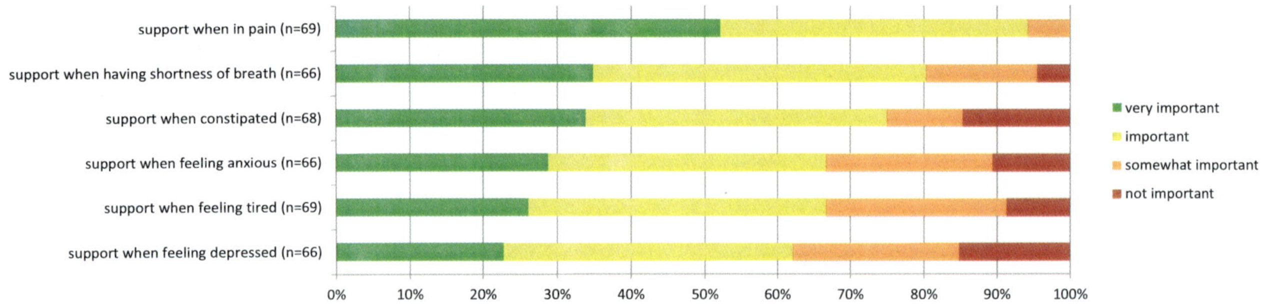

Fig. 1 Perceived importance of aspects of support when having a specific symptom as rated by patients

important did not receive this support or only did so sometimes. For most symptoms the proportion ranged between 20 and 30%. The exceptions were feeling tired, for which almost 50% of the patients did not receive support or only received support sometimes, and being in pain, for which only 13% received no or only occasional support (Fig. 3).

As to respect for autonomy and information provision, most patients indicated that they did indeed receive the care they considered important. The only aspect that a considerable number of patients considered important but did not receive or only received sometimes was information about the expected course of the illness (23% of those who considered it at least somewhat important to receive this information) (Fig. 3).

Discussion

Main findings

Patients with advanced cancer as well as their GPs and home care nurses considered respect for autonomy and information provision to be very important and most patients did indeed receive these aspects of care. Patients considered support when experiencing specific symptoms somewhat less important. However, about a third of those who considered it important to receive support from the GP or home care nurse when they experienced a specific symptom indicated that they did not receive this support or only did so sometimes. For fatigue, this was the case for almost half of the patients. An exception was support when in pain, which patients considered more important

Table 2 Mean importance score (95% CI) for aspects of respect for autonomy and information provision as rated by patients, GPs and home care nurses

Item	Patients	GPs	Home care
Care for physical and psychosocial well-being			
Support when in pain	3.46 (3.32–3.61)	–	–
Support when experiencing shortness of breath	3.11 (2.90–3.31)	–	–
Support when constipated	2.94 (2.69–3.19)	–	–
Support when feeling anxious	2.85 (2.61–3.09)	–	–
Support when feeling tired	2.84 (2.62–3.06)	–	–
Support when feeling depressed	2.70 (2.45–2.94)	–	–
Respect for autonomy			
Patient is involved in decisions about care	3.63 (3.50–3.75)	3.87 (3.78–3.95)	3.96 (3.88–4.04)
Professional caregivers take personal preferences into account	3.58 (3.45–3.71)	–	–
Information provision			
Professional caregivers give consistent information	3.61 (3.48–3.74)	–	–
Patient knows who the contact person is for care	3.56 (3.41–3.70)	3.66 (3.55–3.77)	3.88 (3.75–4.02)
Patient receives information about benefits and risks of treatment	3.51 (3.34–3.69)	3.63 (3.52–3.74)	–
Professional caregivers explain things in a way patient understands	3.51 (3.37–3.66)	–	–
Patient receives information about expected course of the illness	3.39 (3.19–3.58)	3.61 (3.49–3.73)	–

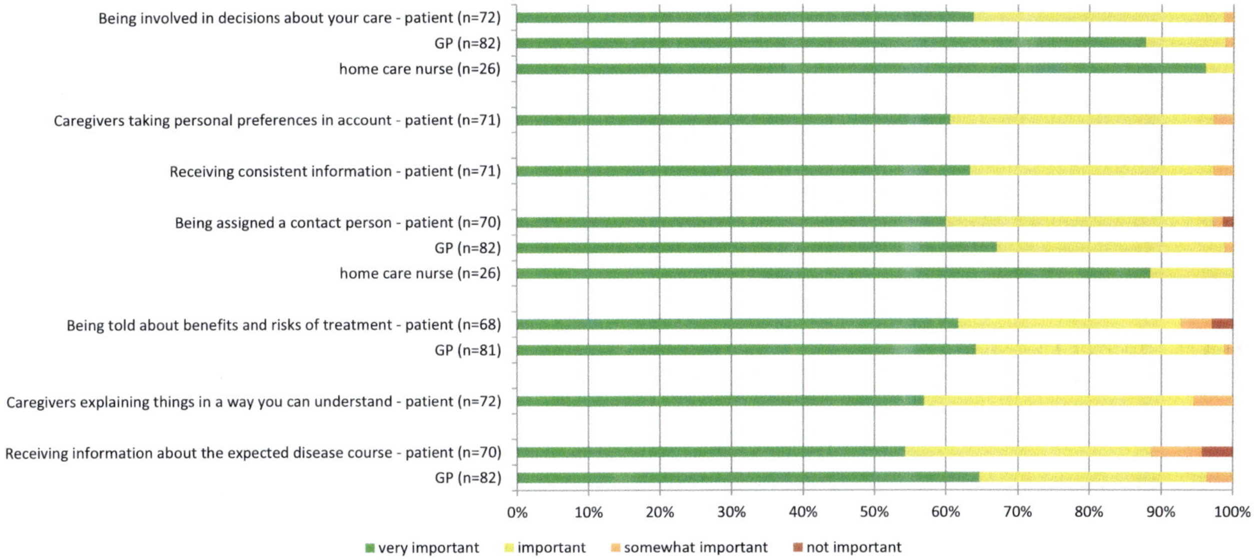

Fig. 2 Importance of aspects of respect for autonomy and information provision as rated by patients, GPs and home care nurses

than support for other symptoms and which they also received more often.

Strengths and limitations

A strength of our study is that we asked patients, their GPs and their home care nurses about their opinions and experiences regarding important aspects of palliative care. This enabled us to compare different points of view. We chose a stepwise inclusion process, first inviting GPs, who then asked patients, who then asked nurses. The advantage was that we could make couples of patients and GPs and GPs were familiar with the situation of the patients and could therefore assess whether patients were able to be contacted and interviewed. However, the stepwise inclusion process may have led to selection bias. Firstly, few GPs responded to the study invitation, the response rate was very low (3%), so we may for example have selected GPs who were specifically interested in the care for advanced cancer patients. Nevertheless, the age and sex profiles of the participating GPs were quite similar to the nationwide figures (mean age of 51 vs. 48 and 42% vs. 48% female) [24]. Secondly, GPs may have selected patients with whom they had a good relationship and patients may have done the same in selecting home care nurses. Our results could therefore be too positive. Thirdly, patients may have felt obliged to respond positively when answering questions about their care that their GP had asked them to answer. However, as patients filled in the questionnaires at home and sent them to the researchers, we think it is not very likely that this influenced the results. An alternative method could have been for instance, to select patients through internet fora, which possibly would have led to lower appreciation for the care received,

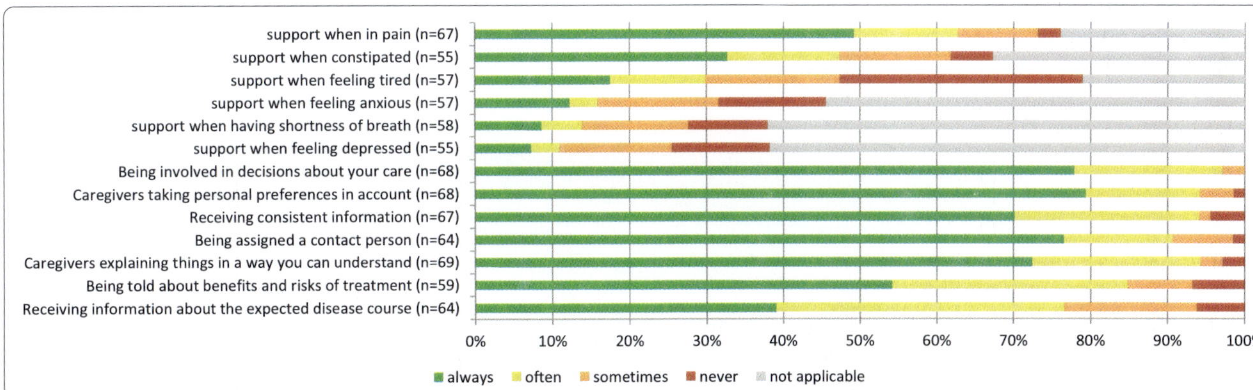

Fig. 3 Received aspects of care rated by patients who find these aspects important*. * patients who rated an aspect as not important were not included

as it is conceivable that patients with negative experiences are more active on these fora. Another alternative inclusion method could have been via the treating specialist, yet, this route would have exclude patients who are no longer being treated by their oncologist, resulting in bias by disease stage.

Another limitation related to our stepwise recruitment is that the number of home care nurses participating in the study was relatively low ($n = 26$). This is because only a limited number of patients were receiving home care delivered by nurses ($n = 32$). As we received questionnaires from most of these nurses, we can assume no selection took place of nurses who were particularly interested in palliative care or had a good relationship with the patient. A validation study using a different sampling method would be interesting.

Interpretation of the study results in relation to existing literature

A comparison of our results with an earlier study of patients' opinions and experiences of palliative care for patients with varying diseases (cancer, chronic obstructive pulmonary disease (COPD), heart failure and other non-cancer diseases) reveals some differences [21]. The patients with advanced cancer in our study considered respect for autonomy as more important than a broader group of patients receiving palliative care (3.58–3.63 vs. 3.46–3.49). Patients in our study considered aspects of support when experiencing specific symptoms to be less important (2.70–3.11 vs. 3.04–3. 36), with the exception of support when in pain, which both samples considered equally important (3.46 vs. 3.51). This may be explained by findings of previous studies that cancer patients have more palliative care, palliative treatments, discussion of end-of-life topics and advance care planning than palliative patients without cancer [6, 25]. Cancer patients may thus have fewer unmet needs as to support from professionals when experiencing symptoms.

In line with the results of our study, previous studies found that most cancer patients had talked to their GPs about life expectancy, possible medical complications and the burden imposed by treatments [6, 25]. GPs are generally better able to foresee imminent death in patients with cancer compared with patients with COPD or chronic heart conditions [26]. This is related to the fact that the disease trajectory is often less variable in cancer than in other chronic life-threatening disease [27], which may facilitate discussing prognosis [28]. This may explain why GPs are more likely to discuss the prognosis with cancer patients. As to support when patients experience physical or psychological symptoms, other studies also reported a need for improvement [18, 29], although it should be stressed that full control of common symptoms like fatigue, shortness of breath and pain may not always be possible.

Implications

Our results indicate potential room for improvement in the support provided by GPs and home care nurses to patients experiencing symptoms, especially fatigue. This could be done by giving more attention to possible symptoms, even if this means acknowledging that full symptom control may not be achievable, particularly in the final phase of the disease. Our results also indicate that it is important that information about the expected course of the illness is tailored to the individual preferences of a patient, as preferences may differ between patients and over time. However, we acknowledge that providing information about the expected course of the illness may be difficult, as this course may not always be predictable. Besides, information provision should be broader than just information about the expected course of the disease. Relating to advance care planning, it should for instance also include the opportunities for good care if a patient suffers from certain symptoms, as well as discussing the patient's perspective on end-of-life decisions about (potentially) life-prolonging or life-shortening treatments.

Conclusions

In conclusion, we found that most patients with advanced cancer receive the care that they consider important. Aspects that could possibly be improved are the support the GPs give when a patient experiences fatigue and discuss with patients whether they want to receive information about the expected course of the illness.

Abbreviations

GP: General practitioner; CQ Index: Consumer quality index; COPD: Chronic obstructive pulmonary disease

Acknowledgements

We would like to thank all patients, GPs and nurses for their participation and Clare Wilkinson for critically revising the English language.

Funding

The study was funded by the Stichting Stoffels-Hornstra. They had no role in study design, data collection, analysis and interpretation of the data, decision to publish, or writing of the manuscript.

Authors' contributions

JH, MR, JK, GD, AF were involved in the conception and design of the study. JH performed the data acquisition, MH performed the data analyses and drafted the manuscript. JH, MR, JK, GD, AF were involved in revising it critically for important intellectual content. All authors gave final approval of the version to be published and agree to be accountable for all aspects of the work.

Competing interests

The authors declare that they have no competing interests.

Author details
[1]Netherlands Institute for Health Services Research (NIVEL), P.O Box 1568, 3500 BN Utrecht, The Netherlands. [2]Amsterdam Public Health research institute, VU University Medical Center, Amsterdam, the Netherlands. [3]Expertise center palliative care, VU University Medical Center, Amsterdam, the Netherlands.

References

1. Australian Institute of H, Welfare. Cancer survival and prevalence in Australia: period estimates from 1982 to 2010. Asia Pac J Clin Oncol. 2013;9:29–39.
2. Baili P, Di Salvo F, Marcos-Gragera R, Siesling S, Mallone S, Santaquilani M, Micheli A, Lillini R, Francisci S, Group E-W. Age and case mix-standardised survival for all cancer patients in Europe 1999-2007: results of EUROCARE-5, a population-based study. Eur J Cancer. 2015;51(15):2120–9.
3. Siegel RL, Miller KD, Jemal A. Cancer statistics, 2016. CA Cancer J Clin. 2016;66:7–30.
4. Siesling S, Visser O, Luth TK, Karim-Kos HE, van de Poll-Franse LV, Aben KK, Damhuis RA. Adult cancer patients are surviving longer in the Netherlands: 5-year survival rate increased by 12% between the periods 1989-1993 and 2004-2008. Ned Tijdschr Geneeskd. 2011;155:A3169.
5. Billingham MJ, Billingham SJ. Congruence between preferred and actual place of death according to the presence of malignant or non-malignant disease: a systematic review and meta-analysis. BMJ Support Palliat Care. 2013;3:144–54.
6. Abarshi E, Echteld M, Donker G, Van den Block L, Onwuteaka-Philipsen B, Deliens L. Discussing end-of-life issues in the last months of life: a nationwide study among general practitioners. J Palliat Med. 2011;14:323–30.
7. Abarshi E, Echteld MA, Van den Block L, Donker G, Bossuyt N, Meeussen K, Bilsen J, Onwuteaka-Philipsen B, Deliens L. Use of palliative care services and general practitioner visits at the end of life in the Netherlands and Belgium. J Pain Symptom Manag. 2011;41:436–48.
8. Abarshi E, Echteld MA, Van den Block L, Donker G, Deliens L, Onwuteaka-Philipsen B. The oldest old and GP end-of-life care in the Dutch community: a nationwide study. Age Ageing. 2010;39:716–22.
9. Meeussen K, Van den Block L, Echteld MA, Boffin N, Bilsen J, Van Casteren V, Abarshi E, Donker G, Onwuteaka-Philipsen B, Deliens L. End-of-life care and circumstances of death in patients dying as a result of cancer in Belgium and the Netherlands: a retrospective comparative study. J Clin Oncol. 2011; 29:4327–34.
10. Donker GA, Slotman FG, Spreeuwenberg P, Francke AL. Palliative sedation in Dutch general practice from 2005 to 2011: a dynamic cohort study of trends and reasons. Br J Gen Pract. 2013;63:e669–75.
11. Rhee JJ, Zwar N, Vagholkar S, Dennis S, Broadbent AM, Mitchell G. Attitudes and barriers to involvement in palliative care by Australian urban general practitioners. J Palliat Med. 2008;11:980–5.
12. Mitchell S, Loew J, Millington-Sanders C, Dale J. Providing end-of-life care in general practice: findings of a national GP questionnaire survey. Br J Gen Pract. 2016;66:e647–53.
13. Ko W, Miccinesi G, Beccaro M, Moreels S, Donker GA, Onwuteaka-Philipsen B, Alonso TV, Deliens L, Van den Block L, Euro I. Factors associated with fulfilling the preference for dying at home among cancer patients: the role of general practitioners. J Palliat Care. 2014;30:141–50.
14. Aabom B, Kragstrup J, Vondeling H, Bakketeig LS, Stovring H. Does persistent involvement by the GP improve palliative care at home for end-stage cancer patients? Palliat Med. 2006;20:507–12.
15. Burge F, Lawson B, Johnston G. Family physician continuity of care and emergency department use in end-of-life cancer care. Med Care. 2003; 41:992–1001.
16. Moens K, Higginson IJ, Harding R, Euro I. Are there differences in the prevalence of palliative care-related problems in people living with advanced cancer and eight non-cancer conditions? A systematic review. J Pain Symptom Manag. 2014;48:660–77.
17. Seymour J, Almack K, Kennedy S. Implementing advance care planning: a qualitative study of community nurses' views and experiences. BMC Palliat Care. 2010;9:4.
18. Hanratty B. Palliative care provided by GPs: the carer's viewpoint. Br J Gen Pract. 2000;50:653–4.
19. Neergaard MA, Olesen F, Jensen AB, Sondergaard J. Palliative care for cancer patients in a primary health care setting: bereaved relatives' experience, a qualitative group interview study. BMC Palliat Care. 2008;7(1)
20. Hofstede JM, Raijmakers NJ, van der Hoek LS, Francke AL. Differences in palliative care quality between patients with cancer, patients with organ failure and frail patients: a study based on measurements with the consumer quality index palliative care for bereaved relatives. Palliat Med. 2016;30:780–8.
21. Claessen SJ, Francke AL, Sixma HJ, de Veer AJ, Deliens L. Measuring patients' experiences with palliative care: the consumer quality index palliative care. BMJ Support Palliat Care. 2012;2:367–72.
22. Yamagishi A, Sato K, Miyashita M, Shima Y, Kizawa Y, Umeda M, Kinoshita H, Shirahige Y, Akiyama M, Yamaguchi T, et al. Changes in quality of care and quality of life of outpatients with advanced cancer after a regional palliative care intervention program. J Pain Symptom Manag. 2014;48:602–10.
23. De Boer D, Hofstede JM, De Veer AJE, Raijmakers NJH, Francke AL. Relatives perceived quality of palliative care: comparisons between care setting where a patient dies. BMC Palliat Care. 2017;16(1):41.
24. Van Hassel D, Kasteleijn A, Kenens R. Cijfers uit de registratie huisartsen: peiling 2015. Utrecht: NIVEL; 2016.
25. Evans N, Pasman HR, Donker GA, Deliens L, Van den Block L, Onwuteaka-Philipsen B, On behalf of E. End-of-life care in general practice: a cross-sectional, retrospective survey of 'cancer', 'organ failure' and 'old-age/dementia' patients. Palliat Med. 2014;28:965–75.
26. Claessen SJ, Francke AL, Echteld MA, Schweitzer BP, Donker GA, Deliens L. GPs' recognition of death in the foreseeable future and diagnosis of a fatal condition: a national survey. BMC Fam Pract. 2013;14:104.
27. Murray SA, Kendall M, Boyd K, Sheikh A. Illness trajectories and palliative care. BMJ. 2005;330:1007–11.
28. Slort W, Schweitzer BP, Blankenstein AH, Abarshi EA, Riphagen II, Echteld MA, Aaronson NK, van der Horst H, Deliens L. Perceived barriers and facilitators for general practitioner-patient communication in palliative care: a systematic review. Palliat Med. 2011;25:613–29.
29. Yamagishi A, Morita T, Miyashita M, Igarashi A, Akiyama M, Akizuki N, Shirahige Y, Eguchi K. Pain intensity, quality of life, quality of palliative care, and satisfaction in outpatients with metastatic or recurrent cancer: a Japanese, nationwide, region-based, multicenter survey. J Pain Symptom Manag. 2012;43:503–14.

Chemotherapy and palliative care near end-of life: examining the appropriateness at a cancer institute for colorectal cancer patients

Ilaria Massa[1], Oriana Nanni[1*], Flavia Foca[1], Marco Maltoni[2], Stefania Derni[3], Nicola Gentili[4], Giovanni Luca Frassineti[5], Andrea Casadei Gardini[5], Martina Valgiusti[5], Dino Amadori[5], Elena Prati[6], Mattia Altini[6], Davide Gallegati[7] and Elisabetta Sansoni[2]

Abstract

Background: Appropriate cessation of chemotherapy and timely referral of patients to hospice services are crucial for the quality of care near death. We investigated the quality of care in our Cancer Institute in very advanced metastatic colorectal cancer patients treated in real life.

Patients and Methods: We performed a retrospective analysis of electronic medical data of patients with metastatic colorectal cancer who were candidates for chemotherapy during the study period (1 January 2007–30 June 2014) and died before 31 December 2014. Quality-of-cancer-care indicators were calculated for the overuse of chemotherapy and referral to hospice. Predictive factors of chemotherapy discontinuation and hospice referral in end-of life care were investigated using parametric and nonparametric methods.

Results: Of the 365 patients who died before 31 December 2014, 26 (7.1%) received chemotherapy in the last 14 days of life and 36 (9.8%) started a new chemotherapy regimen in the last 30 days of life. Factors associated with the overuse of chemotherapy were being < 70 years of age for both indicators and not having received advanced chemotherapy treatments for the former indicator. The majority of patients (74.7%) had access to hospice services, of whom only a small percentage (7.2%) accessed them very near to death.

Conclusions: According to the criteria used, our Institute provides a good quality of cancer care for dying colorectal cancer patients, measured by the use of chemotherapy and referral to hospice in their last days of life.

Keywords: Appropriateness, Chemotherapy, Palliative care, End of life, Indicators

Background

Despite the progress made in cancer care, cancer is still a lethal disease and the use of chemotherapy remains crucial for both curative and palliative purposes. However, the appropriate use of chemotherapy is still unclear near death. The subtle difference between curative and palliative intent when palliative chemotherapy can extend life is under debate [1]. In addition, patient prognosis is complex to predict and the few survival prediction tools available are not easy to use. To date, there has been a lack of international guidelines on the management of cancer patients near death, except for the American Society of Clinical Oncology (ASCO) and the European Society of Medical Oncology [2, 3]. Therefore, the decision to stop a specific treatment in favor of the best palliative care is still incredibly hard and the so-called "therapeutic inertia", i.e. the persistence of inappropriate antitumor treatments in non-responding terminal patients, is frequently used. Such overly aggressive care not only affects a patient's quality of life (QoL) [4] but, from a healthcare system point of view, it raises questions about system sustainability given the

* Correspondence: oriana.nanni@irst.emr.it
[1]Unit of Biostatistics and Clinical Trials, Istituto Scientifico Romagnolo per lo Studio e la Cura dei Tumori (IRST) IRCCS, Meldola, Italy
Full list of author information is available at the end of the article

increasing costs of cancer care (about 20% per year in the U.S. in the period 1990–2020) [5].

Earle et al. identified aggressive care near the end of life (EoL) as a sign of poor quality cancer services [6] and proposed quality indicators of cancer care for external benchmarking. Three major areas were evaluated: a) possible misuse of treatment resulting in high rates of emergency room visits, hospitalization, or intensive care unit admission; b) lack of referral or very late referral to hospice; c) overuse of chemotherapy very near to death [7]. Although numerous studies have meásured some of these indicators, different criteria were used to define populations of interest, making a comparison of results more difficult.

In the present paper we report our data from a retrospective cohort study conducted at our institute (IRST IRCCS) in which we assessed the behavior of physicians towards chemotherapy prescription and the access of terminal colorectal cancer (CRC) patients to hospice care. Our objectives were to gain better knowledge have a better knowledge of the quality of cancer care services in our institute, and a deeper insight into how we manage end-of-life EoL care in a subset of patients. In particular, we aimed to report the frequency of some internationally acknowledged indicators of quality cancer care and to identify whether some factors related to patient characteristics or the organization of services provided can affect the use of chemotherapy and the referral to hospice care at EoL.

Methods

Study design and participants

We conducted a retrospective analysis of the electronic medical data of metastatic CRC patients with candidate to receive chemotherapy. We included all the consecutive patients resident in the catchment area of Forlì (188,357 inhabitants ref. year 2013) and in the adjacent area of Cesena Local Health Authority (AUSL) (209,622 inhabitants ref. year 2013) who were candidates to receive chemotherapy in a metastatic setting from 1 January 2007 to 30 June 2014 and had died before 31 December 2014. The following information was collected for each patient: age of death, gender, number of lines received for advanced disease, date of last cycle of chemotherapy and date of start of last new line of therapy. ECOG Performance Status information was collected on the day of the last chemotherapy line prescription and on the day of the last administration, or in a time range varying from the day of the last administration and 7 days before administration.

With regard to access to palliative care, analysis was possible only for a subgroup of patients who were resident in the Forlì catchment area and who died between February 2009 and December 2014, since registration of access to the palliative care network was recorded from February 2009 onwards. As cancer patients living in the two neighboring areas of Forlì and Cesena are followed by our cancer institute, we were able to verify the homogeneity of the two populations by gender, age, previous treatment for advanced disease, PS ECOG (0 vs. > 1) (data not shown).

The date of the first access to palliative care was retrieved for patients admitted to hospice or home-based hospice care for at least 1 day. Results obtained for this subpopulation can be generalized are representative of the entire population because patient characteristics were the same and all patients were followed at our institute. Patients who had only received best supportive care and patients enrolled in clinical trials were excluded.

Description of indicators

To evaluate appropriate prescription of chemotherapy, we considered 2 indicators proposed by Earle et al. [7] and measured them on the population of patients receiving chemotherapy, as follows:

a) proportion of patients who started a new chemotherapy regimen in the last 30 days of life. The proposed appropriate threshold of $< 2\%$ was set as standard.
b) proportion of patients who received chemotherapy administration in the last 14 days of life.

The proposed appropriate threshold of $< 10\%$ was set as standard by Earle et al. [7].

We considered all types of palliative care interventions which represent constitute the "Local Palliative Care Network (LPCN)". The network is divided into two types of interventions: early palliative care, which is further divided into outpatient and inpatient care for patients undergoing chemotherapy, and EoL palliative care, which is further divided into inpatient hospice care and home-based hospice care mainly for those who are no longer amenable to chemotherapy. Although some authors [8] consider home-based hospice care as a form of early palliative care, we, together with others [9–11], regard it as a form of EoL palliative care, as the average length of stay for patients in this setting is about 60–90 days.

With regard to early palliative care interventions during the study period, oncologists did not systematically refer patients to a palliative care specialist but only requested their intervention for pain and symptom management. We did not thus were unable to analyze the impact of early palliative care on the decision of the oncologist as to whether or not prescribe administer chemotherapy.

We used the following 2 indicators proposed by Earle et al. [7], measured on the population of patients for whom the date of access to palliative care was available, to evaluate appropriate access to hospice services:

- proportion of patients receiving hospice services before death to compare with the proposed appropriate threshold of > 55%;
- proportion of the above-mentioned patients admitted to hospice 3 days before death to compare with the proposed appropriate threshold of < 8%.

The proposed appropriate thresholds were set as standard by Earle et al. [7].

We then compared our data considering both forms of EoL palliative care.

Statistical methods

Categorical variables were expressed as frequencies and percentages, while continuous variables were presented using median and range.

The relationship between demographic and clinical characteristics and patient status based on the considered indicators were analyzed using chi-square, Fisher exact test or Cochran-Armitage test for trend as appropriate. In case of continuous variables, Wilcoxon Mann-Whitney test was used.

Logistic regression was used to investigate the effect explanatory variables (age, gender and previous line of advanced therapy) to evaluate the physician's behavior in the management of cancer patients in the last days of life (last chemotherapy scheme prescription ≤30 days vs. > 30 days to death; last chemotherapy cycle administration ≤14 days vs. > 14 days to death). To describe the association, adjusted odds ratios (OR) with 95% profile likelihood confidence intervals (95%CI) were evaluated. A p-value of < 0.05 was considered statistically significant. Statistical analyses were carried out with SAS Statistical software (version 9.3, SAS Institute, Cary, NC, USA).

Results

Population characteristics

We observed 365 patients with metastatic CRC deceased before 31 December 2014 who had started a new chemotherapy regimen with palliative intent in at our Institute between 1 January 2007 and 30 June 2014. Males were 58.9% and median age was 70 years (33–87) (Table 1). Considering previous treatment features, 245 patients out of 365 (67.1%) had already received at least 1 chemotherapy treatment in metastatic setting.

Use of chemotherapy

Thirty-six (9.8%) patients out of 365 started a new chemotherapy regimen in the last month of life, while 26 (7.1%) patients received last chemotherapy administration within 14 days before death. Out of the former 36 patients receiving a new chemotherapy regimen, 12 (33.3%) received a first-line treatment, 12 (33.3%) a second-line, 8 (22.2%) a third-line, and 4 (11.2%) > third-line.

Results showed that, among the patients receiving aggressive chemotherapy approach in the last month of life, patients aged ≤70 years of age were likely to receive a more aggressive approach (12.8% vs. 6.8%, $p = 0.05$) than older patients. Considering the last chemotherapy administration in the last 14 days of life, age ≤ 70 years

Table 1 Patient characteristics and factors associated to the use of CT in the EoL

	Total No. (%)	New CT scheme prescription > 30 days to death No. (%)	New CT scheme prescription ≤30 days to death No. (%)	p-value	Last CT cycle administration > 14 days to death No. (%)	Last CT cycle administration ≤14 days to death No. (%)	p-value
Overall	365 (100.0)	329 (90.1)	36 (9.8)	–	339 (92.9)	26 (7.1)	–
Gender							
Male	215 (58.9)	190 (88.4)	25 (11.6)	0.18	200 (93.0)	15 (7.0)	0.90
Female	150 (41.1)	139 (92.7)	11 (7.3)		139 (92.7)	11 (7.3)	
Age							
Median (range)	70 (33–87)	71 (33–87)	63.5 (37–83)	0.13	70 (33–87)	62.5 (45–80)	0.09
≤ 70 years	188 (51.5)	164 (87.2)	24 (12.8)	0.05	170 (90.4)	18 (9.6)	0.06
> 70 years	177 (48.5)	165 (93.2)	12 (6.8)		169 (95.5)	8 (4.5)	
Period of study inclusion							
2007–2010	142 (38.9)	129 (90.9)	13 (9.1)	0.72	136 (95.8)	6 (4.2)	0.09
2011–2014	223 (61.1)	200 (89.7)	23 (10.3)		203 (91.0)	20 (8.9)	
Previous treatment for advanced disease							
None	120 (32.9)	108 (90.0)	12 (10.0)	0.95	105 (87.5)	15 (12.5)	< 0.01
At least one	245 (67.1)	221 (90.2)	24 (9.8)		234 (95.5)	11 (4.5)	

(9.6% vs. 4.5%, $p = 0.06$) and not having received previous advanced treatments ($p < 0.01$) were predictive factors for aggressive behavior. Neither gender nor years of treatment (2007–2010 vs. 2011–2014) appeared to influence the chemotherapy approach (Table 1). These results were maintained in the multivariate analysis (Fig. 1).

With regard to ECOG Performance Status (PS) at the start of the last line of chemotherapy (or within the previous 7 days) (data were available for 192 patients out of 365, 52.6%), we observed that 158 (82.3%) patients had either ECOG PS 0 or 1, while 34 patients (17.7%) had either ECOG PS 2 or 3 (Table 2). At the time of the last chemotherapy administration, ECOG PS was available for 129 patients out of 365 (35.3%) and was either 0 or 1 for 91 patients (70.6%), and either 2 or 3 for 38 patients (29.4%). As expected, we found that the distribution of PS of patients who received both a new chemotherapy line in the last month of life and the last chemotherapy administration in the last 14 days of life and those who did not, was different, worsening for the group of patients who received chemo in the last period of life. This factor was not included in the multivariate analysis due to the high amount of missing data. These results are maintained in a multivariate analysis (Fig. 1).

Access to hospice services

Regarding access to LPCN, we found that out of 166 patients resident in the Forlì catchment Local health Authority area, 28 (16.9%) patients had never had a palliative care contact with the LPCN in the advanced setting, while the remaining 138 (83.1%) had had at least one contact. In particular, 73 (44%) patients had at least one early palliative care visit, 124 (74.7%) patients accessed at least one EoL palliative care service (Hospice inpatient admission and Home-Care Hospice Program), and 59 (35.5%) patients accessed both EoL palliative care services. Out of the 124 patients who had access to EoL palliative care, 9 (7.2%) referred to the hospice in the last 3 days of life (Table 3). A higher, albeit not significant, percentage of patients who had had an early palliative consultation (80.8% vs. 69.9%, $p = 0.11$) accessed the hospice. However, no difference in terms of appropriate access (> 3 days from death) to Hospice itself was found among patients.

Discussion

According to Earle's criteria, our Institution carries out an acceptable "therapeutic inertia" in terms of chemotherapy administration in the last 14 days of life (7.1% compared to < 10% proposed by Earle). Nevertheless, improvements should be made concerning the start of a new chemotherapy regimen in the last month of life (9.8% compared to < 2% proposed by Earle). When considering factors predictive of therapeutic inertia, we found that age ≤ 70 years was associated with a more aggressive treatment in both starting a new chemotherapy line in the last 30 days of life and receiving chemotherapy in the last 14 days of life, as confirmed in literature [12–14]. Although this behavior might be acceptable from a psychological point of view, it is not indeed supported by any scientific basis, as highlighted by earlier studies [13]: a more balanced approach is currently being studied.

In this study, female gender and treating physician were no predictor factors, unlike in other studies [15]. Since our Institution is organized into pathology-specific medical teams, an appointed group of physicians regularly meeting to discuss clinical cases is in charge of the management of CRC patients, thus reducing bias of treating physician.

As for the role of PS in the decision making process, we observed that it is likely to be poorer for patients very near death. In fact, as expected, PS is poorer in patients receiving chemotherapy in the last period of life than in patients not receiving any, due to the different timing respect to death in which it was measured.

In clinical studies with chemotherapy, eligibility criteria usually couple a good PS (ECOG 0–1, less frequently 0–2) with a survival prognosis of at least 3 months. Functional activity indexes can correctly evaluate disability, but need to be combined and integrated with other parameters in order to assess prognosis. Recent evidence from Prigerson [4], that combined PS values, chemotherapy administration and QoL near

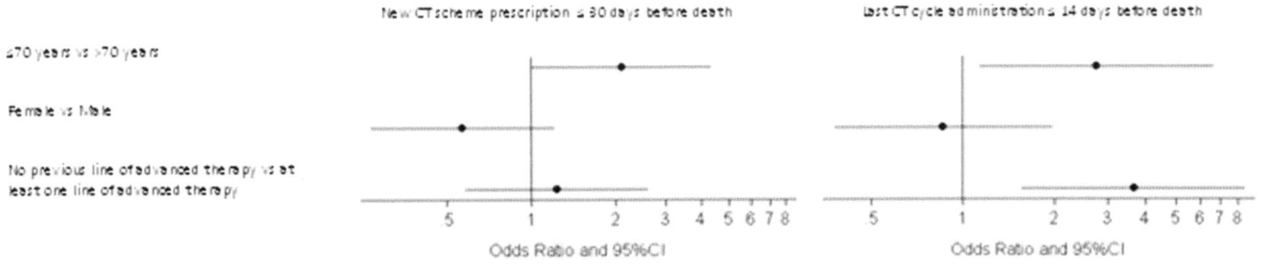

Fig. 1 Clinical factors associated to therapeutic inertia

Table 2 EoL chemotherapy and PS ECOG distribution

	Total No. (%)	New CT scheme prescription > 30 days to death No. (%)	New CT scheme prescription ≤30 days to death No. (%)	*p*-value	Total No. (%)	Last CT cycle administration > 14 days to death No. (%)	Last CT cycle administration ≤14 days to death No. (%)	*p*-value
Overall	192 (100.0)	170 (88.5)	22 (11.5)		129 (100.0)	115 (89.1)	14 (10.9)	
PS (ECOG)								
0	78 (40.6)	75 (96.2)	3 (3.8)	< 0.01	34 (26.4)	32 (94.1)	2 (5.9)	0.01
1	80 (41.7)	74 (92.5)	6 (7.5)		57 (44.2)	51 (89.5)	6 (10.5)	
2	28 (14.6)	18 (64.3)	10 (35.7)		35 (27.1)	30 (85.7)	5 (14.3)	
3	6 (3.1)	3 (50.0)	3 (50.0)		3 (2.3)	2 (66.7)	1 (33.3)	

death, showed that chemotherapy administration did not improve QoL for patients with poor PS. On the contrary, it can be detrimental on QoL for patients with good PS. Prognosis in advanced cancer patients is a highly debated topic. For this reason, some tools have been studied in palliative care. Among them, the Palliative Prognostic Score (PaP Score) [16–18] has been an accurate tool in several independent terminally ill cancer case series, classifying the studied population into 3 subgroups according to life expectancy and demonstrating that it could help clinicians to better select those patients who could actually benefit from a palliative chemotherapy. Pap Score could be assessed at every cycle of chemotherapy together with ECOG PS.

Some methodological issues on therapeutic inertia near death are noteworthy. Many publications [12, 19, 20] have measured these indicators in different types of cancer and settings in a non-homogeneous way, changing criteria to define the population of interest, so that it is almost impossible to compare data from different institutions.

We could compare our population, representing the entire population in the catchment area of our Cancer Institute, with a Canadian study [21] and an Australian study [15]: our percentage for treatment in the last 14 days is lower than in Canada, while it is similar to Australia. It is worth mentioning that, like in Australia but unlike in Canada, we restricted our analysis to CRC patients, excluding hematological malignancies which are usually more aggressively treated. In Earle's publications, indicators were evaluated on a cohort monitored by one of the SEER (Surveillance, Epidemiology and End Results) registry whose Medicare population was > 65 years old, thus not allowing for wide comparability of percentages.

Focusing on "EoL palliative care interventions" within LPCN, we found that about 74.7% of our patients that died of cancer had received EoL palliative care. Overall, as only 16.9% of colorectal cancer patients had no access to LPCN during their cancer history, palliative care was guaranteed to the vast majority of the cancer population in this setting, and referring to EoL palliative care services, they were accessed in a timely and appropriate manner. We found also that referral to early palliative care consultation can aid subsequent referral to EoL hospice care.

In order to better understand the role of early palliative care (EPC) on patient outcome and QoL, our Institute carried out a randomized clinical trial on patients with advanced pancreas cancer, confirming that systematic EPC significantly improved QoL with respect to on-demand EPC. A positive impact was also observed for some indicators of EoL treatment aggressiveness, including the administration of chemotherapy during the last 30 days of life [22, 23]. These data confirmed the findings of Temel, Bakitas and ASCO Provisional Clinical Opinion, all of which highlighted the benefits of palliative care combined with standard anticancer therapies [24–26].

The main limitations of the present study include its retrospective design and the collection of data performed in a wide time range in a non-homogeneous way leading to a suboptimal completeness of retrieved data (i.e. ECOG PS). Moreover, as it was impossible to establish the reasons for chemotherapy discontinuation, we

Table 3 Relationship between early PC consultation and access to EoL-PC (*n* = 166)

	Total	Access to EoL Palliative Care			
		None	At least one	Before ≤3 days to death	Within ≤3 days to death
	No. (%)	No. (%)	No. (%)	No. (%)	No. (%)
Overall	166 (100.0)	42 (25.3)	124 (74.7)	115 (92.8)	9 (7.2)
Access to early PC consultation					
None	93 (56.0)	28 (30.1)	65 (69.9)		
At least one	73 (44.0)	14 (19.2)	59 (80.8)		

assumed it was due to progression of disease. Another limitation is that we hypothesized that death had always been cancer-related without, however, linking data to a death registry, which may have resulted in an underestimation of deaths. Despite these limitations, we used real-world clinical data, as the best informative way that can change clinical practice. An essential tool for this research was the Electronic Health Records (EHR), which allow to conduct a variety of research projects, from retrospective studies to monitoring programs like this one, that involve all treated patients for estimating the value of healthcare. Despite the lengthy adoption time of EHRs, we believe that data collection will improve over time both quantitatively and qualitatively, overcoming the limitations of using administrative data only. Our Institute has recently set up an operative taskforce, involving clinicians, methodologists, cost management specialists, and the healthcare direction to regularly verify clinical outcomes, appropriateness and costs, so that health resources can be employed to the best.

Conclusions

In conclusion, our assessment of the frequency of some indicators of cancer care quality shows that, according to the criteria used, our institute provides a good quality of care to the CRC patients included in this study. For the Palliative Care Community, our experience can contribute to the "culture of measuring" that needs to be enhanced in EoL care, in order to improve the quality of care. In this vision, multicenter experiences must be promoted, including also cost evaluations for a more complete picture of EoL cancer care.

Abbreviations

ASCO: American Society of Clinical Oncology; AUSL: Local Health Authority; CI: Confidence interval; ECOG PS: Eastern cooperative oncology group performance status; EHR: Electronic Health Record; EoL: End of life; EPC: Early palliative care; IRST IRCCS: Istituto Scientifico Romagnolo per lo Studio e la Cura dei Tumori (IRST) IRCCS; LPCN: Local Palliative Care Network; OR: Odds ratio; PaP Score: Palliative prognostic score; QoL: Quality of life; SEER: Surveillance Epidemiology and End Results

Acknowledgements

The authors wish to thank Grainne Tierney and Veronica Zanoni for editing the manuscript.

Funding

This project was partially funded by MoH RF-2011-02350971 (ministerial project).

Authors' contributions

IM, ON, MA and MM conceived and designed the study, SD, ES, GLF, ACG and MV provided the study materials, IM, FF, EP and NG collected the data, IM, FF, ON and MM did the data analysis and interpreted the results, IM, FF, ON and MM prepared the manuscript, DA and DG revised it and all the authors finally approved the manuscript and agreed to be accountable for all aspects of the work.

Competing interests

The authors declare that they have no competing interests.

Author details

[1]Unit of Biostatistics and Clinical Trials, Istituto Scientifico Romagnolo per lo Studio e la Cura dei Tumori (IRST) IRCCS, Meldola, Italy. [2]Palliative Care Unit, Istituto Scientifico Romagnolo per lo Studio e la Cura dei Tumori (IRST) IRCCS, Meldola, Italy. [3]Palliative Care Unit, AUSL Romagna, Forlì, Italy. [4]IT Unit, Istituto Scientifico Romagnolo per lo Studio e la Cura dei Tumori (IRST) IRCCS, Meldola, Italy. [5]Department of Medical Oncology, Istituto Scientifico Romagnolo per lo Studio e la Cura dei Tumori (IRST) IRCCS, Meldola, Italy. [6]Healthcare Administration, Istituto Scientifico Romagnolo per lo Studio e la Cura dei Tumori (IRST) IRCCS, Meldola, Italy. [7]Planning and Control, Istituto Scientifico Romagnolo per lo Studio e la Cura dei Tumori (IRST) IRCCS, Meldola, Italy.

References

1. Harrington SE, Smith TJ. The role of chemotherapy at the end of life: "when is enough, enough?". JAMA. 2008;299:2667–78.
2. Peppercorn JM, Smith TJ, Helft PR, Debono DJ, Berry SR, Wollins DS, Hayes DM, Von Roenn JH, Schnipper LE. American Society of Clinical Oncology statement: toward individualized care for patients with advanced cancer. J Clin Oncol. 2011;29:755–60.
3. Cherny NI, Catane R, Kosmidis P. ESMO takes a stand on supportive and palliative care. Ann Oncol. 2003;14:1335–7.
4. Prigerson HG, Bao Y, Shah MA Paulk ME, LeBlanc TW, Schneider BJ, Garrido MM, Reid MC, Berlin DA, Adelson KB, Neugut AI, Maciejewski PK. Chemotherapy use, performance status, and quality of life at the end of life. JAMA Oncol. 2015;1:778–84.
5. Sullivan R, Peppercorn J, Sikora K, Zalcberg J, Meropol NJ, Amir E, Khayat D, Boyle P, Autier P, Tannock IF, Fojo T, Siderov J, Williamson S, Camporesi S, McVie JG, Purushotham AD, Naredi P, Eggermont A, Brennan MF, Steinberg ML, De Ridder M, McCloskey SA, Verellen D, Roberts T, Storme G, Hicks RJ, Ell PJ, Hirsch BR, Carbone DP, Schulman KA, Catchpole P, Taylor D, Geissler J, Brinker NG, Meltzer D, Kerr D, Aapro M. Delivering affordable cancer care in high-income countries. Lancet Oncol. 2011;12:933–80.
6. Earle CC, Landrum MB, Souza JM, Neville BA, Weeks JC, Ayanian JZ. Aggressiveness of cancer care near the end of life: is it a quality-of-care issue? J Clin Oncol. 2008;26:3860–6.
7. Earle CC, Neville BA, Landrum MB, Souza JM, Weeks JC, Block SD, Grunfeld E, Ayanian JZ. Evaluating claims-based indicators of the intensity of end-of-life cancer care. Int J Qual Health Care. 2005;17:505–9.
8. Davis MP, Temel JS, Balboni T, Glare P. A review of the trials which examine early integration of outpatient and home palliative care for patients with serious illnesses. Ann Palliat Med. 2015;4:99–121.
9. Maltoni M, Derni S, Innocenti MP, Rinaldi A, Amadori D. Description of a home care service for cancer patients through quantitative indexes of evaluation. Tumori. 1991;77:453–9.
10. Hughes SL, Cummings J, Weaver F, Manheim L, Braun B, Conrad K. A randomized trial of the cost effectiveness of VA hospital-based home care for the terminally ill. Health Serv Res. 1992;26:801–17.
11. Jordhøy MS, Fayers P, Saltnes T, Ahlner-Elmqvist M, Jannert M, Kaasa S. A palliative-care intervention and death at home: a cluster randomised trial. Lancet. 2000;356:888–93.
12. Numico G, Trogu A, Cristofano A, Mozzicafreddo A, Courthod G, Franco P, Silvestris N. Active treatment given in the last weeks of life: poor quality cancer care or justifiable behavior? Support Care Cancer. 2014;22:2813–9.
13. Yun YH, Kwak M, Park SM, Kim S, Choi JS, Lim HY, Lee CG, Choi YS, Hong YS, Kim SY, Heo DS. Chemotherapy use and associated factors among cancer patients near the end of life. Oncology. 2007;72:164–71.

14. Gonçalves JF, Goyanes C. Use of chemotherapy at the end of life in a Portuguese oncology center. Support Care Cancer. 2008;16:321–7.
15. Kao S, Shafiq J, Vardy J, Adams D. Use of chemotherapy at end of life in oncology patients. Ann Oncol. 2009;20:1555–9.
16. Maltoni M, Nanni O, Pirovano M, Scarpi E, Indelli M, Martini C, Monti M, Arnoldi E, Piva L, Ravaioli A, Cruciani G, Labianca R, Amadori D. Successful validation of the palliative prognostic score in terminally ill cancer patients. Italian Multicenter Study Group on Palliative Care. J Pain Symptom Manage. 1999;17:240–7.
17. Pirovano M, Maltoni M, Nanni O, Marinari M, Indelli M, Zaninetta G, Petrella V, Barni S, Zecca E, Scarpi E, Labianca R, Amadori D, Luporini G, Italian Multicenter and Study Group on Palliative Care. A new palliative prognostic score: a first step for the staging of terminally ill cancer patients. J Pain Symptom Manage. 1999;17:231–9.
18. Tassinari D, Montanari L, Maltoni M, Ballardini M, Piancastelli A, Musi M, Porzio G, Minotti V, Caraceni A, Poggi B, Stella A, Aielli F, Scarpi E. The palliative prognostic score and survival in patients with advanced solid tumors receiving chemotherapy. Support Care Cancer. 2008;16:359–70.
19. Zdenkowski N, Cavenagh J, Ku YC, Bisquera A, Bonaventura A. Administration of chemotherapy with palliative intent in the last 30 days of life: the balance between palliation and chemotherapy. Intern Med J. 2013; 43:1191–8.
20. Sezgin Goksu S, Gunduz S, Unal D, Uysal M, Arslan D, Tatlı AM, Bozcuk H, Ozdogan M, Coskun HS. Use of chemotherapy at the end of life in Turkey. BMC Palliat Care. 2014;13:51.
21. Barbera L, Paszat L, Chartier C. Indicators of poor quality end-of-life cancer care in Ontario. J Palliat Care. 2006;22:12–7.
22. Maltoni M, Scarpi E, Dall'Agata M, Schiavon S, Biasini C, Codecà C, Broglia CM, Sansoni E, Bortolussi R, Garetto F, Fioretto L, Cattaneo MT, Giacobino A, Luzzani M, Luchena G, Alquati S, Quadrini S, Zagonel V, Cavanna L, Ferrari D, Pedrazzoli P, Frassineti GL, Galiano A, Casadei Gardini A, Monti M, Nanni O, Early palliative care Italian study group (EPCISG). Systematic versus on-demand early palliative care: A randomised clinical trial assessing quality of care and treatment aggressiveness near the end of life. Eur J Cancer. 2016; 69:110–8.
23. Maltoni M, Scarpi E, Dall'Agata M, Zagonel V, Bertè R, Ferrari D, Broglia CM, Bortolussi R, Trentin L, Valgiusti M, Pini S, Farolfi A, Casadei Gardini A, Nanni O, Amadori D, Early palliative care Italian study group (EPCISG). Systematic versus on-demand early palliative care: results from a multicentre, randomised clinical trial. Eur J Cancer. 2016;65:61–8.
24. Temel JS, Greer JA, Muzikansky A, Gallagher ER, Admane S, Jackson VA, Dahlin CM, Blinderman CD, Jacobsen J, Pirl WF, Billings JA, Lynch T. Early palliative care for patients with metastatic non-small-cell lung cancer. N Engl J Med. 2010;363:733–42.
25. Bakitas M, Lyons KD, Hegel MT, Balan S, Brokaw FC, Seville J, Hull JG, Li Z, Tosteson TD, Byock IR, Ahles TA. Effects of a palliative care intervention on clinical outcomes in patients with advanced cancer: the project ENABLE II randomized controlled trial. JAMA. 2009;302:741–9.
26. Smith TJ, Temin S, Alesi ER, Abernethy AP, Balboni TA, Basch EM, Ferrell BR, Loscalzo M, Meier DE, Paice JA, Peppercorn JM, Somerfield M, Stovall E, Von Roenn JH. American society of clinical oncology provisional clinical opinion: the integration of palliative care into standard oncology care. J Clin Oncol. 2012;30:880–8.

16

Exploring the meaning and practice of self-care among palliative care nurses and doctors

Jason Mills[1,2,3*], Timothy Wand[2] and Jennifer A. Fraser[2]

Abstract

Background: Self-care practice within the palliative care workforce is often discussed, yet seemingly under-researched. While palliative care professionals are required to implement and maintain effective self-care strategies, there appears little evidence to guide them. Moreover, there is an apparent need to clarify the meaning of self-care in palliative care practice. This paper reports qualitative findings within the context of a broader mixed-methods study. The aim of the present study was to explore the meaning and practice of self-care as described by palliative care nurses and doctors.

Methods: A purposive sample of 24 palliative care nurses and doctors across Australia participated in semi-structured, in-depth interviews. Interviews were digitally recorded and transcribed prior to inductive qualitative content analysis, supported by QSR NVivo data management software.

Results: Three overarching themes emerged from the analysis: (1) *A proactive and holistic approach to promoting personal health and wellbeing to support professional care of others*; (2) *Personalised self-care strategies within professional and non-professional contexts;* and (3) *Barriers and enablers to self-care practice.*

Conclusions: The findings of this study provide a detailed account of the context and complexity of effective self-care practice previously lacking in the literature. Self-care is a proactive, holistic, and personalised approach to the promotion of health and wellbeing through a variety of strategies, in both personal and professional settings, to enhance capacity for compassionate care of patients and their families. This research adds an important qualitative perspective and serves to advance knowledge of both the context and effective practice of self-care in the palliative care workforce.

Keywords: Palliative care, Self-care, Self-compassion, Positive emotions, Workforce

Background

The concept of relentless self-care is well known to those in the field of palliative social work [1]. Interest in self-care is growing within the nursing and medical disciplines [2, 3], and its importance to all palliative care professionals is evident internationally through a suite of quality standards, core competencies, and practice standards in which self-care practice is mandated [4–10]. But what does self-care mean?

Self-care is broadly defined by Sherman [11] as 'the self-initiated behaviour that people choose to incorporate to promote good health and general well-being'. Despite this health-promoting emphasis on good health and wellbeing, the palliative care literature focuses largely on coping strategies in the context of occupational stressors such as burnout or compassion fatigue [12]. Clearly, management of stress is very important; however, there are other important aspects of promoting good health and wellbeing that extend beyond the scope of coping with stress. In many cases there also appears to be conflation between the terms coping strategy and self-care strategy. Further confusion about the meaning of self-care was highlighted in an Australian survey of palliative

* Correspondence: jm.mills@qut.edu.au
[1]Institute of Health and Biomedical Innovation, Queensland University of Technology, Kelvin Grove, QLD, Australia
[2]Susan Wakil School of Nursing and Midwifery, The University of Sydney, Camperdown, NSW, Australia
Full list of author information is available at the end of the article

care professionals [13]. Beyond academic definitions, there is a need to understand and articulate the meaning of self-care in a palliative care practice context. Given that some palliative care professionals have reported low levels of self-care ability, there is also an urgent need to explore barriers and enablers to self-care, and identify examples of effective self-care strategies used in practice. In reviewing the literature [12], significant gaps are apparent in the current evidence base for self-care practice and education.

To advance knowledge in these areas, this study aimed to explore the meaning and practice of self-care as described by palliative care nurses and doctors. Specifically, the following research questions were addressed:

1. What is the meaning of self-care, as described by palliative care nurses and doctors?
2. How do palliative care nurses and doctors describe effective self-care practice?

Methods

Research design

Given the nature of the research questions, a qualitative research design was employed [14]. An interview guide (see Table 1) was developed to address the study aim in consideration of gaps identified from the literature. The initial guide was refined in response to feedback received from a small group of palliative care professionals not involved in this study. Open questions were used to elicit deeper exploration of meaning and experience within a flexible yet focused discussion about participants' self-care practice [15].

A purposive sample was recruited into this qualitative research from a pool of palliative care nurses and doctors who had completed a self-care survey as part of a broader mixed-methods study [13]. Consistent with the purpose of obtaining relevant and rich data from an appropriate source, eligible participants were nurses and doctors practising in Australia with palliative care as their main area of practice. Informed written consent was obtained from all participants through initial email contact prior to being interviewed via telephone. A total of 24 semi-structured, in-depth interviews were conducted over a six-month period in 2015, with recruitment ending once data saturation was reached. That is, when the collection of additional data served only to repeat existing rather than generate new content, as identified from the use of field notes and iterative analysis. The first author, an experienced qualitative researcher, conducted all interviews and recorded field notes to support a process of iterative analysis throughout the data collection period. The average duration of interviews was approximately 50 min, with audio content digitally recorded, transcribed verbatim, and de-identified. Gender-appropriate pseudonyms were randomly allocated to each respondent.

Table 1 Interview Guide

- In the context of palliative care practice, what does self-care mean to you?
- From your experience, how would you describe effective self-care practice?
- Tell me about the self-care strategies you find to be most effective
- What supports your self-care practice?
- What, if anything, gets in the way of your self-care practice?

Data analysis

Interview transcripts were initially read and re-read to make note of key words and phrases before importing them into QSR NVivo 11 data management software for open coding and qualitative content analysis. Qualitative content analysis is a widely used method for interpreting the content of textual data through a process of systematic classification, coding, and identification of patterns or themes [16]. As recommended by Graneheim and Lundman [17], a number of decisions were made to guide content analysis and ensure trustworthiness.

First, it was decided that a conventional approach to content analysis would be adopted [16]. That is to say, the analysis was inductive and focused on latent content, or words and sentences that required an interpretation of underlying meaning. Second, whole participant interviews were discerned to be the most appropriate unit of analysis in terms of providing a context for meaning units during the analytical process [17]. Finally, it was decided that these meaning units would comprise interrelated words, sentences and paragraphs from interview transcripts. In this way, interview data were analysed inductively through the generation of codes, grouping and collapsing of codes into common categories, and subsequent abstraction to identify overall themes that represent the raw data in an aggregated form [18, 19]. Figure 1 outlines the thematic coding and category content generated from the content analysis.

Sample

The sample of 24 participants comprised 12 nurses and 12 doctors working in community, inpatient, or consult palliative care services located in both metropolitan and regional/rural settings across six of the eight States and Territories in Australia. These were clinical nurse specialists, nurse educators, clinical nurse consultants, nurse practitioners, nurse unit managers, senior medical officers, consultant physicians, and heads of department. They had an average of 15 years' experience working in either adult, aged, or paediatric palliative care settings. Most were female, aged between 40 and 49, and worked in full-time roles. See Table 2 for detailed participant demographics.

A proactive and holistic approach to promoting personal health and wellbeing to support professional care of others

- ***Meaning***
  - Relational context
  - Balancing care for others with care for self
  - Promotion of health and wellbeing
  - More than just a tick-box checklist

Maintain a range of personalised self-care strategies within professional and non-professional contexts

- ***Self-care strategies used inside the workplace setting***
  - Reflective practice
  - Accessing other staff support
  - Boundaries
  - Regulation of workload
  - Work-life harmony
  - Team-care/healthy team
  - Laughter and use of humour
- ***Self-care strategies used outside the workplace setting***
  - Separating work from home
  - Meditation
  - Spiritual practice
  - Positive social relationships
  - Rest and relaxation
  - Preventative health behaviours
  - Accessing support from health care professionals
- ***Shared responsibility***
  - Individual self-care practice
  - Staff support from employer
- ***Self-care as a personalised and ongoing practice***
  - Practised according to the individual and context
  - Ongoing nature

Manage barriers and enablers to self-care practice

- ***Facilitators of self-care***
  - Recognising importance of self-care
  - Planning and prioritising self-care in a preventative approach
  - Self-awareness
  - Supportive work culture and leadership
  - Leadership/role models to normalise self-care
  - Positive emotions and relationships
  - Character strengths
- ***Impediments to self-care***
  - Unsupportive work culture and environment
  - Stigma
  - Busyness
  - Lack of planning/prioritising self-care
  - Inadequate boundaries between work and home
  - Self-criticism and low self-worth

Fig. 1 Thematic coding and category content

Results

Three overarching themes emerged from the analysis in relation to the meaning and practice of self-care: (1) *A proactive and holistic approach to promoting personal health and wellbeing to support professional care of others*; (2) *Personalised self-care strategies within professional and non-professional contexts*; and (3) *Barriers and enablers to self-care practice.* Figure 2 illustrates the application of these as the meaning and practice of self-care. Thematic data from these themes are reported in Tables 3, 4, and 5, in the form of participant quotations to ensure trustworthiness [20].

Theme 1: A proactive and holistic approach to promoting personal health and wellbeing to support professional care of others

The meaning of self-care was described in terms of its positive relational context with self and others. Although self-care was focused primarily on individual needs, it was informed by the broader clinical context of capacity

Table 2 Participant Demographics and Professional Characteristics ($N = 24$)

Demographic	n (%)
Gender	
Female	15 (63)
Male	9 (37)
Age Group	
30–39 years	4 (17)
40–49 years	11 (46)
50–59 years	7 (29)
≥ 60 years	2 (8)
Population Focus	
Adult Palliative Care	19 (79)
Paediatric Palliative Care	2 (8)
Aged Palliative Care	3 (13)
Work Status	
Full-time	14 (58)
Part-time	10 (42)
Years Worked in Palliative Care	
1–5 years	1 (4)
6–10 years	3 (13)
11–15 years	12 (50)
≥ 16 years	8 (33)

Table 3 Theme 1

A proactive and holistic approach to promoting personal health and wellbeing to support professional care of others	
Prudence	*Through self-care, what we are doing is developing a relationship with ourselves – which actually supports us in developing relationships with everybody else.*
Gwendolen	*Self-care - it's looking after me to look after patients, so to speak; if I'm not of a good healthy physical state or emotional state, I'm hardly likely to be able to support someone.*
Darrell	*You can't look after dying patients without looking after yourself, really, can you? And do a good job of that, in a compassionate way?*
Felicity	*Balancing care for yourself and others is essential.*
Patrick	*It's part of a holistic approach… if you're not caring for yourself then you're less able to care for others.*
Merilyn	*[It's about] maintaining a good balance between body and mind… being able to stay fit and healthy.*
Winston	*You look after your own health so that you can deliver patient-centred care.*
Prudence	*That's what self-care is; it's a way of living, it's a way of living every moment.*
Mason	*The thing is, [self-care] is not a tick-box commodity.*

to engage in positive and therapeutic relationships to provide patient care. Self-care meant fulfilling a fundamental part of palliative care practice, with one participant commenting that self-care *is intrinsic to the work itself.*

Self-care also meant balancing care for others with care for self, with the promotion of personal health and wellbeing central to its meaning. Self-care was described as a conscious and deliberate practice that meant much more than just a 'tick-box' checklist to be completed within a set of allocated tasks.

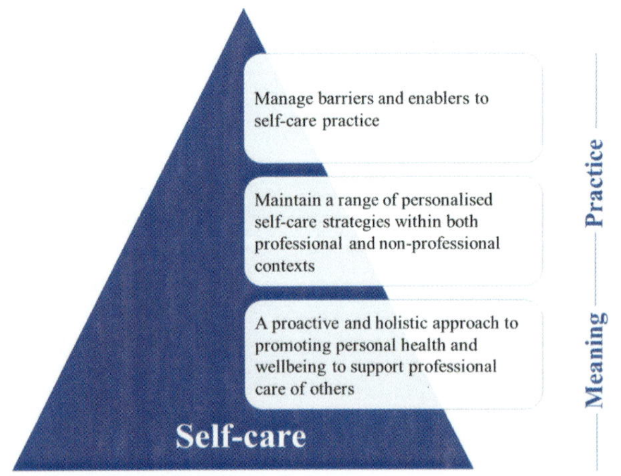

Fig. 2 The meaning and practice of self-care

Theme 2: Personalised self-care strategies within professional and non-professional contexts

Effective self-care practice was described as a personalised and ongoing endeavour. In the words of one participant, *it's a constant work in progress.* Participant descriptions of effective self-care practices were consistently characterised by a variety of self-care strategies that were maintained both within, and external to, workplace settings.

Self-care in personal settings

Effective self-care strategies used outside of the workplace settings included a range of health behaviours, meditation and spiritual practice. A healthy diet, adequate sleep, and moderation of alcohol intake were considered important. In addition to exercising for fitness, other physical activities such as yoga and massage were found to be effective self-care strategies. Rest and relaxation at home in a bath were described as effective self-care strategies when feeling overwhelmed or needing to wash away (metaphorically) thoughts of the workplace. Socialising and maintaining positive relationships with friends and family was both supportive and meaningful. Meditation practice was also an effective self-care used within both personal and professional contexts. A variety of meditation practices were used by participants, including loving kindness

Table 4 Theme 2: Personalised self-care strategies within professional and nonprofessional contexts

Philis	*It's really not formulaic; it's really quite individual, and so everybody has to find their own way of doing it.*
Carmel	*You not only need self-care strategies in the workplace - but also in your personal life.*
Felicity	*I do try and exercise a reasonable amount and I try and get to bed on time because I have to get up at a reasonable time… and diet's important.*
Gwendolen	*I regularly exercise, do yoga and have a regular massage as well.*
Abbie	*[Having] a bath; it's almost like I'm washing the hospital off me.*
Larissa	*I have an extremely supportive, very good husband and I have an extremely good network of friends, so… spending time with family and friends.*
Doreen	*Maintaining relationships with family; making sure I'm spending a reasonable amount of time with my children makes me feel that all is right in the world.*
Abbie	*Meditate for half an hour a day; that's all I actually need to do to function well - I'm great at work, I'm calm with [son]. But if I don't do that, then I get irritable [and] I don't have as much to give at work. With just half an hour of meditation a day as my top priority for the day, I'm just better all round.*
Lucas	*I'm quite involved in my Church, and faith is actually a big anchor [that keeps me grounded].*
Reece	*…my spiritual practice which, for me, is a very reliable tool; Buddhist practices… to do with strengthening my connection with compassion or loving kindness for self and others.*
Deanna	*Work-life balance is really important.*
Sandra	*There's no such thing as work-life balance, it's rubbish.*
Cathi	*If it's after five o'clock: (a) I won't be [at work]; and (b) my diary will be sitting on my desk with my mobile phone on it turned off, with my name tag sitting on it. My computer will be off. [It's] about making certain that work is at work, so I don't take my mobile phone home. I don't take my diary home [to follow up on things]; no, sorry that's work, and it will wait… work stays at work.*
Felicity	*I take the train… I can only arrive at a certain time and leave at a certain time – those boundaries are actually very helpful. I've never been very good at placing boundaries, so I actually have to do this physical boundary of 'Right, the train's leaving, and I have to go' - and that's worked quite well.*
Deanna	*My de-escalating time is driving home and when I walk in the door at home, work stays at work… and I find that something to be really important to me actually – that the two don't intermix.*
Winston	*It's not sustainable to give out more than you really can on an ongoing basis… absolutely [regulating work demands is important].*
Cathi	*I take regular holidays. I'm not somebody who's got an annual leave balance; I always take my meal breaks, take my days off, and sick leave when ill.*
Larissa	*I chose [to work] part-time.*
Scott	*It's very difficult to do self-care without [team] support, and so you support each other in doing self-care at work, definitely.*
Doreen	*A mindful activity, just grounding yourself …this conscious thing of 'Okay, what can I see? What can I feel? What am I touching?*
Carmel	*Supervision [provides] a safe and guided reflective space that allows you to talk about your practice; to think about what is meaningful to you, about a time, something you did, something you've been experiencing recently… allow yourself to really drill into - not just the story - but how did it make you feel… how did you behave… what would you change?*
Darrell	*[informal debriefing] is a sign of a healthy team because that's… self-initiated, as opposed to organised or imposed.*
Deanna	*It's Friday, I'm tired. A lot has gone on, and I'm giving a handover. I get half-way through the ward and then I start wrapping up. And they go, 'What are you doing? There's still the other half of the ward to go yet,' and I'm like, 'Oh, damn'! So, being able to [make a mistake] and be able to laugh about it was important. Being kind and being compassionate about that. Being able to accept that you are human.*
Abbie	*We've all got a very black sense of humour, so it works really well.*

meditation. Spiritual practice was also considered an effective self-care strategy.

Finding harmony between personal and professional roles was consistently described as an effective self-care strategy. Some described this harmony in terms of work-life balance. Interestingly, others found the concept of work-life balance to be problematic in practice. Given the elusive nature and individual context of what constitutes a balance between work and life, most considered it more important to acknowledge that different life-domains require varying degrees of attention at any given time; and that finding individual harmony between personal and professional roles was a key strategy towards flourishing in life. One participant explained:

> *It's never like you've got this nice balance - where work finishes, then you've got an hour to sort of wind down before the rest of life begins... [it's more about] just trying to keep all the different areas of life flourishing* (Darrell).

Establishing and maintaining boundaries between home and the workplace was considered an effective self-care strategy. Some boundaries involved commuting to the

Table 5 Theme 3: Barriers and enablers to self-care practice

Cathi	*There's too many patients and you can't get enough done… busyness contributes to poor self-care because you actually don't stop to go 'How has this affected me? What can I do? What do I need to make me 'okay' about it?'*
Patrick	*There is an expectation that people won't take holidays, but how are people supposed to recharge so they can keep working?*
Scott	*There's this… culture sometimes where you just sort of 'soldier on' and do what's expected – take work home.*
Merilyn	*It just follows you home and it can really impact on your home life and your health, because you're just… stressing about things*
Gordon	*The biggest hindrance to self-care is organisational culture.*
Larissa	*There's a big culture shift that needs to ha in order for people to be able to look after themselves properly.*
Winston	*There is still a lot of stigma around having feelings or accepting feeling or being vulnerable… we do see confronting things but there is still that superhero, you know, not letting it affect you.*
Peggie	*People are considered to be selfish if they do something for themselves… you know, if you take a day off because you're on a mental health day people think 'Oh, she's so selfish because she's let her team down'*
Prudence	*Lack of self-worth and self-value is a bit of an issue… I can see that in how my colleagues - how people treat themselves, and that's not a judgment - it's an observation coming from someone doing pretty much the same kind of thing.*
Sandra	*Self-care always get shoved down to the bottom… that self-worth thing of… you know, something else always being much more important.*
Philis	*I certainly used to be quite critical about myself… which isn't a particularly helpful thing to do really… [most of us] just beat ourselves up emotionally and physically… and then eventually work out why you can't keep doing that for the rest of your life.*
Carmel	*Self-care goes down the toilet when it's random… there's no effective random self-care.*
Peggie	*I'm very conscious of [self-care] because I've been a in bad spot before with palliative care… I really didn't cope very well, so I'm [now] highly vigilant about self-care.*
Gordon	*I was 'young and bullet-proof'… and I found [that] to be a fairly unpleasant experience; 'young and bullet-proof' didn't work very well. But it took me about seven years to work that out, and I became significantly burnt out… So, having burnt out… taken time off, and readjusted… I'm now very conscious of how important self-care is.*
Abbie	*When I do [prioritise self-care] I'm calm and I'm more compassionate.*
Winston	*Preventative maintenance… Yeah, well it is [like having a regular check-up and a tune-up]*
Reece	*I have written self-care plans for myself… but I don't approach that in a sense of, you know, at six months – 'now I need to redo my self-care plan'. An ongoing planning process is the critical element rather than just the piece of paper.*
Carmel	*Leadership. It's got to come from the top. You can't have someone at the top who thinks that people who need to go for counselling are 'poor little things'. Seriously, it's not going to work*
Kaleb	*Having a reasonable degree of self-awareness is hugely important [for effective self-care], particularly in our line of work.*
Cathi	*Finding the positive in situations… also taking account of things that have negatively impacted me [but still finding] something positive.*
Doreen	*…intentionally choose how I want to be each morning, and how I want to leave work, and respond to events; having a mindset of gratitude.*
Reece	*Practising self-compassion is a really important enabler – without that I'm not really sure how authentic my self-care would be.*
Gordon	*Being realistic about your limitations is central to self-care… self-care involves being honest about a whole host of things, and it's primarily being honest with yourself - and being prepared to take that up with other people where you need to - but it's about being honest with yourself in relation to your limitations.*
Lucas	*Contemplating my own mortality is very important in terms of self-care. I have to have confronted that; there but for the Grace of God go I… and this could be me [dying]… Really puts things into perspective and helps you to live and enjoy your life to the full.*

workplace via modes of transport that prevented overworking, while for others the commute time itself constituted a process of unwinding from work so as to separate from it when arriving home.

Self-care in workplace settings

Boundaries were also relevant to effective self-care within the workplace. Awareness of boundaries in this context was supportive in terms of not over-working due to resource limitations, whilst also ensuring clarity of expectations for multiple stakeholders. In the words of one participant:

The amount of resources [allocated to the] palliative care service - that actually creates a certain set of boundaries within which I can work - I'm not going to step over those boundaries; if they want additional work, they need to increase the resourcing... It's about managing expectations around what I will do and what I won't do - and being able to be very upfront in relation to that... with management... with staff that I work with, so [they] are aware of what we can do, and what we can't; but more importantly, with patients and their families, so there's a very clear set of expectations around what can reasonably be done for them (Gordon).

Self-regulation of workload was important, but often difficult to achieve. It involved being assertive about one's capacity in relation to workload and wellbeing. Taking meal breaks, taking recreation leave for regular holidays, and taking personal leave during illness were also considered effective self-care strategies. For some, choosing to work part-time was an effective self-care strategy that provided ongoing regulation of workload in relation to other competing demands.

Self-regulation as a self-care strategy was often supported by other members of the team. In this way, team-care was considered an aspect of effective self-care that contributed to a healthy team. One participant described an example of team-care in terms of checking in with colleagues about how they are feeling, as a reminder and invitation to attend to self-care.

Having a cohesive team was important and this contributed to a supportive working environment. Mindfulness exercises were an effective self-care strategy in the workplace, both in individual and group contexts. A sense of allowing oneself to be human, in the context of displaying emotion in the clinical setting, was also part of effective self-care practice.

Reflective practice, especially through participation in clinical supervision, was described by many as an effective self-care strategy, although formal supervision was not available in all participants' workplace. Importantly, respect and confidentiality were important components for clinical supervision to be effective. But formal supervision was not necessarily helpful for everyone, with many finding informal debriefing with peers to be effective. However, this also required trust among colleagues. While the use of informal debriefing among colleagues was considered a sign of a healthy team, formal, structured debriefing was also common in some workplaces to support self-care. Use of humour and laughter was also an effective self-care strategy used in the workplace, with laughter often expressing a sense of acceptance, kindness and compassion for oneself rather than self-judgement during times when feelings of inadequacy arise.

Participants reported accessing a variety of professional supports as part of effective self-care practice. These ranged from Employee Assistance Programs and private counsellors to psychologists, general practitioners and other medical specialists. For doctors, it was considered especially helpful to seek objective medical advice from a general practitioner. Interestingly, choice of employer was a self-care consideration in terms of gauging organisational commitment to support staff with workplace self-care activities such as clinical supervision. Finally, effective self-care practice was described as a shared responsibility between palliative care professionals and the health services in which they practised. However, there can be a lack of clarity with regards to this shared responsibility.

Theme 3: Barriers and enablers to self-care practice

Participants described the ongoing need to manage self-care barriers and enablers as part of maintaining self-care strategies in both personal and professional contexts.

Self-care barriers

Multiple impediments to self-care were identified in the workplace including busyness. For some, this workload was compounded by limited opportunity to take holidays from work. Workplace culture was also identified as problematic, where it was not conducive to self-care. In some workplace cultures there was a stigma associated with self-care, making it difficult for individuals to engage in self-care practice without feeling judged as being selfish. Bringing work home was described as a barrier to self-care, and related to workplace culture and expectations. Self-worth was also discussed as a common concern for effective self-care, where self-criticism and a lack of self-worth undermined self-care as an important priority. Finally, a lack of planning for self-care, or otherwise adopting a solely ad hoc approach was considered a barrier to effective self-care.

Self-care enablers

Several factors were described as facilitators of effective self-care. Recognising the importance of self-care was considered an important enabler by all. Some became conscious of this through previous experiences of illness or being unwell after having initially neglected self-care. Prioritising self-care was an important enabler which correlated with noticeable benefits. Adopting a preventative approach to self-care was important, whilst recognising that additional strategies may need to be implemented, as required, according to context. While formal self-care plans were used by some, for most participants it was more important to engage in reflection and self-assessment as part of an ongoing planning process, rather than have a static document.

Positive workplace cultures supportive of self-care were described as vital to effective self-care practice. Where a supportive culture was absent, the normalisation of self-care within workplaces was considered a key enabler, requiring leadership from the top-down to effect positive change towards a culture more supportive of self-care. One participant explained:

> *Normalisation... the reason I bang on about [self-care] is because I think, yes, you do need to normalise it. I think the key thing is the ethos of the unit, and I think*

that's set firstly through the medical head but then also the administrative or hierarchal structure [helps] - if it's normalised and supported from the top then I think that flows down through the service... [from my observation] it is the leadership group of the team, and unfortunately that is still medical, who set the ethos of the unit. So, if you want to change the culture of the place, my approach would be to get the most senior consultants on board, (Winston).

Leadership and positive role models were considered key enablers to effective self-care. This also related to the allocation of reasonable workloads. Other facilitators of effective self-care were more intrapersonal. These included having a positive outlook, self-awareness and positive emotions. Self-awareness was described as central to effective self-care practice. Gratitude and taking a positive perspective, even in the face of negative circumstances, enabled self-care. Self-compassion was considered essential to self-care, and relational to compassion for others - as expressed through patient care. One participant explained:

Self-care is built on self-compassion. If your compassion does not include yourself, it is not complete; it extends to yourself and to your clients equally. And if you're not doing that, then something's not working (Carmel).

Importantly, self-compassion did not necessarily come naturally, and in many cases had to be learned. For some, self-compassion was viewed as an emotion that became more apparent later in life, and when career achievement was less of a priority. Authenticity and courage were also described as self-care enablers. These encompassed self-advocacy and self-acceptance – in terms of being realistic about limitations; and being, in the words of one participant, *authentically human.* Lastly, reflecting on and having an appreciation of one's own mortality was considered important and enabling for self-care practice.

Discussion

This study explored the meaning and practice of self-care as described by palliative care nurses and doctors. These findings contribute new knowledge in several ways, with implications for clinical practice, research and education.

A proactive and holistic approach to promoting personal health and wellbeing to support professional care of others

The holistic nature of self-care as revealed in this study is consistent with the discourse analysis conducted by Breiddal [21]. Findings from the present study extend this existing knowledge by providing new insight into the meaning of self-care, and also through further evidence of the relational context in which self-care is practised, as voiced by practitioners in the field. For palliative care professionals, self-care is not a selfish endeavour apathetic to the needs of others; rather, it is a proactive and relational practice cognisant of practitioners' health and human needs, and motivated by the professional context of sustaining compassionate care in therapeutic relationship with patients and their families. This was especially evident in the words of one participant: *...if you don't feed yourself, you've got nothing to give; much of what we do in palliative care is about human connectedness.* It also supports Kearney and colleagues' [22] assertion that self-care is not a selfish luxury, but is instead essential to clinicians' therapeutic relationship with patients.

Personalised self-care strategies within professional and non-professional contexts

While most research has to date focused on strategies used to cope with occupational stressors [12]; these findings, situated in the broader context of self-care, reveal not only the variety of effective strategies employed, but also the challenges and complexities involved with maintaining effective self-care strategies in practice. The need for reflective practice to build self-awareness, as well as the management of multiple barriers and enablers to self-care practice, clearly demand ongoing attention from practitioners and palliative care services.

That mindfulness exercises were used spontaneously by participants in practice settings suggests that the benefits of formal mindfulness training initiatives extend beyond the training room and into the clinical milieu [23, 24]. Clinical supervision was effective for many, but not for others; and in many instances, it was not available at all. This seems to reflect, in part, a different attitude to clinical supervision within the nursing and medical disciplines; when compared to other disciplines such as social work, in which supervision has long been a cornerstone. As a social worker, Firth [25] explains that many nurses may feel threatened by supervision, whilst doctors have traditionally avoided it. Given the potential benefits to self-awareness and staff wellbeing, the provision of supervision should nonetheless be considered; perhaps with an emphasis on the restorative aspects of clinical supervision [25–27].

Formal and informal debriefing was consistently described as an effective self-care strategy, and thus should be encouraged. Similarly, laughter and the use of humour formed a fundamental part of self-care, and should be fostered as appropriate. Laughter has long been considered a coping strategy to manage stress in palliative care settings [28]; however, this finding extends a new context in terms of self-care behaviours to support health and wellbeing. Indeed, there is evidence to suggest not only psychological, but also physiological health benefits from laughter, including enhanced cardiac and immune function [29–31].

Establishing and maintaining effective boundaries within and outside of the workplace was an effective self-care strategy for participants in this study, as was work-life harmony. Whilst so-called work-life balance was discussed by some, and has also featured in other palliative care research into coping mechanisms [32]; this concept was incongruous to the experience of others. Overall, it was important to acknowledge that different life-domains require varying degrees of attention at any given time, and finding one's individual harmony between personal and professional roles was thus a key strategy towards flourishing in life. This is consistent with McMillan and colleagues' [33] definition of work-life harmony as 'an individually pleasing, congruent arrangement of work and life roles that is interwoven into a single narrative of life'. It also corresponds with recent research findings that work-life interference, or conflict, is associated with higher levels of burnout in nurses and predicts intention to leave an organisation or the nursing profession [34]. Thus, work-life harmony is an important aspect of effective self-care. Given this finding, future self-care education might usefully incorporate this new emphasis on work-life harmony over the common parlance of 'work-life balance' which is ill-defined and otherwise problematic in practice for some [33].

Another interesting finding related to participants electing to work part-time as a self-care strategy. While only 42% of participants worked part-time in the present study, the majority of participants who had earlier completed a survey worked part-time. Given these and earlier research findings [32], working a part-time load appears to be a common self-care strategy for palliative care professionals. Indeed, one participant suggested that part-time roles should perhaps be encouraged in favour of a full-time load, given the emotionally demanding nature of palliative care. However, this would need to be weighed up by the individual in relation to feasibility of lower income and potentially limited opportunities for career advancement in roles where full-time work is required.

Barriers and enablers to self-care practice

While positive workplace cultures were discussed as enablers of self-care, there were many who described their current workplace culture as a barrier to effective self-care, in that it was not supportive of self-care practice. This finding is alarming, yet not altogether surprising when taken in the context of self-care being highly stigmatised – as either selfish or weak – in some participants' workplaces. Perhaps more concerning, is that this stigma may serve to not only impede effective self-care practice in the workplace; it could also discourage palliative care professionals from taking personal leave or seeking professional support when they become unwell. As described by Hill [35], a paediatric palliative care physician, showing vulnerability or seeking help is often viewed as a sign of weakness; and acknowledging one's shared humanity and vulnerability through self-compassion is vital to self-care behaviours. Understanding factors that contribute to supportive workplace cultures and facilitate self-care is therefore essential. Some palliative care services in Australia might benefit from the experience of their counterparts in Canada and the United Kingdom, who have focused on leadership to foster workplace cultures of self-awareness, self-care, and staff support [36, 37].

Several enabling factors to self-care practice were identified in this study, both interpersonal and environmental. Authenticity, courage, and leadership were highlighted by participants. Being authentically human in acknowledging one's own vulnerability; having the courage to challenge stigma or be assertive in saying 'no', when acquiescing to additional workload may compromise one's own wellbeing; and leading by example in supporting and normalising self-care as an essential aspect of palliative care practice. Authenticity, courage, and leadership have been recognised as character strengths that can be measured and cultivated [38]. Development of these character strengths in palliative care teams should therefore be encouraged to assist in transforming any unsupportive workplace cultures.

In this study, positive emotions such as gratitude and self-compassion enabled self-care. This is consistent with a growing field of positive psychology research, in which positive emotions not only have a biological basis for physiological health benefits; but have also been shown to broaden repertoires of positive thoughts and actions which, in turn, help to build personal and social resources that lead to wellbeing and flourishing [39–43]. Whilst, in the context of psychological flexibility, negative emotions are not necessarily to be avoided [44]; awareness of, and capacity for the cultivation of, positive emotions should thus be fostered as part of self-care practice. This may serve to promote resilience and emotional intelligence both individually and across the palliative care team [45, 46].

That self-compassion was considered enabling to self-care, corresponds with findings from a recent correlational study [47] in which perceived self-care ability was significantly associated with increased self-compassion in palliative care nurses and doctors. Indeed, as highlighted by Vachon [48], self-compassion entails knowing and caring for oneself. The self-care barriers identified in the present study provide a valuable context which may also explain the low levels of self-care ability identified in some doctors and nurses from the previous study. Building from emerging evidence to support compassion-oriented training interventions in palliative care teams [24], future research should therefore investigate any causal relationship between these variables longitudinally. Potential studies could incorporate interventions that draw upon loving kindness meditation or other compassion training programs which have been shown to enhance compassion for self and others, and may therefore contribute positively to both self-care and compassionate care of others [49–53].

In other research [13, 54], palliative care professionals' reported self-care practices have corresponded with physical, social, and inner domains of self-care. Importantly, findings from the present study underscore the imperative that strategies from these self-care domains are implemented and maintained in both personal and workplace settings. Findings from this study can thus inform the self-care education and training interventions recently called for [55], especially in relation to self-care planning, work-life harmony, and management of identified barriers and enablers to effective self-care practice. Educational resources might usefully draw upon this qualitative evidence previously lacking in the literature, to articulate and foster the meaning and practice of effective self-care in the palliative care workforce. For example, clarifying staff confusion about the shared responsibility for self-care practice – as identified in this study.

The issue of balance between individual and organisational responsibility is multi-faceted and requires careful consideration by palliative care services. Clearly, an organisation cannot practise self-care on behalf of its workforce; however, it can enable and enhance self-care through corporate leadership and a variety of structural supports to foster positive workplace cultures that are conducive to effective self-care practice [36, 37]. At the same time, individual practitioners carry a personal responsibility for self-care to maintain their health and capacity for professional practice. This was highlighted by one participant, who stated: *It's the responsibility of every team member to look after themselves, but having management or organisational strategies in place to support someone doing self-care is incredibly important... it's a dual process.* This collaborative approach to promoting health and wellbeing in workplace contexts is reflected in the World Health Organisation's (WHO) [56] Healthy Workplace Framework.

While individual responsibility relates to implementing and maintaining self-care strategies, organisational responsibility is thus oriented towards supporting staff in effective self-care practice to promote health and wellbeing. This support represents an investment, with a host of potential organisational benefits including increased patient and family satisfaction, increased staff retention and reduced absenteeism, improved staff morale and job satisfaction [27]. Conflict between colleagues can be a common source of staff stress, and is an important workplace concern where all parties must take some responsibility. While the degree of responsibility will vary according to context, the use of employee assistance programs and adoption of the WHO Healthy Workplace Framework can provide support and guidance in this area.

Clarity may also be lacking with regards to shared responsibility for self-care practice where clinicians experience chronic illness and or disability. Health services, as institutions, have the potential to promote health and wellbeing not only for health care consumers; but also for health care professionals [57]. Indeed, some argue that hospitals should serve as exemplars of healthy workplaces [58]. Given this context, a collaborative approach encompassing individual self-management and organisational support would be consistent with the WHO Healthy Workplace Framework, which recommends that workplaces be supportive of employees living with chronic disease and disability [56]. Palliative care services might usefully draw upon this or similar approaches.

Given the highly personalised nature of self-care, palliative care services should also consider ways in which a variety of self-care strategies can be supported. For example, providing opportunities for both informal debriefing and formal clinical supervision – depending on individual preference; as well as scope for the supported development of individual self-care plans for those who feel they would benefit from them.

A novel finding from this study was the concept of team-care to promote a healthy team. As an encouraging sign of positive workplace cultures, this highlights an additional dimension to the relational context of self-care practice, whilst underscoring the importance of supporting interdisciplinary teamwork as an integral part of the philosophy of palliative care. It also contributes to the literature on positive relationships and workplace wellbeing in the context of self-care and positive health [59]. Taken together, the practice of team-care as an antecedent to a healthy team in palliative care represents a potential avenue of qualitative inquiry for future research. This would be enhanced with the inclusion of participant observation and patient-reported outcomes on any perceived benefits to the quality of care provided.

Limitations

Limitations to this study should be noted. Socio-cultural considerations were not represented in the demographic data collected or subsequent analysis. Whilst, to our knowledge, any significant impact of culture on self-care has not featured in the literature to date, we acknowledge that palliative care professionals from culturally and linguistically diverse backgrounds may understand and approach self-care practice in ways other than as described in this study sample. Additionally, the sample was somewhat limited in terms of participants' geographical location. While the study recruited participants from metropolitan and inner or outer (rural) regional locations of nearly all Australian States and Territories, remote area locations were not represented. The meaning and practice of self-care may have unique characteristics in remote area practice, thus transferability of findings from this study should be gauged by remote area practitioners. Despite these limitations, which may be addressed in the future by discrete population-specific studies, this research has generated new knowledge in line with the study aim.

Conclusions

The findings of this study reveal a context and complexity of effective self-care practice previously lacking in the literature. Taken together, the findings of this research provide new insight to support palliative care practice and education. Self-care is a proactive and personalised approach to the promotion of health and wellbeing through a variety of strategies, in both personal and professional settings, to support capacity for compassionate care of patients and their families. Importantly, it is a shared responsibility between palliative care professionals and the palliative care services in which they work, with staff support and positive workplace cultures required to manage various barriers and enablers to effective self-care practice. This research adds an important qualitative perspective and serves to advance knowledge of both the context and effective practice of self-care in the palliative care workforce.

Acknowledgements

The authors gratefully acknowledge the palliative care nurses and doctors who generously shared their time and candour as participants in this study. JM's PhD Candidature was supported by an Australian Postgraduate Award from the University of Sydney.

Funding

This research received no specific grant from any funding agency in the public, commercial, or not-for-profit sectors.

Authors' contributions

JM and JF contributed to the initial conception and design of the study, whilst TW contributed to its refinement and finalisation. JM conducted the data collection and analysis with guidance from JF and TW. JM drafted the manuscript; JW and TW made critical revisions to the paper for intellectual content. All authors approved the final manuscript.

Competing interests

The authors declare that they have no competing interests.

Author details

[1]Institute of Health and Biomedical Innovation, Queensland University of Technology, Kelvin Grove, QLD, Australia. [2]Susan Wakil School of Nursing and Midwifery, The University of Sydney, Camperdown, NSW, Australia. [3]School of Nursing, Faculty of Health, Queensland University of Technology, Kelvin Grove, QLD 4061, Australia.

References

1. Renzenbrink I. Relentless self-care. In: Berzoff J, Silverman PR, editors. Living with dying: a handbook for end-of-life healthcare practitioners. New York: Columbia University Press; 2004. p. 848–67.
2. Mills J, Chapman M. Compassion and self-compassion in medicine: self-care for the caregiver. Australas Med J. 2016;9(5):87–91.
3. Mills J, Wand T, Fraser JA. On self-compassion and self-care in nursing: selfish or essential for compassionate care? Int J Nurs Stud. 2015;52(4):791–3.
4. American Academy of Hospice and Palliative Medicine (HPM Competencies Project Work Group). Hospice and Palliative Medicine Core Competencies - Version 2.3. 2009. http://aahpm.org/uploads/education/competencies/Competencies%20v.%202.3.pdf. Accessed 20 Jan 2018.
5. Canning D, Yates P, Rosenberg JP. Competency standards for specialist palliative care nursing practice. 2005. http://www.pcna.org.au/images/documents/competystds.pdf. Accessed 20 Jan 2018.
6. Downing J, Ling J, Benini F, Payne S, Papadatou D. A summary of the EAPC white paper on core competencies for education in paediatric palliative care. Eur J Palliat Care. 2014;21(5):245–9.
7. Gamondi C, Larkin P, Payne S. Core competencies in palliative care: an EAPC white paper on palliative care education – part 2. Eur J Palliat Care. 2013; 20(3):140–5.
8. Hospice New Zealand. Hospice New Zealand Standards for Palliative Care. 2012. http://www.hospice.org.nz/cms_show_download.php?id=647. Accessed 20 Jan 2018.
9. Palliative Care Australia. Standards for providing quality palliative care for all Australians. 2005. http://palliativecare.org.au/wp-content/uploads/2015/07/Standards-for-providing-quality-palliative-care-for-all-Australians.pdf. Accessed 20 Jan 2018.
10. Palliative Care Nurses New Zealand. A National Professional Development Framework for Palliative Care Nursing in Aotearoa New Zealand. 2014. http://www.health.govt.nz/system/files/documents/publications/national-professional-development-framework-palliative-care-nursing-practice-nz-oct14.pdf. Accessed 20 Jan 2018.
11. Sherman D. Nurses' stress & burnout: how to care for yourself when caring for patients and their families experiencing life-threatening illness. Am J Nurs. 2004;104(5):52.
12. Mills J, Wand T, Fraser JA. Palliative care professionals' care and compassion for self and others: a narrative review. Int J Palliat Nurs. 2017;23(5):219–29.
13. Mills J, Wand T, Fraser JA. Self-care in palliative care nursing and medical professionals: a cross-sectional survey. J Palliat Med. 2017;20(6):625–30.
14. Payne S. Qualitative methods of data collection and analysis. In: Addington-Hall JM, Bruera E, Higginson IJ, Payne S, editors. Research methods in palliative care. New York: Oxford University Press; 2007.
15. Doody O, Noonan M. Preparing and conducting interviews to collect data. Nurse Researcher. 2013;20(5):28–32.
16. Hsieh H-F, Shannon SE. Three approaches to qualitative content analysis. Qual Health Res. 2005;15
17. Graneheim UH, Lundman B. Qualitative content analysis in nursing research: concepts, procedures and measures to achieve trustworthiness. Nurse Educ Today. 2004;24(2):105–12.

18. Elo S, Kyngäs H. The qualitative content analysis process. J Adv Nurs. 2008; 62(1):107–15.
19. Vaismoradi M, Turunen H, Bondas T. Content analysis and thematic analysis: implications for conducting a qualitative descriptive study. Nurs Health Sci. 2013;15(3):398–405.
20. Elo S, Kääriäinen M, Kanste O, Pölkki T, Utriainen K, Kyngäs H. Qualitative content analysis: a focus on trustworthiness. SAGE Open. 2014;4(1):1–10.
21. Breiddal SMF. Self-care in palliative care: a way of being. Illn Crisis Loss. 2012;20(1):5–17.
22. Kearney MK, Weininger RB, Vachon MS, Harrison RL, Mount BM. Self-care of physicians caring for patients at the end of life: "being connected . . . A key to my survival". JAMA. 2009;301(11):1155–64.
23. O'Connor M, Peyton S. Mindfulness for resilience - a self-care strategy for staff working with emotionally distressed individuals. Eur J Palliat Care. 2015; 22(2):64–7.
24. Orellana-Rios CL, Radbruch L, Kern M, Regel YU, Anton A, Sinclair S, et al.. Mindfulness and compassion-oriented practices at work reduce distress and enhance self-care of palliative care teams: a mixed-method evaluation of an "on the job" program. BMC Palliative Care. 2017;17(1):3.
25. Firth P. Clinical supervision and relective practice in palliative care: luxury or neccessity? In: Renzenbrink I, editor. Caregiver stress and staff support in illness, dying and bereavement. Oxford: Oxford University Press; 2011. p. 170–7.
26. Edmonds KP, Yeung HN, Onderdonk C, Mitchell W, Thornberry K. Clinical supervision in the palliative care team setting: a concrete approach to team wellness. J Palliat Med. 2015;18(3):274–7.
27. Kearney M, Weininger R. Whole person self-care: self-care from the inside out. In: Hutchinson TA, editor. Whole person care. New York: Springer; 2011. p. 109–25.
28. Dean RA. Occupational stress in hospice care: causes and coping strategies. Am J Hosp Palliat Care. 1998:151–4.
29. Bennett MP, Lengacher C. Humor and laughter may influence health IV. Humor and immune function. Evid Based Complement Alternat Med. 2009; 6(2):159–64.
30. Berk LS, Felten DL, Tan SA, Bittman BB, Westengard J. Modulation of neuroimmune parameters during the eustress of humor-associated mirthful laughter. Altern Ther Health Med. 2001;7(2):62–76.
31. Miller M, Fry WF. The effect of mirthful laughter on the human cardiovascular system. Med Hypotheses. 2009;73(5):636.
32. Zambrano SC, Chur-Hansen A, Crawford GB. The experiences, coping mechanisms, and impact of death and dying on palliative medicine specialists. Palliat Support Care. 2014;12(4):309–16.
33. McMillan HS, Morris ML, Atchley EK. Constructs of the work/life Interface: a synthesis of the literature and introduction of the concept of work/life harmony. Hum Resour Dev Rev. 2011;10(1):6–25.
34. Moloney W, Boxall P, Parsons M, Cheung G. Factors predicting registered nurses' intentions to leave their organization and profession: a job demands-resources framework. J Adv Nurs. 2018;74(4):864–75
35. Hill AB. Breaking the stigma — a Physician's perspective on self-care and recovery. N Engl J Med. 2017;376(12):1103–5.
36. Dechamps A. Leadership and staff care, self-care and self-awareness: reflections from St Christohpher's hospice, London. In: Renzenbrink I, editor. Caregiver stress and staff support in illness, dying and bereavement. Oxford: Oxford University Press; 2011. p. 127–38.
37. Wainwright W, Breiddal S. Staff support: a shared responsibility at Victoria hospice society, British Columbia, Canada. In: Renzenbrink I, editor. Caregiver stress and staff support in illness, dying and bereavement. Oxford: Oxford University Press; 2011. p. 111–9.
38. Peterson C, Park N. Classifying and measuring strengths of character. In: Lopez SJ, Snyder CR, editors. Oxford handbook of positive psychology. New York: Oxford University Press; 2009. p. 25–33.
39. Cohn MA, Fredrickson BL. Positive emotions. In: Lopez SJ, Snyder CR, editors. The Oxford handbook of positive psychology. 2 ed. Oxford: Oxford University Press; 2009. p. 13–24.
40. Fredrickson BL. What good are positive emotions? Rev Gen Psychol. 1998; 2(3):300–19.
41. Fredrickson BL. The role of positive emotions in positive psychology: the broaden and build theory of positive emotions. Am Psychol. 2001; 56(3):218–26.
42. Kreibig SD. Autonomic nervous system aspects of positive emotions. In: Tugade MM, Shiota MN, Kirby LD, editors. Handbook of positive emotions. New York: Guilford Press; 2014. p. 133–58.
43. McCraty R, Rees RA. The central role of the heart in generating and sustaining positive emotions. In: Lopez SJ, Snyder CR, editors. Oxford handbook of positive psychology. New York: Oxford University Press; 2009. p. 527–36.
44. Kashdan TB, Ciarrochi J, editors. Mindfulness, acceptance, and positive psychology: the seven foundations of well-being. Oakland: New Harbinger; 2013.
45. Tugade MM, Fredrickson BL. Resilient individuals use positive emotions to bounce back from negative emotional experiences. J Pers Soc Psychol. 2004;86(2):320–33.
46. Tugade MM, Fredrickson BL. Positive emotions and emotional intelligence. In: Barrett LF, Salovey P, editors. The wisdom in feeling: psychological processes in emotional intelligence. New York: Guilford Press; 2002. p. 319–40.
47. Mills J, Wand T, Fraser JA. Examining self-care, self-compassion, and compassion for others: a cross-sectional survey of palliative care nurses and doctors. Int J Palliat Nurs. In Press
48. Vachon MLS. Targeted intervention for family and professional caregivers: attachment, empathy, and compassion. Palliat Med. 2016;30(2):101–3.
49. Fredrickson BL, Cohn MA, Coffey KA, Pek J, Finkel SM. Open hearts build lives: positive emotions, induced through loving-kindness meditation, build consequential personal resources. J Pers Soc Psychol. 2008;95(5):1045–62.
50. Jazaieri H, Jinpa T, McGonigal K, Rosenberg E, Finkelstein J, Simon-Thomas E, et al. Enhancing compassion: a randomized controlled trial of a compassion cultivation training program. J Happiness Stud. 2013;14(4):1113–26.
51. Jazaieri H, Lee IA, McGonigal K, Jinpa T, Doty JR, Gross JJ, et al. A wandering mind is a less caring mind: daily experience sampling during compassion meditation training. J Posit Psychol. 2015:1–14.
52. Jazaieri H, McGonigal K, Jinpa T, Doty J, Gross J, Goldin P. A randomized controlled trial of compassion cultivation training: effects on mindfulness, affect, and emotion regulation. Motiv Emot. 2014;38(1):23–35.
53. Neff KD, Germer CK. A pilot study and randomized controlled trial of the mindful self-compassion program. J Clin Psychol. 2013;69(1):28–44.
54. Sansó N, Galiana L, Oliver A, Pascual A, Sinclair S, Benito E. Palliative care professionals' inner life: exploring the relationships among awareness, self-care, and compassion satisfaction and fatigue, burnout, and coping with death. J Pain Symptom Manag. 2015;50(2):200–7.
55. Linzitto JP, Grance G. Health professionals' quality of life in relation to end of life care. Curr Opin Support Palliat Care. 2017;11(4):306–9.
56. World Health Organisation. Healthy Workplace Framework and Model. 2010. http://www.who.int/occupational_health/healthy_workplace_framework.pdf. Accessed 8 Apr 2018.
57. Whitehead D. Health promoting hospitals: the role and function of nursing. J Clin Nurs. 2005;14(1):20–7.
58. Russell LM, Anstey MHR, Wells S. Hospitals should be exemplars of healthy workplaces. Med J Aust. 2015;202(8):424–6.
59. Seligman MEP. Positive health. Appl Psychol Int Rev. 2008;57:3–18.

Negative pain management index scores do not necessarily indicate inadequate pain management

Naoki Sakakibara[1,2*], Takahiro Higashi[1], Itsuku Yamashita[3], Tetsusuke Yoshimoto[4] and Motohiro Matoba[5]

Abstract

Background: The Pain Management Index (PMI) is widely used in the assessment of pain management, and negative scores are traditionally considered to indicate inadequate pain management. However, it is not known whether negative PMI scores are always problematic.

Methods: In this prospective observational study, we examined the data of 1156 patients with cancer and pain who were hospitalized in a cancer care hospital in Japan from July 2012 to January 2015 and compared the proportion of patients with PI across various PMI scores in this cohort. We further evaluated the predictive validity of PMI scores for PI using different cutoffs. This study aimed to examine the association between PMI scores and the proportion of patients whose pain interferes with their daily lives (i.e., pain interference [PI]).

Results: We found that lower PMI scores were generally associated with a higher percentage of patients with PI. A smaller proportion of patients with PMI scores of − 1 (567/1550, 36.6%) reported PI compared with those with PMI scores of 0 (788/1505, 52.4%). The sensitivities of PMI scores < -1 and < 0 for predicting PI were 0.16 and 0.37 and the corresponding specificities were 0.95 and 0.71, respectively.

Conclusions: These findings suggest that PMI scores are inversely associated with the proportion of patients with PI. However, PMI scores of − 1 do not always indicate inadequate pain management; pain management should therefore be evaluated from multiple perspectives.

Keywords: Cancer pain, Pain management index (PMI), Quality indicator, Pain interference, Palliative care

Background

A substantial proportion of patients with cancer experience pain [1], which sometimes interferes with their daily lives and affects their mental health [2, 3]. As stated in the World Health Organization (WHO) guidelines on pain relief and palliative care, assessment of pain and providing appropriate treatment for it are important aspects of pain management [4]. Systematic evaluation is indispensable for ensuring appropriate pain management.

The Pain Management Index (PMI) is used worldwide to evaluate cancer pain management [5]. The PMI evaluates pain management by reflecting the balance between the class of the most potent analgesics used/prescribed and the patient's reported pain intensity. Analgesic drugs and pain intensity are assigned scores of 0 to 3; subtracting the latter from the former provides the PMI. Thus, when the score for pain intensity is larger than the analgesic drug score, the PMI is negative; this has traditionally been considered to indicate inadequate pain management [6]. In a systematic review published in 2008, the prevalence of negative PMI scores among patients with cancer was reported as 43% worldwide, and higher in Asia [5]. A more recent report, published in 2014, showed slight improvement, the prevalence of negative PMI scores being 31.8% [7]. However, according to conventional criteria, this means that approximately

* Correspondence: nsakakib@ncc.go.jp; nsakaki@luke.ac.jp
[1]Division of Health Services Research, Center for Cancer Control and Information Services, National Cancer Center, 5-1-1 Tsukiji, Chuo-ku, Tokyo 104-0045, Japan
[2]Department of Palliative Care, St. Luke's International Hospital, 9-1 Akashicho, Chuo-ku, Tokyo 104-8560, Japan
Full list of author information is available at the end of the article

one third of patients still do not receive pain medication that is proportional to their pain intensity [7].

Another indicator for evaluating pain management is pain interference [PI], defined as whether pain interferes with daily life. The Brief Pain Inventory (BPI), another popular instrument for assessing pain, assesses the intensity of pain and interference from pain in seven areas of daily life [8]. PMI and BPI scores are often used to assess patients' pain status and the adequacy of analgesia [3]. The intensity of pain reflects only the pain, whereas the PI assesses the effectiveness of pain management by using measures like the PMI.

According to Deandrea et al., the process–outcome link is an important validity check for any performance measure [5]. However, the relationship between PMI and PI scores in patients with cancer has not been evaluated since the PMI was first developed in 1994, when Cleeland et al. compared PI scores between patients with negative PMI scores and those with scores of ≥zero [6]. However, a non-negative PMI value does not necessarily mean that the patient's pain management is appropriate, because PMI only looks at the analgesic classes and the levels of pain. [9–11]. The further steps of analgesic choice and appropriate dosage are necessary to achieve appropriate pain management. In addition, negative PMI scores may not indicate inadequate pain management in patients without PI. This possibility was raised during the process of practice reviews of pain management in our institution. Several clinicians whose pain management practice was considered inadequate based on the PMI are opposed to the criteria, claiming that "inadequate pain management" is a false accusation because patients whose PMI scores were – 1 are not necessarily troubled by pain.

We performed this study to test these clinicians' claims by analyzing in more detail the overall trend in PI scores across various PMI and PI scores. We aimed to assess the performance of the PMI as an indicator of the quality of pain management by relating the scores to PI, an outcome measure of pain management. We also expected that differences in prevalence of PI across PMI scores would provide insights on the how PMI scores should be used to assess quality of pain management.

Methods

Setting, participants, and data collection

Participants were recruited for this study from patients with cancer who were hospitalized at Aomori Prefectural Central Hospital, a general hospital in rural northern Japan, between July 2012 and January 2015. This hospital has approximately 700 beds and provides care to approximately 1200 new patients with cancer annually. All patients aged 20 years and older with a diagnosis of cancer who had cancer-related pain or had taken any analgesic medications in the past 24 h were invited to participate, provided their primary physicians assessed that they were capable of participating in the study. Participants were asked by staff nurses about pain and cancer-related PI as part of routine care during morning rounds every day. The patients' reports on pain status during hospital days 1 to 7 were analyzed. Medications used were recorded by a staff nurse, who also documented the cause of pain (e.g., cancer- or treatment-related).

Measures and definitions of variables

Pain and pain interference [PI]

Patients who had experienced cancer-related pain or taken any analgesic drugs in the past 24 h were eligible for the study. Given that patients with cancer can experience pain caused by various factors, including cancer itself, treatment, and coexisting illness [12], patients with pain other than cancer-related pain were excluded.

PI was defined as cancer pain that resulted in the patient feeling troubled or being incapable of doing something. Participants were asked a single question "Do you have trouble with pain or is there anything you cannot do because of pain?" They could respond "yes" or "no" [13].

Pain management index

Pain intensity can be determined at its strongest, as the average amount of pain in the past 24 h, or at rest and in motion. The strongest pain in the past 24 h was chosen as the basis for the PMI, in accordance with the original method of Cleeland et al. [6]. Pain intensity was reported on a numerical rating scale (NRS) from 0 to 10, with zero denoting no pain and 10 the worst pain imaginable. Information on prescribed analgesics (name, dose, frequency, and routes of administration) was collected from the medical record and patients' responses to the staff nurses' questions.

PMI scores were calculated by subtracting the pain score from the analgesics score as in the WHO pain relief ladder [6]. An NRS was used to ascertain the worst pain intensity and these scores used to create the following four categories of pain intensity: no pain (pain score 0; 0 on NRS); mild pain (pain score 1; 1–4 on NRS), moderate pain (pain score 2; 5 or 6 on NRS), and severe pain (7–10) [14]. An analgesic score based on the most potent analgesic prescribed to the patient at the time of the survey was assigned according to the WHO pain relief ladder as follows: 0, no analgesic medication; 1, non-opioid analgesics, such as non-steroidal anti-inflammatory drugs or acetaminophen; 2, weak opioids; and 3, strong opioids. Analgesics not classified in the WHO pain relief ladder were assigned an analgesic score of "0".

Data analysis

The proportion of patients with PI for each PMI score from − 3 to + 3, overall, and stratified by hospital day were calculated, after which the trend in proportion of patients with PI for each PMI score was assessed by using the Cochran–Armitage test. A P value of less than 0.05 was considered to indicate statistical significance. To further clarify the relationship between PMI scores and PI, the distribution of pain intensity experienced within each PMI score category was calculated. For the comparison of proportions of patients with the PI across categories, Pearson's chi-square test was used. Because the ultimate target of pain management is to eliminate PI, the PMI can be viewed as a tool that tests "inadequate pain management" and thus assesses the process of achieving this target. Therefore, sensitivities and specificities of PMI < − 1 and PMI < 0 for predicting PI were computed. Although PMI < 0 is the conventional criterion for inadequate pain management, a PMI of − 1 is a looser criterion. The sensitivity of the PMI score was defined as the proportion of patients with PI who actually scored positive (i.e., PMI < − 1 or PMI < 0), and the specificity was defined as the proportion of patients without PI who scored negative (i.e., PMI > = − 1 or PMI > =0). All analyses were performed with Stata version 13.1 (StataCorp LP, College Station, TX, USA).

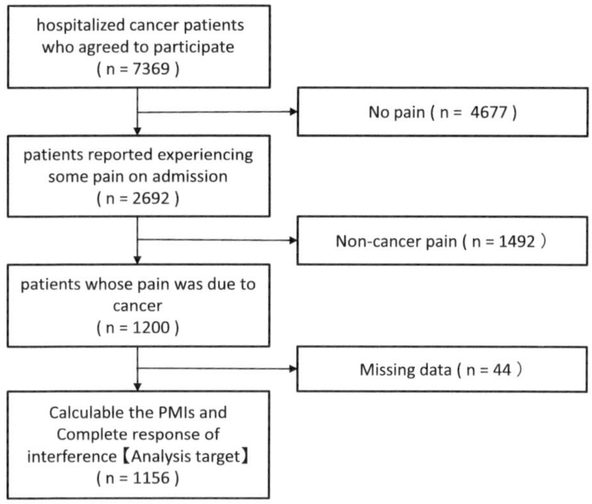

Fig. 1 Flow diagram of the study

Results

Characteristics of study patients

Of 7369 patients with cancer who agreed to be screened for pain as potential participants in the study, 2692 reported experiencing some pain on admission. Among the 1200 patients whose pain was attributable to cancer, 1156 reported pain on the NRS and were eligible for analysis. A total of 6732 responses about pain from these 1156 patients were analyzed (Fig. 1. On average, patients reported pain on the NRS 5.8 times). Table 1 presents these patients' characteristics and condition on the first hospital day. Their mean age was 62.9 years (SD, 11.6 years) and 500 (43.3%) were women, 71.9% of them had a performance status of 0 or 1, 33.8% of them were not given prescriptions for analgesics, a little less than half of whom (41.2%) reported mild pain and 20.1% no pain. The average NRS value of patients with PI was 5.2, whereas that of patients without was 2.0 ($P < 0.001$).

Relationship between PMI scores and PI

Figure 2 shows the proportions of patients who reported PI according to PMI score. Overall, there was a significant trend toward lower PMI being associated with a higher proportion of patients with PI ($P < 0.001$). A large proportion of patients with PMI scores of − 2 or − 3 reported PI, whereas this proportion was much smaller among those with PMI scores of − 1, approximating the proportions of those with positive PMI scores of 1 or 2; no patients with positive PMI scores of 3 reported PI. The proportion of patients with PI was lower for those with PMI scores of − 1 than for those with PMI scores of 0 ($P < 0.001$). Figure 3 shows the same analyses as Fig. 2, stratified by hospital day (1–7); the graphs are of similar shape as that in Fig. 2. Except for on days 3 and 6, the proportion of patients reporting PI was greater in those with PMI scores of − 3 than in those with PMI scores of − 2; on days 3 and 6 the findings for these PMI scores were reversed.

Distribution of pain intensity and PI according to category of PMI scores

Figure 4 shows the distribution of pain intensity in patients with PMI scores ≤0. Most (78.7%) patients with PMI scores of − 1 had mild pain; 18.2% and 3.2% and had moderate and severe pain, respectively. However, 38.0% of patients with PMI scores of 0 had severe pain (38.0%). Table 2 shows the proportion of patients with PI according to category of PMI score or pain intensity group. At the same levels of PMI scores, there was a larger proportion of patients with greater pain intensity reported PI, indicating correct estimation of PI.

The sensitivities of PMI scores < − 1, < 0 and < 1 for predicting PI were 0.16, 0.37, and 0.67, respectively; the corresponding specificities being 0.95, 0.71, and 0.53, respectively.

Discussion

Negative PMI scores are widely accepted as indicating inadequate management of pain, whereas non-negative

Table 1 Relevant clinical characteristics ($n = 1156$)

Age — mean ± *SD*	62.9 ± 11.6
Female sex — no. (%)	500 (43.3)
Hospitalized Department no. (%)	
Surgery	227 (19.6)
Gastroenterology	400 (34.6)
Respiratory Meds	213 (18.4)
Hematology	87 (7.5)
ENT	71 (6.1)
Urology	58 (5.0)
Gynecology	86 (7.4)
Other	14 (1.4)
Analgesics[a] — no. (%)	
None	391 (33.8)
Non opioids	321 (27.8)
Mild opioids	47 (4.1)
Strong opioids	397 (34.3)
Performance Status — no. (%)	
0	456 (39.5)
1	374 (32.4)
2	159 (13.8)
3	118 (10.2)
4	49 (4.2)
Treatment history — no. (%)	
Surgery	463 (40.1)
Chemotherapy	671 (58.0)
Radiation therapy	244 (21.1)
NRS — no. (%)	
0 (No pain)	232 (20.1)
1–4 (Mild pain)	476 (41.2)
5–6 (Moderate pain)	191 (16.5)
7–10 (Severe pain)	257 (22.2)

[a]Classification according to the WHO's pain relief ladder. Non-opioids included non-steroidal anti-inflammatory drugs or acetaminophen. Analgesics not classified in the WHO's pain relief ladder, such as adjuvant analgesics, were assigned to "none" in this study
NRS numerical rating scale

(0 to 3) scores are thought to denote acceptable pain management [5, 7, 11, 15, 16]. Indeed, we found a trend toward the proportion of PI decreasing as PMI scores increased, and that a large proportion of patients with PMI scores of – 2 or – 3 reported PI. However, we found that a larger proportion of patients in the group with PMI scores of 0 reported PI than in the group with PMI scores of – 1. This finding indicates that patients with a PMI score of – 1, traditionally considered as "treated inadequately", were experiencing less interference with daily living than those with PMI scores of 0, usually considered as receiving "acceptable pain management".

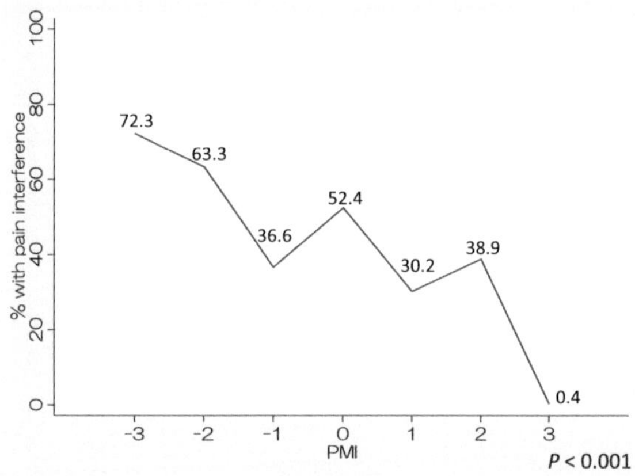

Fig. 2 Relationship between PMI scores and pain interference (sum of all days). The percentages are of patients with PI at each level of PMI score. *P* value: Cochrane-Armitage test for trend was performed

This finding suggests caution must be exercised when evaluating pain management using the PMI. A PMI score of – 1 should be considered as ambiguous, rather than denoting inadequate pain management, and treated differently according to the purpose of the evaluation. When the aim is to identify definitively inadequate care, PMI scores of – 2 and – 3 should be considered, and not scores of – 1. However, when the aim is to broadly capture potentially deficient care for further evaluation, patients with scores of 0 and – 1 should be included. In previous studies that used the PMI to evaluate the quality of pain management, all negative PMI scores were considered to denote inadequate pain management [5, 7, 11, 15, 16]. Thus, the criteria may need to be re-assessed according to the purpose of administering the PMI. Additionally, to take the other perspective, non-negative PMI scores do not necessarily indicate acceptable care: a substantial proportion of patients with PMI scores of 0–2 reported PI. Although we do not have information on the severity of that PI, these patients warrant attention [9–11].

The explanation for fewer persons with PMI scores of – 1 having PI than those with PMI of 0 may relate to the difference in distribution of pain intensity experienced by these patients. Most patients with PMI scores of – 1 had untreated mild pain, whereas those with PMI scores of 0 had a more balanced distribution of mild and severe pain. A possible reason for this finding is that patients with some mild pain decline pain medications because they have no PI, or because of cost or other reasons; this may be true of the group of patients with PMI scores of – 1 in our study. Scenarios such as patients with mild pain receiving no analgesics versus patients with moderate or severe pain taking appropriate classes of analgesics require more attention when exploring how to improve pain management. Assessment of quality of

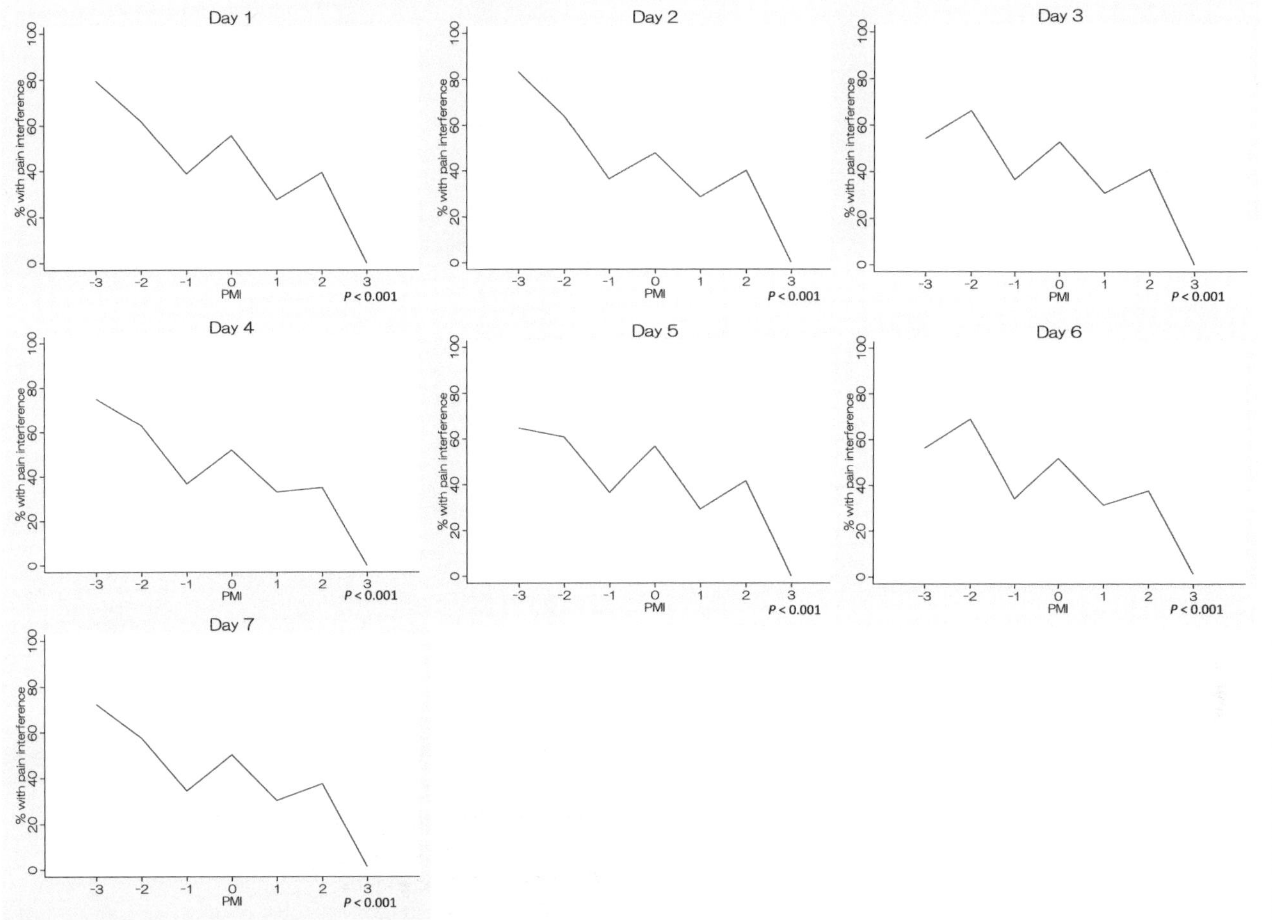

Fig. 3 Relationship between PMI scores and pain interference (each PMI level stratified by hospital day). *P* value: Cochrane-Armitage test for trend was performed

pain management by the PMI at best reflects only one aspect of the multidimensional factors involved in pain and pain management.

Our study has several limitations. First, it was conducted in a single facility in rural Japan, is a cancer care hospital that plays a central role in cancer diagnosis and treatment in a prefecture of Japan. Most of the patients with cancer were in the early stages and receiving active anti-tumor treatment. Thus, our results may not be generalizable to other settings, such as hospitals in large cities that have a higher proportion of patients receiving end-of -life care. However, even in different types of settings, we consider that not all negative PMI scores indicate inadequate pain management. Evaluation needs to be more comprehensive and consider various factors. Second, we used PI as a dichotomous variable, that is, we did not take into account the extent of PI. PI may be more severe in patients with large negative PMI scores than those with other scores. Assessing only the proportion of patients reporting PI may have resulted in missing some important aspects of the problems. Additionally, the simplicity of the single question used to assess PI meant that it did not go through as rigorous a validation process as when developing the measurement tool. It is possible that some patients misunderstood the PI question. However, the mean value of the NRS of pain in the no PI patients was substantially lower (mean 2.0) than that of patients with PI (5.4). Third, PI is a subjective measure and can therefore be affected by patients' personal perceptions of pain, expectations of their own function, their ability to coping with their pain, and lifestyles. An example of this is that bedridden patients may have low expectations concerning function and may therefore report no interference by pain. Additionally, PI has the limitation that patients sometimes have difficulty in distinguishing interference by pain itself from limitation by other factors, such as their general physical condition. Furthermore, similar to other outcome measures (e.g., survival), PI is an inclusive measure of care, and is sometimes influenced by factors other than care. Finally, in the present study PI was assessed from the patient's response to a single question. This could account for slight differences in results

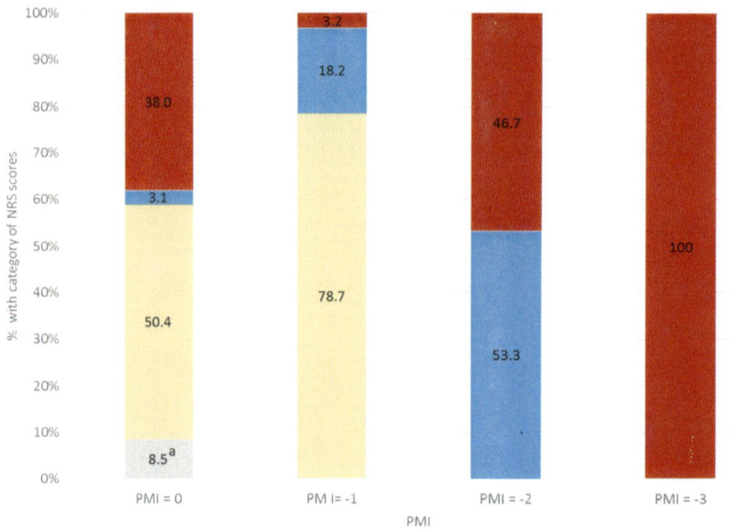

Fig. 4 Distribution of patients in categories of PMI scores and pain intensity. "a", percentage of patients whose pain was relieved by adjuvant analgesics or by analgesics that are not classified in the WHO pain relief ladder. NRS, Numeric Rating Scale. NRS scores range from 0 to 10, lower scores indicating less severe pain, scores grouped into four categories

between this study and other studies that assessed PI by other means.

Conclusions

Lower PMI scores predict a large proportion of patients who experience interference with their daily lives by pain. However, negative PMI scores do not necessarily indicate that pain is interfering with a patient's daily life, and non-negative PMI scores do not necessarily indicate adequate pain management. The PMI is a useful tool for quickly assessing pain management. However, it captures only one aspect of pain management, namely the balance of pain intensity and analgesics used. The PMI misses other important factors that may affect patients' wellbeing, such as dosage of analgesics and response to breakthrough pain. Our findings also indicate that judging the quality of pain management solely on PMI scores is an oversimplification of a complex issue. The PMI is effective in promoting assessment of care in broad settings; however, detailed interpretation by other means would facilitate further improvement in assessment of pain management.

Table 2 Proportion of patients experiencing PI according to category of PMI scores and pain intensity

pain intensity (NRS)/PMI	PMI = 0	PMI = −1	PMI = −2	PMI = −3
NRS = 0 (no pain)	0 /128 (0%)			
NRS = 1–4 (mild pain)	278/758 (36.7%)	339/1219 (27.8 %)		
NRS = 5–6 (moderate pain)	30 /47 (63.8%)	191/282 (67.7%)	122/234 (52.1%)	
NRS = 7–10 (severe pain)	480/572 (83.9%)	37/49 (75.5%)	156/205 (76.1%)	136/188 (72.3%)
Total	788/1505 (52.4%)	567/1550 (36.6%)	278/439 (63.3%)	136/188 (72.3%)

Note: The numbers of each cell are shown, the denominator is the number of patients who experienced cancer pain, and the numerator is the number of patients who had pain interference due to cancer. *NRS* numerical rating scale. The numbers in this table are cumulative number because it contains Days 1–7 including patients who were discharged in fewer than 7 days

Abbreviations

BPI: The Brief Pain Inventory; NRS: A Numerical Rating Scale; PI: Pain Interference; PMI: The Pain Management Index

Acknowledgments

We thank the patients and health professionals and everyone who cooperated and participated in this study.

Funding

This study was funded by a grant-in-aid from the Ministry of Health, Labour and Welfare, Japan. [H26-GANSEISAKU-IPPAN-003].

Author contributions

NS, TH, and MM designed the study; NS and TY conducted literature review; IY and TY were responsible for recruitment and data generation; NS and TH carried out the data analysis; All authors contributed to the manuscript preparation. All authors read and approved the final manuscript.

Competing interests

The authors declare that they have no competing interests.

Author details
[1]Division of Health Services Research, Center for Cancer Control and Information Services, National Cancer Center, 5-1-1 Tsukiji, Chuo-ku, Tokyo 104-0045, Japan. [2]Department of Palliative Care, St. Luke's International Hospital, 9-1 Akashicho, Chuo-ku, Tokyo 104-8560, Japan. [3]Department of Palliative Care, Aomori Prefectural Central Hospital, 2-1-1 Higashitsukurimichi, Aomori City, Aomori 030-8553, Japan. [4]Department of Palliative and Supportive Care, Chukyo Hospital, 1-1-10 Sanjo, Minami-ku, Nagoya City, Aichi 457-8510, Japan. [5]Department of Palliative Care, Japan Red Cross Medical Center, 4-1-22 Hiroo, Shibuya-ku, Tokyo 150-0012, Japan.

References

1. van den Beuken-van Everdingen MH, de Rijke JM, Kessels AG, Schouten HC, van Kleef M, Patijn J. High prevalence of pain in patients with cancer in a large population-based study in the Netherlands. Pain. 2007;132(3):312–20.
2. Lee YP, Wu CH, Chiu TY, Chen CY, Morita T, Hung SH, Huang SB, Kuo CS, Tsai JS. The relationship between pain management and psychospiritual distress in patients with advanced cancer following admission to a palliative care unit. BMC Palliat Care. 2015;14(1):69.
3. Te Boveldt N, Vernooij-Dassen M, Burger N, Ijsseldijk M, Vissers K, Engels Y. Pain and its interference with daily activities in medical oncology outpatients. Pain Physician. 2013;16(4):379–89.
4. World_Health_Organization. Pain Relief and Palliative Care. In: Organization WH, editor. National cancer control programmes : policies and managerial guidelines - 2nd ed. Geneva: World Health Organization; 2002. p. 84.
5. Deandrea S, Montanari M, Moja L, Apolone G. Prevalence of undertreatment in cancer pain. A review of published literature. Ann Oncol. 2008;19(12):1985–91.
6. Cleeland CS, Gonin R, Hatfield AK, Edmonson JH, Blum RH, Stewart JA, Pandya KJ. Pain and its treatment in outpatients with metastatic cancer. N Engl J Med. 1994;330(9):592–6.
7. Greco MT, Roberto A, Corli O, Deandrea S, Bandieri E, Cavuto S, Apolone G. Quality of cancer pain management: an update of a systematic review of undertreatment of patients with cancer. J Clin Oncol. 2014;32(36):4149–54.
8. Daut RL, Cleeland CS, Flanery RC. Development of the Wisconsin brief pain questionnaire to assess pain in cancer and other diseases. Pain. 1983;17(2): 197–210.
9. Mercadante S. Comments on Wang et al., PAIN, 67 (1996) 407-416. Pain. 1998;74(1):106–7.
10. Mercadante S, Bruera E. Good...but Bad News. J Clin Oncol. 2015;33(18):2119.
11. Mercadante S, Guccione C, Di Fatta S, Alaimo V, Prestia G, Bellingardo R, Gebbia V, Giarratano A, Casuccio A. Cancer pain management in an oncological ward in a comprehensive cancer center with an established palliative care unit. Support Care Cancer. 2013;21(12):3287–92.
12. Twycross RG, Fairfield S. Pain in far-advanced cancer. Pain. 1982;14(3):303–10.
13. Sakakibara N, Higashi T, Yamashita I, Miura H, Yoshimoto T, Yoshida S, Hayasaka Y, Komatsu H, Matoba M. Current status of pain control for older cancer patients in comparison to younger patients in outpatient and inpatient settings: a report from one prefectural cancer care hospital. Palliative Care Research. 2015;10(2):135–41.
14. Serlin RC, Mendoza TR, Nakamura Y, Edwards KR, Cleeland CS. When is cancer pain mild, moderate or severe? Grading pain severity by its interference with function. Pain. 1995;61(2):277–84.
15. Mitera G, Fairchild A, DeAngelis C, Emmenegger U, Zurawel-Balaura L, Zhang L, Bezjak A, Levin W, McLean M, Zeiadin N, et al. A multicenter assessment of the adequacy of cancer pain treatment using the pain management index. J Palliat Med. 2010;13(5):589–93.
16. Mitera G, Zeiadin N, Kirou-Mauro A, DeAngelis C, Wong J, Sanjeevan T, Sinclair E, Danjoux C, Barnes E, Tsao M, et al. Retrospective assessment of cancer pain management in an outpatient palliative radiotherapy clinic using the pain management index. J Pain Symptom Manag. 2010;39(2):259–67.

A public health approach to palliative care in the response to drug resistant TB: an ethnographic study in Bengaluru, India

Joseph M. Sawyer[1*], Rahul Asgr[2], Florence N. Todd Fordham[1] and John D.H. Porter[3]

Abstract

Background: The treatment of Multidrug-Resistant Tuberculosis represents one of the most significant challenges to global health. Despite guidance on improving treatment outcomes, there is little focus on how to support individuals in their suffering. Palliative care is therefore proposed as a necessary component in the global strategy to fight Tuberculosis. We aim to describe the informal resources and networks available to persons affected by Multidrug-Resistant Tuberculosis, how they are accessed and how they are integrated into everyday lives.

Methods: In-depth ethnographic research was conducted in Bengaluru, India. Informal interactions and observations were recorded across a range of palliative care and tuberculosis treatment providers over a month-long period. In addition, ten individuals with Multidrug-Resistant Tuberculosis were asked for in-depth interviews, and five agreed.

Results: Multidrug-Resistant Tuberculosis caused a dynamic chain of events that transgress through physical and psychological domains to cause human suffering. Participants utilised support from their family and friends to build a network of care that was of therapeutic benefit. Informal care networks were similar to the holistic model of care practice by specialist palliative care services and represent an underused resource with enormous potential.

Conclusion: Patient suffering is poorly addressed in current Tuberculosis treatment programmes. A community-based palliative care approach may extend peoples' support networks, helping to alleviate suffering. Further research on existing support structures and integration of these services into Tuberculosis control programmes is required.

Keywords: TB, MDR-TB, Palliative care, Suffering, Drug resistance

Background

Tuberculosis (TB) is amongst the top 10 causes of death worldwide and in 2017 it caused an estimated 1.3 million deaths, the highest from any single infectious agent [1]. Attempts to control the disease reflect both advancements in medicine but also how society cares for its most vulnerable. Indeed, the UK achieved a steep decline in the burden of TB before effective chemotherapy became available, indicating the importance of socio-economic factors in disease control [2]. A dominant pharmacological approach has seen these matters take a back seat whilst problems relating to access and adherence to treatment have grown [3]. The world is now facing TB in its resistant form, with the situation described as a global public health crisis [1].

Multidrug-resistant-TB (MDR-TB), defined as resistance to at least isoniazid and rifampicin, is a life-threatening condition posing an international threat to public health. In 2017, the WHO estimated 558,000 incident cases of Rifampicin resistant (RR) TB worldwide, of these an estimated 82% had MDR-TB, resulting in 230,000 deaths [1]. MDR-TB has a global treatment success rate of 55%, whilst extensively drug resistant TB (XDR-TB), a subset of MDR-TB with added resistance to fluoroquinolones and second line injectable drugs, is at 34% [1]. These statistics only partially tell the story as many people are left

* Correspondence: joseph.sawyer@ucl.ac.uk
[1]Marie Curie Palliative Care Research Department, UCL, 6th Floor, Wing B, Maple House, 149 Tottenham Court Road, London W1T 7NF, UK
Full list of author information is available at the end of the article

undiagnosed, are lost to follow up or do not have their treatment outcomes evaluated.

India has the largest burden of TB related disease however the true effect of M/XDR-TB is difficult to quantify in part due to a lack of specialist drug sensitivity testing. Of the 558,000 MDR-TB cases globally almost half (47%) were in India, China and the Russian federation [1]. In 2016 there was an estimated incidence of 147,000 cases of RR/MDR-TB in India, with a treatment success rate of 46% for MDR-TB and 29% for XDR-TB [4]. As such the country is a major focus for TB prevention and control programmes.

As we face the challenge of finding new drugs and improving diagnostics, we must not neglect the care needs of those suffering from potentially terminal disease. This is acknowledged in the WHOs End TB strategy which outlines a vision of zero deaths, disease and suffering due to TB [5]. This bold vision requires innovative approaches that work in conjunction with communities whilst promoting human rights, ethics and equity [6]. With this in mind, the WHO have advocated for palliative care in the global response to MDR-TB [7–9]. Palliative care provides a holistic network of support with a focus on human suffering that spans physical, psychological, social and spiritual needs [10]. Fundamental to the specialty is the concept of 'total pain' which takes into consideration not just physical distress but also mental, emotional and social pain [11].

For a long time, palliative care has been associated with care of the terminally ill towards the end-of-life. However, there is a growing recognition that its services can have profound impact when integrated alongside curative treatments in non-terminal conditions [12]. Many larger hospice organisations now offer palliative care for serious, non-terminal conditions for the purpose of improving quality of life and aiding the recovery process for both the individual and their family. With the evolution of cancer treatments many malignant diseases are now curable yet the need for palliative care services continues to grow. The focus of care has shifted from purely end-of-life care towards complex symptom management and emotional support in order to support people through the ordeals of chemotherapy and into the survivorship phase where people are often left with untreated chronic symptoms that have a dramatic impact on health. There are direct parallels with this and the treatment of tuberculosis and as such the role of palliative care warrants further evaluation.

Specialist palliative care has been present in India since the 1990s although coverage remains poor [13]. This is a problem facing palliative care globally; in response, a public health approach has been proposed.

First outlined by Kellehear, the movement is characterised by social efforts designed to build cohesive community networks that provide person centred holistic care [14] [15]. These networks are often described as 'compassionate communities' [16–18]. Networks may either be formal, composed of professionally facilitated links within a healthcare setting or informal, compromising an individual's personal social networks and support structures built up over time. Under this model, issues such as those seen in TB; loneliness, stigma and inequitable care access, are community issues best tackled by its constituent members rather than healthcare professionals alone.

This approach has led to a wave of community-motivated interventions. From the mobilisation of resources through naturally-existing or externally-facilitated social networks, to the direct support and training of volunteers, there is now an international movement to promote health at the end-of-life [19]. This work is potentially transferable to MDR-TB and could address issues around treatment adherence, infection control at home, nutritional support and treatment withdrawal.

The concept of 'compassionate communities' in India is relatively new, however developments have occurred In Kerala, where there is a community-led initiative aiming to provide home-based palliative care [20–22]. How this model is integrated across a culturally diverse nation with the added influence of traditional healing systems has not been explored.

Aims and objectives

We explore the context of disease and disease management from the individual's perspective. Using this as a backdrop, we aim to describe the informal resources and networks available to people with MDR-TB, how they are accessed and integrated into everyday lives at a cross-section in time. Framing this in the context of a public health approach to palliative care, we hope to provide evidence for the development of a community-led supportive care programme specific to MDR-TB.

Methods

Conceptual framework and literature review

A conceptual framework was created to guide the study and data analysis (see Fig. 1). This was based upon the initial literature review, which demonstrated the structural components of a palliative care programme and how these may accommodate the different modalities of suffering experienced. The following search terms were used across Medline and Embase; exp. Tuberculosis, Multidrug-resistant/ or exp. Extensively drug resistant Tuberculosis/ or exp. Tuberculosis/ or exp. Mycobacterium tuberculosis AND Palliative Care OR palliat* care or palliat* medicine or hospice or Psychol* support or spirit* support or Soc* support. After eliminating duplicates and reviewing documents available in full text, a

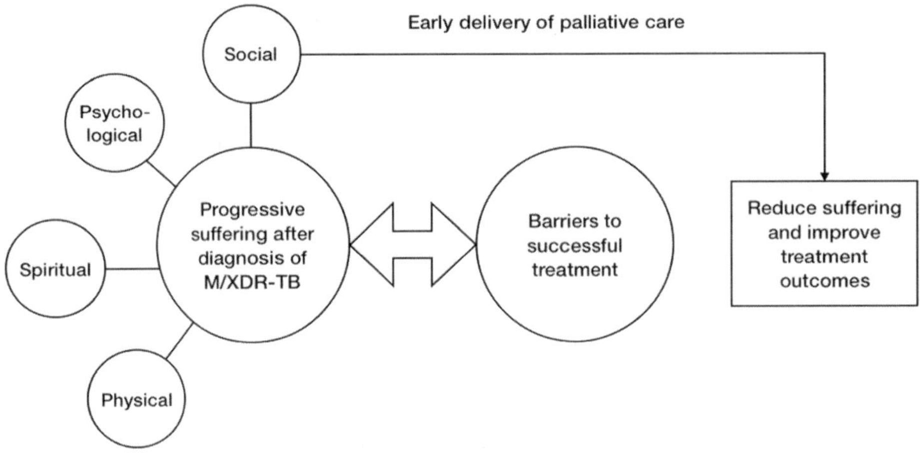

Fig. 1 Conceptual framework

total of 57 relevant articles were identified. The search was updated in 2018 with the same terms and revealed a total of 61 relevant articles.

Study setting

The study was conducted in Bengaluru (Bangalore), India where urbanisation has brought an influx of migrants from neighbouring states resulting in rich linguistic and cultural diversity. Healthcare is predominantly provided by a westernised privately funded system. However, Bengaluru is also home to AYUSH (Department of Ayuverda, Yoga and Naturopathy, Unani, Siddha and Homeopathy). These traditional Indian healing systems offer a holistic approach to disease prevention and cure and have a significant but poorly quantified impact on the delivery of healthcare in India [23]. Formal networks of care were provided through institutions of healthcare including those private and state funded. Informal networks of care were more subtle and ranged from family and community support to the care received from religious institutions and the local environment.

Study design

This study used qualitative ethnographic methods. In-depth interviews and informal observations formed the main data collection methods.

Interviews

Interviewees were selected by convenience sampling. They were recruited from the respiratory clinic attached to St Johns Medical Centre (SJMC), Bengalaru, India. Telephone contact was made by the lead nurse who was familiar with all participants. A preliminary meeting was arranged to introduce the research team and discuss consent prior to interview (see Table 1 for research team).

Interviews were conducted in the summer of 2014 with the use of a topic guide created following a literature review. A pilot interview was held on arrival to the study site and the topic guide refined. Interviews were conducted by team members 1 and 2. Interviews were conducted in the participants' preferred language: Kannada, English, Tamil or Hindi. Where the interviews were not conducted in English, translations were verbatim and conducted in real-time. Interviews occurred in clinics or participant's homes and lasted up to an hour. Interviews were audio-recorded and transcribed in English; emerging themes were recorded in a contact summary form on the day of interview. The audio-recording and written translations were subsequently reviewed by the original translator and discrepancies corrected. Reflexivity is key when conducting ethnographic methods, and thus the social background and personal assumptions of the translator were considered when reviewing transcripts.

Ten participants were approached to take part. One withdrew after interview, four declined to take part and one participant did not have capacity to consent. The remaining participants are summarised in Table 2. The interview with participant four was done in conjunction with his wife (participant 5). A significant theme that hindered recruitment centred on the process of consent and the various cultural forces that impact on this process.

The principle of autonomy, as understood by the Western bioethics, forms the cornerstone to informed consent. In the Indian context, paternalism and patriarchy may influence decision making. Whilst this is perhaps more common in the rural setting, Bengaluru has a diverse population representing great breadth in cultural norms and this issue was frequently encountered. In addition, many participants who were suffering with advanced and disabling disease were too fatigued and fearful to take part. One participant in particular, who was

Table 1 Research team members and their background

Team member	Role	Background/qualifications
Researcher 1	Lead researcher and instigator of conceptual design. Author of field notes and observational study. Present during interview and recruitment process, contributed probing questions via interpreter. Lead for data analysis and coding. Introduced to participants as the lead for research alongside information sheet.	Native to UK and foreign to the studied environment. UK based general medical training and fully qualified clinician at the time of study. Basic training in social science methodology.
Researcher 2	Translator for interview and recruitment process. Helped conduct interviews using topic guide. Provided valuable reflections and insights that contributed to data analysis.	Native to India. Fluent in all local dialects. Indian based medical training and fully qualified clinician. Basic social science training and public health training.
Researcher 3	Supervisory role, contributed to theoretical development of the study and data analysis through discussion of data and evaluation of themes.	Native to UK. Medical training in the UK, public health training in the USA and UK. Extensive experience in public ethics of TB treatment. Knowledge and experience of AYUSH.

from a low socio-economic background, became concerned that involvement in the study would impact negatively on his family, disrupt his treatment options and the relationship with his treating medical team.

"I have met with X twice to discuss the study, each time there appear to be new concerns. Today X was fearful of having his treatment withdrawn as a consequence of speaking to me...not even the local DOTS (Directly Observed Treatment, Short-course) provider [whom X was friendly with] could pacify X's concerns...." *Excerpt from field diary: 5th July 2014.*

Ethical issues surrounding the consent process were discussed with the wider supervisory team who provided valuable insights into issues around cross-cultural social dynamics as well as research and trust ethics. These discussions contributed to the analytic phase.

Informal observations

Informal observations were conducted across the sites mentioned in Table 3. Healthcare professionals were shadowed in their work and informal conversations were held when opportunity arose. Data was collected in the form of field notes. Informal observation facilitates a deep review of the social world in which the study is situated. However, this method also raises issues of subjectivity and researcher bias. This is pertinent as the study was conducted in Bengaluru, where language barriers and cultural considerations positioned the researcher in a new social context. Therefore, it is important to reflect on the research process, the challenges of reflexivity and the influence of researcher perceptions.

Haraway states that self-reflexivity is defined by an "introspective stance" towards one's own conception of information, provoking an awareness of a researcher's positionality [24]. With respect to this study the lead researcher was foreign to the studied environment. The work also required a transition from a western biomedical approach towards more holistic constructs. In order to achieve this, a period of two weeks was spent meeting members of SOCHARA (Society for Community Health Awareness Research and Action) and learning about traditional Indian healing practices. SOCHARA is an innovative community of professionals and activists who facilitate community health and well-being using an

Table 2 Patient demographics and Interview Code: MP = Male Participant, FP = Female Participant, FPFM Female participant, Family member

Characteristics	Participant 1	Participant 2	Participant 3	Participant 4	Participant 5
Age (years)	50–60	20–30	20–30	40–50	40–50
Sex	Male	Female	Female	Male	Female
Treatment stage	Completed	Completed	Continuous phase	Continuous Phase	N/A
Previously treated for TB	Yes	Yes	Yes	Yes	N/A
Socio-economic status	Low	Middle	Middle	Upper	Upper
Living arrangement	Joint family	Nuclear family	Nuclear family	Nuclear family	Nuclear family
Marital status	Married	Single	Single	Married	Married
Language spoken	Kanada	English/Kanada	Tamil	Hindi/English	Hindi/English
Occupation	Labourer	Student	Student	Office worker (IT)	Housewife
Religion	Hindu	Christian	Atheist	Christian	Christian
Educational status	No formal education	Formally educated	Formally educated	Formally educated	Formally educated
Interview code	MP1	FP2	FP3	MP4	FPFM5

Table 3 Description of study sites

Site	Description
Site 1	A large Catholic funded private hospital practicing western medicine. Discussions were held informally with doctors and observations of MDTs, the ward environment and outpatient services were conducted.
Site 2	An autonomous institute specialising in western medical treatments of respiratory disease. Informal observations were held during a visit designed for recruitment purposes.
Site 3	An interdisciplinary resource group of community health professionals utilising multiple pathways to facilitate and promote the goal of Health for All. It focuses on public health system development, action on the social determinants of health and community action for health with a social justice perspective. Constituent members had a range of expertise spanning the social sciences, allopathic medicine, traditional holistic Indian healing systems (AYUSH). Observations were conducted over a month long period and informal conversation held with constituent members on issues ranging from the impact of AYUSH, the relevance of palliative care to TB and the impact of trust ethics on recruitment to the study. This helped enable me as the primary researcher to become more embedded in the culture and traditional practice.
Site 4	A traditional hospice based on the UK model. Practice included western medicine, social work and chaplaincy and spiritual support. Informal conversations were held with members of each of these disciplines during a day visit.
Site 5	A traditional hospice based on the UK model. Conversations were held with nursing staff and observations conducted during a day visit.
Community health centres	Patients were met and consented for recruitment at various community health centres scattered across the city. The process of consent would often take several meetings during which observations were conducted.
Churches	Local Churches of catholic denomination were visited and observations held. The role of spirituality was discussed informally with the community of brothers.
Temples	Small temples were scattered throughout the city and visited for the purposes of observation only.
Community settings	On several occasions people were visited at home to discuss enrolment in the study. Observations of their living environment and surrounding area were conducted.

equity, rights and health determinants perspective. Spending time here allowed the principal researcher to become aware of themes that arose in forthcoming data collection.

To further counter the effects of positionality, and the potential influence on the construction of knowledge, a field diary was kept to critically and constantly analyse researcher perceptions. This reflexive fieldwork practice prompted a more conscious encounter with the multi-faceted aspects of the study site, whilst still acknowledging the situatedness of the researcher, giving rich insights into the doctor-patient relationship in the context of overarching professional structures of care in Bengaluru.

Data analysis

To analyse the ethnographic field notes, a traditional approach of immersion in the text through repeated reading was used. Interviews were analysed via a process of coding based on recurring meanings and ideas [25]. NVivo was used to support a preliminary framework analysis to gain familiarity with the data before developing more detailed thematic analysis.

During thematic analysis coding groups were built up in an iterative process across the whole dataset. This allowed integration between the field notes and interview data. Recurring ideas were grouped together into higher-level themes [25].

Ethical considerations

The study was approved locally by the St Johns Medical Centre ethics committee of Bengaluru, India (ref 78/2014, June 2014) and by the London School of Hygiene & Tropical Medicine Research Ethics Committee (ref 7617, June 2014). Each participant was asked to read an information sheet and given opportunity to ask questions before giving written consent to take part in the study. Where participants could not read, this was read to them in their preferred language. All participants have given written consent for the publication of anonymised results.

Results

The findings are discussed according to the themes identified. The first section explores the human context in which biomedical disease management occurred. The second section explores the informal networks people established and how they were integrated into everyday life.

Human context of disease

Realms of suffering

The medical management of MDR-TB was found to occur in the context of profound human suffering. This theme emerged through discussion and observation.

"Physically X looks very weak and X must be very frightened" *Excerpt from field diary: 5th July 2014.*

Interview data revealed suffering to occur according to a disturbance in human connection, either with the self, with others or within a spiritual network.

Inevitable thoughts on death created an uneasy relationship with 'the self' as participants began to examine their existence in the context of MDR-TB. This ranged from inner turmoil to thoughts of suicide.

"I didn't know what else to do so I thought killing myself was the best thing" *MP1.*

This led to a breakdown in relationships within the family or wider social network.

"...because he can't share his stress with some other [person], he is speaking [only] with me, maybe fighting with me" *FPFM5.*

In search of stability people sought solace in religion, whereas others found this to be another source of uncertainty and grief.

"So when I was not able to get up my sister took me to the church in Madivalla, they said a prayer and I was able to stand" *MP1.*

"He lost a little trust in God...faith was reduced" *FPFM5.*

This lead to the understanding that spiritual suffering was not restricted to religion, instead representing an unmet human need that encompasses and transcends the traditional bio-psycho-social model. Imbalance within someone's spiritual network was a principal theme within the data and represented a disturbance in the connection people felt with themselves, others around them, and their living environment.

"...my elder sister had two children. I missed to kiss them and hug them, really I missed it. I keep wanting to kiss and hug them but I am worried [about disease transmission], I maintain the distance, I do not kiss her, I do not share food or anything..." *FP2.*

Points of suffering

The relationship of human suffering to the context of biomedical treatment models highlighted three themes upon which suffering was noticeably triggered or accentuated; prognostic uncertainty, vulnerability in disease disclosure and the trauma of drug treatment.

Prognostic uncertainty caused spiralling doubt that would permeate through anticipated major life events. All patients had been told their disease was 'definitely' curable however limited information had been given beyond this.

"...no council was done they just made a diagnosis..." FPFM05.

This fed into the aura of uncertainty that would lie on the path ahead, creating anxiety and apprehension.

"I don't know, I believe that it will be curable, I have been told that there is a 100% cure, I have been taking the treatment so I believe that it will be cured, I really don't know, you should ask the doctor or the sister about this..." *FP03.*

"...it is common for respondents to convey a sense of positivity with respect to their prognosis, however when given the opportunity to ask questions to me everyone wants to know why it [MDR-TB] has affected them, the likelihood of it coming back and the chance of cure..." *Excerpt from field diary: 5th July 2014.*

This theme later developed across the whole data set:

"I keep on thinking whether it is curable or not. Then marriage will come and I am worried about it..." *FP2.*

In disclosing their diagnosis, participants faced a range of reactions that varied according to social context. Themes included disdain, pity, fear and aggression.

"So they scold me because they know that I am having the disease, but what can I do? I just move away if they tell me to go, I cannot do anything about it..." *MP1.*

Vulnerability was also detected at the doctor-patient interface. In the context of privately-funded healthcare, participants were often subject to long in-patient admissions. This often represented a lack of participant involvement in decision making which came at a physical, psychological and financial cost.

"Actually, no, hospital is not that clever, because they will think maybe it's something else [not TB] and they will ask him to stay [in the hospital]...That made him feel even more stressed..." *FPFM5.*

Whilst TB chemotherapy was seen as the cure, it was in itself a source of suffering. Side effects range from disturbance in vision to lethargy, nausea and vomiting. In some cases, the cure became as much of a burden as the disease. One interviewee highlighted that as a parent, watching your child endure this suffering could lead to a vacillating appreciation of what may be right or wrong.

"She [participant's mother] kept telling me don't worry. She is also crying, when they put [administer] the injections I will be crying and my mum also is crying" *FP2.*

Resources, practices and support networks

Recognition of the importance of holistic care, and the role of the community in providing it, arose through observational data collected during a SOCHARA workshop:

"...I am fascinated to learn of the concept of community health and it strikes me as being incredibly relevant yet almost completely unspoken of in the [UK based] National Health Service. The work done in communities here implies that medical services are not just a model or structure for consumerist use but embody a fluid process that enables/empowers people for collective action and care. Here the community is able to maintain health and provide health within its own means...this is a radically different approach that is well characterised by their 'paradigm shift' i.e. moving away from professional 'control', moving from a medical model to a social model, from patients to

the individual, disease to health, providing to enabling, drugs and technology to knowledge and process..." *Excerpt from field diary 16th June 2014.*

Interview data developed this theme, highlighting participants reliance on their family and friends to provide supportive care. This ranged from practical help, such as transport and food, to a deeper level of care that embodied themes of compassion and love. This was demonstrated by one participant who could not cope with the sight of her tablets. Her father collected her tablets from hospital and her mother prepared them daily in a specially made box.

"Yeah, she [Participant's mother] only cuts my tablets and gives it to me. I did not see anything...So my mum gave me separate in the box also. That was the main thing; yeah I didn't see a bunch of tablets..." *FP2.*

The assiduous nature of a mother's care, combined with the sense of normality conveyed by family-led care, was vital to the participant's well-being and ability to continue treatment.

In search of support of this kind, participants would explore human connections - both physical and metaphysical. This was demonstrated by a participant explaining how he survived feelings of self-harm and suicide:

"So going to the church helped reduce that thought of killing myself, I was also admitted for two/three months in the hospital and this reduced that thought also... When I was in the hospital the doctors used to come and take care of me, give me tablets, the food was also free, I used to not think so much about the house and also there used to be five or six other patients in the ward and I used to talk to them and my time would pass so all these thoughts [of suicide] would not come" *MP1.*

From this, it became apparent that support structures were interdependent. This represented holistic care and, as a concept, was fundamental in addressing a state of equilibrium that we may call 'health'. The holistic care observed was similar in construct and theory to that provided by a specialist palliative care service.

"Because of all the support I am well now, without the support it would have been difficult" *MP1.*

In contrast to observed community support networks, medical structures of care promoted fear amongst the community, whilst demonstrating coercion as a means of control.

"...sometimes when I didn't come to the hospital the doctor used to come and give me the tablets, so if the doctor used to come home with the tablets the neighbours used to scold me saying that you have this disease, so from that day onwards I always used to come to the hospital and take the tablets myself." *MP1.*

Importantly, community-led care occurred naturally and was initiated and provided for by lay people. In the hospice environment, the intervention was creating an environment where community support could flourish, thereby promoting and strengthening social networks. Observational data from hospices highlighted how the environment held and supported staff and patients alike.

"...I was struck by the importance of the environment in creating a positive and healthy atmosphere. This was mirrored by the staff who were engaged and enthusiastic about their work...it became clear that the medical consultation was only one step in the chain of support that assisted patients and their families back into the community or in the case of those with end stage disease, through the process of death...."

"After sharing lunch with the staff, we walked back through the grounds where X mentioned how they had built the surrounding gardens from scratch, he spoke of the positive atmosphere this created for him which resonated with my initial feelings on arrival." *Excerpts from field diary 16th June 2014.*

These findings were in contrast to experiences from hospitals which were often overcrowded and fearful places.

"I waited to speak to the Doctor for an hour and half, during this time I was surrounded by TB patients...Many were emaciated, some barely conscious...this felt like an isolating and fearful place full of pain." *Excerpt from field diary: 4thJuly 2014.*

"...actually they asked him to stay [in the hospital]...the environment he didn't like because all the other patients are more severe [severely unwell], he was just started [on treatment]...he got even more scared around them..." *FPFM5.*

It was found that structures valuing human connections as therapeutic were of fundamental importance. Peoples' individual stories, their resources, practices and networks of care, were brought together and integrated into everyday life through the creation of a social platform, be that a hospital ward, a park, a place of worship or a cinema.

"I speak with my friends also like going to movies and things like that." *FP2.*

"I like to go to temples, I feel comfortable, I express my feelings with God..." *FP2.*

"So I used to go and sit and parks, also I used to go and walk around" *MP1.*

Being able to 'connect' in the broadest sense of the word allowed for the development of a network that encouraged self-care and community-led care.

Discussion

Main findings

This study describes informal networks of care that are responsive and reflexive to the multi-dimensional human suffering caused by MDR-TB. Community based care networks were found to be theoretically similar to the model of holistic care enacted by specialist palliative care services. Participants built supportive networks through existing social platforms that intervened at focal points of accentuated suffering. This network appeared to work independently and sometimes at odds with a medical management programme that focussed on technology, drug treatments and specialist biomedical knowledge.

These findings suggest that in order to achieve the vision for 'zero suffering' outlined as part of the WHOs End TB strategy there must be a robust capacity for delivering large scale, context specific and community centred palliative care services. Applying the principles of a public health approach to holistic palliative care allows human suffering to become the central focus as opposed to the disease. What follows is a recognition of the interdependence between supportive structures allowing them to realign and work in unison to help bring about meaningful outcomes at both the individual and population level (See Fig. 2 for schematic representation).

Strengths and limitations

The rising calls for TB treatment programmes to integrate palliative care into their services have been met with a growing evidence base [26] [27]. Currently this focusses on symptom burden giving strong evidence for the integration of specialist palliative care alongside potentially curative options [26]. By describing human suffering in the context of MDR-TB we found suffering was poorly acknowledged by professional structures of care thus giving weight to this argument. In addition, we propose three focal points to suffering upon which interventions could be designed. These relate to a disturbance in human connection, either with the self, with others or within a greater, all-encompassing, spiritual network. The overarching domain of spiritual care represented the bond between individuals, families, communities and their natural environment whilst encompassing themes of love and compassion. This research was embedded in a culture of traditional holistic networks of care and is therefore culture and context specific.

Interviews were conducted and analysed with an explicit interest into how social networks and community structures related to the suffering experienced. Participants were found to depend on a network of family, friends and community members. Rather than compromising care, this was found to add quality and enhance relationships whilst allowing people to overcome physical and psychological barriers to treatment. This was in part due to care being individualised and person specific. This is congruent to the theories proposed by Kellehear in the development of 'compassionate communities' [18]. Most existing research is framed within advanced or incurable disease. Our results suggest there is scope to integrate this approach alongside curative interventions in order to tackle issues such as access and adherence to medications.

Traditionally, palliative care has utilised professional knowledge and skills to deliver such a service. However, in the context of limited resources, our study suggests that non-specialist measures from friends and family were used to good effect. There is an argument that the standard of care delivered by an attentive family, supplemented with access to relevant knowledge and information, would provide a standard of care greater than that achieved by professionals alone.

It is important to acknowledge the inherent methodological limitations to the study. As a non-native researcher entering an intensely emotional and culturally foreign context, researcher bias is an issue. As such, reflexivity during field work and during the evaluative process was of vital importance. Cross-cultural group discussion and cultural integration allowed the principal researcher to reflect upon his personal beliefs, values and professional identity and how they influenced the research process. It is also recognised that some themes will have been left uncovered in the study. With such cultural breadth in Bengaluru it was not possible to uncover the complexities in each unique social network with 5 participants from predominantly middle and higher socio-economic backgrounds. This combined with the highly personal and emotionally challenging nature of the interviews and the inherent language barriers, meant that some issues may have been left uncovered. Using the same translator who was native to the culture and briefed in the study objectives helped limit this impact.

What this study adds

Our research adds weight to the call for integration of palliative care services into MDR-TB treatment programmes. By demonstrating the importance of community networks, and evaluating how they are accessed, we suggest a potential mechanism by which a sustainable palliative care service may be integrated into this specific setting. A public health approach to palliative care is growing a significant evidence base and palliative care as a speciality is ideally placed to drive forward such interventions [19]. Further research is required to understand the impact of social networks in this particular disease context across a range of settings.

Conclusion

The findings from this study suggest that under the WHO's End TB Strategy there is scope to integrate palliative care practice at local, national and international levels [9]. If we are to acknowledge the report's ambition to reach zero deaths, disease and suffering whilst

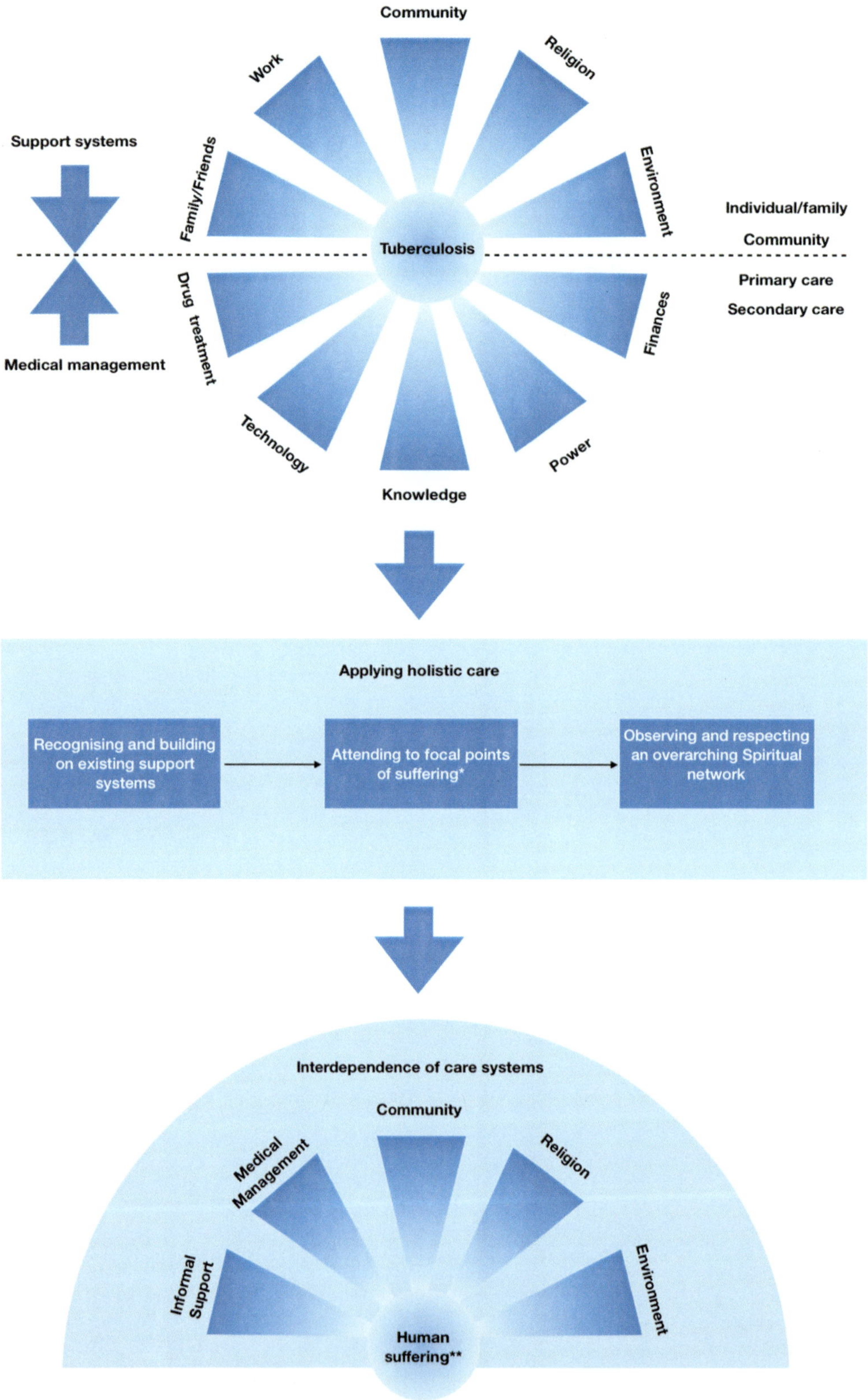

Fig. 2 Schematic representation of themes and subthemes. *prognostic uncertainty, vulnerability in disease disclosure and the trauma of drug treatment. ** a disturbance in human connection, either with the self, with others or within an overarching spiritual network

addressing the complex ethical issues surrounding treatment there is a desperate need for community empowered palliative care services to support on the issues raised throughout this paper.

Further research into existing support networks for both patients and carers is required in order to build a robust capacity for delivering palliative care in MDR-TB. To further understand this, longitudinal studies looking at how and why social networks evolve and adapt around an individual with tuberculosis over the course of treatment and beyond are essential. This must run in conjunction with attempts to influence society's perceptions and reactions to death and dying. By recognising and empowering the work done by communities we can build an economically sustainable model of palliative care with a level of quality and continuity that is in tune with peoples cultural and social needs.

Abbreviations

AYUSH: Ayuverda, Yoga and Naturopathy, Unani, Siddha and Homeopathy; MDR-TB: Multi-drug resistant TB; RR-TB: Rifampicin resistant TB; SJMC: St. Johns Medical Centre; SOCHARA: Society for Community Health Awareness Research and Action; TB: Tuberculosis; WHO: World Health Organisation; XDR-TB: extensively drug resistant TB

Acknowledgements

I would like to acknowledge the support of Dr. Solomon Salve who assisted in developing my skills in qualitative methodology; he also reviewed the initial interview guide and provided recommendations. On arrival in Bengaluru Dr. George D'Souza provided academic supervision. He provided contact with the local DOTS (Directly Observed Therapy, Short-Course) centre and provided advice over cultural issues around the consent process. Members of SOCHARA provided regular practical advice, I am particularly grateful to Dr. Adithya Pradyumma, Dr. Thelma Narayan and Dr. Ravi Narayan for their support during challenging situations and their overall guidance, which provided direction to my work.

Declaration of conflicting interests

The author(s) declared no potential conflicts of interest with respect to the research, authorship, and/or publication of this article.

Funding

J.S. received funding from the LSHTM for transport to the research site. Both J.S and F.TF are supported in their current academic posts by Marie Curie core funding.

Authors contributions

J.S conceived, designed and conducted this study. R.A provided support with interviews, recruitment, translation and interpretation of results, F.TF provided methodological support. J.P provided academic supervision and input at all stages of design and reporting, and contributed to the analyses. J.S, F.TF, J.P. contributed to the drafting and approval of the manuscript.

Competing interests

The authors have no competing interests.

Author details

[1]Marie Curie Palliative Care Research Department, UCL, 6th Floor, Wing B, Maple House, 149 Tottenham Court Road, London W1T 7NF, UK. [2]Society for Community Health Awareness Research and Action, Public Health, Bengaluru, Karnataka, India. [3]Departments of Clinical Research and Global Health and Development, London School of Hygiene and Tropical Medicine, Keppel Street, London WC1E 7HT, UK.

References

1. World Health Organization, "Global Tuberculosis Report 2018," 2018.
2. Cohen T, Dye C. "Clinical tuberculosis," 5th ed., P. Davies, S. Gordon, and G. Davies. Florida: CRC Press; 2014. p. 19–36.
3. Coker RJ. From Chaos to coercion: detention and the control of tuberculosis: St. Martin's Press; 2000.
4. WHO. Global Tuberculosis Report 2017. Global Tuberculosis Report. 2016; 2016:5–130.
5. World Health Organization. The end TB. Strategy. 2015.
6. Uplekar M, Weil D, Lonnroth K, Jaramillo E, Lienhardt C, Dias HM, Falzon D, Floyd K, Gargioni G, Getahun H, Gilpin C, Glaziou P, Grzemska M, Mirzayev F, Nakatani H, Raviglione M. WHO's new end TB strategy. Lancet. 2015; 385(9979):1799–801.
7. Harding R, Foley KM, Connor SR, Jaramillo E, Harding R, Foley KM, Connor SR, Jaramillo E. Palliative and end-of-life care in the global response to multidrug-resistant tuberculosis. *Lancet Infect. Dis 2012*. 2012;12(8):643–6.
8. R. Laniado-labor, M. G. B. Spanevello A., D'Ambrosio L., Centis R., R. K. Laniado-Laborin R., Laniado-Laborin R. Kiy R. Spanevello A. D'Ambrosio L. Centis R. Migliori GB., Connor S. Foley K. Harding R. Jaramillo E., J. E. Connor S., Foley K., Harding R., and M. G. B. Laniado-Laborin R., Kiy R., Spanevello A., D'Ambrosio L., Centis R., "Declaration on palliative care," Int J Tuberc Lung Dis, vol. 16, no. 10, pp. 1418–1419, 2012.
9. World Health Organization. Global strategy and targets for tuberculosis prevention , care and control after 2015. In: no. November 2013, pp. 1–23; 2015.
10. "WHO | WHO Definition of Palliative Care".
11. Bond VA, Tihon V, Muchimba M, Godfrey-Faussett P. Kuyendela odwala TB'--visiting TB patients: the widening role of home-based care organisations in the management of tuberculosis patients in Lusaka Zambia. *Int J Tuberc Lung Dis*. 2005;9(3):282–7.
12. Traue DC, Ross JR. Palliative care in non-malignant diseases. J R Soc Med. 2005;98(11):503–6.
13. McDermott E, Selman L, Wright M, Clark D. Hospice and palliative care development in India: a multimethod review of services and experiences. J Pain Symptom Manag. Jun. 2008;35(6):583–93.
14. A Karapliagkou and A Kellehear, "Public Health Approaches to End of Life Care: A toolkit," 2014.
15. Kellehear A. Health promoting palliative care. Melbourne: Oxford University Press; 1999.
16. WHO, "The Ottawa Charter for health promotion," 1986.
17. Wegleitner K, Heimerl K, Kellehear A. *Compassionate communities: case studies from Britain and Europe*. Abingdon: Routledge; 2015.
18. Kellehear A. Compassionate cities. London: Routledge; 2005.
19. Sallnow L, Richardson H, Murray SA, Kellehear A. The impact of a new public health approach to end-of-life care: a systematic review. Palliat Med. 2016;30(3):200–11.
20. Sallnow L, Chenganakkattil S. The role of religious, social and political groups in palliative care in northern Kerala. Indian J Palliat Care. 2005;11(1):10.
21. Khosla D, Patel FD, Sharma SC. Palliative care in India: current progress and future needs. Indian J Palliat Care. Sep. 2012;18(3):149–54.

22. Thayyil J, Cherumanalil JM. Assessment of status of patients receiving palliative home care and services provided in a rural area-Kerala, India. Indian J Palliat Care. Sep. 2012;18(3):213–8.
23. Rudra S, Kalra A, Kumar A, Joe W. Utilization of alternative systems of medicine as health care services in India: evidence on AYUSH care from NSS 2014. PLoS One. 2017;12(5):1–20.
24. D. J. Haraway, Simians, cyborgs, *and women : the reinvention of* Nature .
25. Corbin J, Strauss A. Basics of qualitative research: techniques and procedures for Developeing grounded theory. 2nd ed. London: Sage Publications; 1998.
26. Harding R, Defilippi K, Cameron D. What palliative care–related problems do patients with drug-resistant or drug-susceptible tuberculosis experience on admission to hospital? A cross-sectional self-report study. Palliat Med. 2016; 30(9):862–8.
27. University Research Co. Comprehensive guidelines for TB and DR- TB palliative care and support. In: no. May; 2015.

19

Allow natural death versus do-not-resuscitate: titles, information contents, outcomes, and the considerations related to do-not-resuscitate decision

Sheng-Yu Fan[1*], Ying-Wei Wang[2] and I-Mei Lin[3]

Abstract

Background: As the "do not resuscitate" (DNR) discussion involves communication, this study explored (1) the effects of a title that included "allow natural death", and of information contents and outcomes of the decision; and (2) the information needs and consideration of the DNR decision, and benefits and barriers of the DNR discussion.

Methods: Healthy adults ($n = 524$) were presented with a scenario with different titles, information contents, and outcomes, and they rated the probability of a DNR decision. A questionnaire including information needs, consideration of the decision, and benefits and barriers of DNR discussion was also used.

Results: There was a significantly higher probability of signing the DNR order when the title included "allow natural death" ($t = -4.51$, $p < 0.001$), when comprehensive information was provided ($F = 60.64$, $p < 0.001$), and when there were worse outcomes ($F = 292.16$, $p < 0.001$). Common information needs included remaining life period and the prognosis. Common barriers were the families' worries and uncertainty about future physical changes.

Conclusion: The title, information contents, and outcomes may influence the DNR decisions. Health-care providers should address the concept of natural death, provide comprehensive information, and help patients and families to overcome the barriers.

Keywords: Allow natural death, Barriers, Cardiopulmonary resuscitation, Do not resuscitate, Information needs

Background

Cardiopulmonary resuscitation (CPR) is an emergency procedure that has been developed to stop cardiopulmonary bypass caused by accidents [1]; however, CPR is not appropriate for patients with a terminal illness or who are dying. It cannot cure the diseases but causes harms [2]. In Taiwan, the Hospice Palliative Act was passed in 2000 and adults can sign a "do not resuscitate" (DNR) order to refuse futile medical treatment when a person is dying.

Some surveys have revealed that most patients are willing to participate in an DNR discussion [3, 4]. However, decision-making is not easy and the timing of the decision may be close to death [5]. While, in Taiwan, terminal patients who received hospice care had to have DNR orders [6], and around 65% patients in intense care units had DNR orders [7]. Less than 2% of the healthy adults had decided DNR orders for themselves, and older adults do not have it [8].

The predictors of a DNR order include older age [9, 10], a cancer diagnosis or poor prognosis [10], poor health condition [9], poor activities of daily living [10], terminal illness with pain symptoms [11], and awareness of prognosis and the survival time following CPR [12]. A study used scenarios with various conditions, and the results showed that patients tended to accept a DNR order under the conditions with older age, pain symptoms, and dementia; and for incurable conditions, better quality of life was an important consideration of DNR [13]. In addition, people with relevant experience, such as experience of caring for

* Correspondence: shengyu@mail.ncku.edu.tw
[1]Institute of Gerontology, College of Medicine, National Cheng Kung University, Tainan, Taiwan
Full list of author information is available at the end of the article

patients with a terminal illness and dying patients [14], and those with knowledge [15], tended to sign the DNR order.

The decision of DNR involves specific medical knowledge and legal regulations, and discussing DNR is a process of communication between the patient and physicians. Several variables may influence their understanding. The first variable is the title; using the term "DNR" that includes "do not" may hint that they should give up or that the medical staff should not give any treatment [16]. Meyer (2002) suggested using the term "allow natural death" (AND) to replace DNR, which addresses the fact that death is natural and that the goal of care in the dying phase is for the patient to be comfortable rather than suffering unnecessarily [17]. A study that used scenarios with DNR and AND showed that a higher ratio of nurses and nursing students signed the permissions with AND compared to those with DNR [18]. Physicians and nurses also had more positive perceptions about AND than DNR [19].

The second variable is the contents. The success rate of CPR can influence the participants' decision; it decreases the decision of receiving CPR when they realize its low success rate [20]. However, people may misunderstand the effect of CPR [21] and do not comprehend the information adequately [22]. In addition, descriptions that are too negative [23] and that have too much or too little information [24] decrease the likelihood of signing the DNR. Few studies have explored the potential effects of the title and contents on the DNR decision in a healthy population.

Better quality of communication about DNR was related to higher satisfaction with care [25]. However, there are problems with the DNR communication: (1) the DNR discussion may be too little and the patients' preferences may not be respected, (2) the timing of the discussion is too late for the patients to participate, (3) the medical staff do not provide appropriate information for decision-making, and (4) the medical staff inappropriately assume that patients with the DNR orders did not want any treatments [26]. The barriers in patients include that the patients do not understand their diagnosis or prognosis well, are not ready to talk, and are afraid of death [27]. Exploring people's information needs and their consideration of DNR is important that medical staff could provide the essential information and talk about the individual persons' needs in relation to DNR decisions.

Therefore, the aims of this study were to explore: (1) how "allow a natural death" versus "do not resuscitate" and specific scenarios and outcomes, influence the willingness to sign a DNR order; and (2) the information needs and consideration of the DNR decisions, and the benefits and barriers of the DNR discussion, in the general population.

Methods

Participants and research design

A cross-sectional survey with convenience sampling was conducted. The participants were healthy adults (age > 20 years) who could read and complete the questionnaire. The participants were recruited from the communities and a clinic of family medicine in eastern Taiwan. Ethical approval was obtained before the beginning of the study (Buddhist Tzu Chi General Hospital IRB102–46) and the participants who joined the study gave informed consent before data collection. The participants were given the paper questionnaire and then completed on their own. A research assistant was available to answer questions if necessary.

Data collection

The data collection included three parts: demographic characteristics and experience of DNR, a scenario, and consideration of the DNR.

Demographic characteristics and experience of DNR

The demographic characteristics included gender, age, job, education level, marriage, religion, and self-rated health. Previous experience of DNR was also collected, including if they had heard about DNR, signed a DNR, one day will sign or not, the appropriate timing of discussion, would like to participate in the discussion, and who should make the decision.

Scenario

The following scenario was presented: "Mr. W is 80 years old and he was diagnosed with lung cancer five years ago. He has received several surgeries and chemotherapy. There was a period of remission. However, recently, the physician has found that the disease has progressed to stage IV with brain and bone metastasis. His education level is senior high school and his previous work was as a government employee. Since retirement, he has lived with his oldest son who is taking care of him now." The participants were asked to rate the likelihood of signing the DNR document that had different titles, information contents, and outcomes, by using a scale ranging from 0 (never) to 10 (definitely yes).

Title The official DNR document of the Ministry of Health and Welfare was presented and another document was presented that was exactly the same except for the title being changed to "AND." Two documents were rated, and in order to balance the sequence effect, a counterbalanced design was used in which half of the participants rated the DNR document first and the other half rated the AND document first.

Information contents The following information was given in sequence: (1) terminal illness: the physician said that the disease has progressed to the end stage and no curative treatment can be provided; (2) goal: the physician said that the goal of DNR is to enable patients to die smoothly and peacefully; (3) success rate: the physician said that the success rate of CPR in patients with a terminal illness is less than 1%, and even though CPR could extend life, there would be only several days of survival time; and (4) harm: the physician said that the CPR procedure includes endotracheal intubation, chest presses, and defibrillation, which may cause harm.

The arrangement of the information was that: bad news was delivered first so that the participants could understand that the disease could not be cured; and then the goal of letting the patient die smoothly and peacefully was presented; in the end, the success rate and side effects of CPR for terminal patients were provided. The participants rated four times when they got information.

Outcomes Different outcomes based on the level of functional impairment and dependence were given. The following consequences of CPR were stated: (1) the patient has to stay in an intensive care unit and he will die within two weeks; (2) the patient has an endotracheal intubation and lives with a ventilator; (3) the patient is in a vegetative state and unconscious; (4) the patient is clearly conscious but cannot take care of himself, and has to rely on others; (5) the patient may have a tracheostomy tube but can take care of himself/herself; and (6) the patient will completely recover.

Consideration of the DNR

A standardized survey was used that included the information needs (11 items), the important factors related to the DNR decision (10 items), the benefits of a DNR discussion (five items), the barriers of a DNR discussion with you (seven items), and the barriers of a DNR discussion with families who have a severe disease (eight items). The items were developed from a previous qualitative study [28]. A dichotomous scale (yes/no) was used to rate whether they needed the specific information, and whether the DNR discussion brought the benefits, and whether they had the barriers.

Statistical analysis

Descriptive statistics were used to present the demographic characteristics and previous experience of DNR. A repeated measures one-way analysis of variance was employed to examine whether there were significant differences in the likelihood of signing the DNR order between the different titles, information contents, and outcomes. The percentage was used to present the importance of the consideration of the DNR.

Results

A total of 524 participants were recruited. The mean age was 39.19 years ($SD = 14.34$), 312 were female, more than half had a college or university degree, and 39.31% rated their health as good. Regarding DNR experience, 84.16% had heard about DNR, 24.43% had signed a DNR order, 95.23% would like to participate in the DNR discussion, and 50.76% would accept the order one day. Regarding the appropriate timing of the discussion, the first was "when the disease had progressed to the terminal stage" (30.34%) and the second was "when the patient was healthy" (27.48%). In addition, 54.39% agreed that patients and their families should make the DNR decision together and share the responsibility, and 35.50% stated that the patients should make the decision by themselves (see Table 1).

Regarding the title, there was a significantly higher probability of signing when using the AND document than when using the DNR document ($t = -4.51$, $p < 0.001$). Regarding the information contents, there were significant differences in the likelihood of signing the DNR order between the four different information contents ($F = 60.64$, $p < 0.001$), and the post-hoc analysis showed that the higher probability was related to more information. Regarding the outcomes, there were significant differences ($F = 292.16$, $p < 0.001$), and the post-hoc analysis showed that "the patient was in a vegetative state and unconscious" outcome had the highest probability and that "the patient has to stay in an intensive care unit and will die within two weeks" and "the patient has an endotracheal intubation and lives with a ventilator" had the second highest probability. This was followed by "the patient is clearly conscious but cannot take care of himself/herself, and has to rely on others," "the patient may have a tracheostomy tube but can take care of himself/herself," and "the patient will completely recover" in sequence (see Table 2).

The most common information needs were "remaining life period" (75.57%), "the prognosis of the disease" (74.43%), "future symptoms" (70.80%), "hospice and palliative care" (67.56%), "the diagnosis of the disease" (66.60%), and "CPR procedure" (63.93%). The important factors when making the DNR decision included "the consequence of the CPR procedure" (88.93%), "patients' willingness" (88.55%), "patients' current physical conditions" (87.40%), "suffering when receiving CPR" (85.88%), and "still having other curative treatments" (83.97%).

The benefits of a DNR discussion included "reducing suffering" (72.90%), "arrangement of medical care as wished" (72.52%), and "reduction of the families' burden" (70.80%). The barriers related to the participants not wanting to discuss DNR included "families' worries" (50.95%) and "uncertainty about future physical changes" (46.76%). The barriers related to a discussion about DNR

Table 1 Demographic characteristics and experience of "do not resuscitate"

Variables	N (%)
Age (years)	Mean = 39.19 (SD = 14.34, range = 20–88)
Gender	
Male	212 (40.46)
Female	312 (59.54)
Job	
Full-time	327 (62.40)
Part-time	48 (9.16)
None	149 (28.44)
Education	
None	11 (2.10)
Elementary school	29 (5.53)
Junior high school	46 (8.21)
Senior high school	99 (18.89)
College and university	277 (52.86)
Postgraduate	62 (11.83)
Marriage	
Single	222 (42.37)
Married	262 (50.00)
Divorced	19 (3.63)
Widowed	14 (2.67)
Others	7 (1.34)
Self-rated health	
Very good	98 (18.70)
Good	206 (39.31)
Usual	192 (36.64)
Not good	20 (3.82)
Very bad	8 (1.53)
Have heard about DNR?	
Yes	441 (84.16)
No	83 (13.84)
Have had a DNR order?	
Yes	128 (24.43)
No	396 (75.57)
One day, will you accept a DNR order?	
Definitely yes	266 (50.76)
Not sure	241 (45.99)
Definitely no	17 (3.24)
The appropriate timing of discussing DNR	
Healthy	144 (27.48)
Just been diagnosed	68 (12.98)
Disease progressed	105 (20.04)
Terminal stage of the disease	159 (30.34)
Facing death/dying	48 (9.16)
Would you like participate in the DNR discussion?	
Yes	499 (95.23)
No	25 (4.77)
Who should make the DNR decision?	
Self	186 (35.50)
Families	12 (2.29)
Medical staff	5 (0.95)
Self and families	285 (54.39)
Self and medical staff	31 (5.92)
Self, families, and medical staff	5 (0.95)

DNR Do Not Resuscitate

with families who had a severe disease included "worry that they cannot handle the topic" (58.59%), "they do not know when the appropriate timing is" (41.22%), "they do not know how to discuss it with them" (36.64%), and "they do not know the progress of the disease" (35.88%) (see Table 3).

Table 2 The probability of signing a "do not resuscitate" order with a different title, information contents, and outcomes

	Mean (SD)	F/p
Titles		
DNR	7.81 (2.19)	$t = -4.51$,
AND	8.11 (1.96)	$p < 0.001$
Information contents		
(1) terminal illness	7.86 (2.24)	$F = 60.64$,
(1) + (2) goal	8.09 (2.19)	$p < 0.001$
(1) + (2) + (3) success rate	8.52 (2.01)	4 > 3 > 2 > 1
(1) + (2) + (3) + (4) harm	8.62 (2.03)	
Outcomes		
(1) The patient has to stay in an intensive care unit and will die within two weeks.	7.29 (2.51)	$F = 292.16$, $p < 0.001$
(2) The patient has an endotracheal intubation and lives with a ventilator.	7.33 (2.60)	3 > 2 = 1 > 4 > 5 > 6
(3) The patient is in a vegetative state and unconscious.	7.63 (2.82)	
(4) The patient is clearly conscious but cannot take care of himself/herself, and has to rely on others.	6.58 (2.89)	
(5) The patient may have a tracheostomy tube but can take care of himself/herself.	4.96 (2.96)	
(6) The patient will completely recover.	2.76 (3.51)	

AND Allowed Natural Death, *DNR* Do Not Resuscitate

Table 3 Information needs, benefits, and barriers of the "do not resuscitate" discussion

	N (%)
Information needs	
Remaining life period	396 (75.57)
The prognosis of the disease	390 (74.43)
Future symptoms	371 (70.80)
Hospice and palliative care	354 (67.56)
The diagnosis of the disease	349 (66.60)
CPR procedure	335 (63.93)
Cannot continue curative treatments	292 (55.73)
Dying symptoms and death situation	192 (36.64)
Artificial nutrition	162 (30.92)
New clinical trial	149 (28.44)
Other physicians and hospitals (second opinion)	77 (14.969)
Important factors related to the DNR decision	
The consequence of the CPR procedure	466 (88.93)
Patients' willingness, such as whether they have expressed an opinion about DNR	464 (88.55)
Patients' current physical conditions, such as pain, uncomfortable symptoms, and suffering	458 (87.40)
Suffering when receiving CPR	450 (85.88)
Still have other curative treatments, such as operations or medicine	440 (83.97)
The diagnosis of the disease	438 (83.59)
Patients' age	432 (82.44)
Future care task, such as taking patients to the hospital and care	406 (77.48)
Future care expenditure	387 (73.85)
Other families' opinions about DNR	281 (53.63)
Benefits of the DNR discussion	
Reduction of suffering	382 (72.90)
Arrangement of medical care as wished	380 (72.52)
Reduction of families' burden	371 (70.80)
Arrangement of funeral as wished	304 (58.02)
Arrangement of property as wished	214 (40.84)
Barriers that stopped you wanting to discuss DNR	
Families' worries	267 (50.95)
Uncertainty about future physical changes	245 (46.76)
No one to discuss it with	80 (15.27)
Families' opinions	64 (12.21)
Worries that physicians gave up treatment	58 (11.07)
Families can understand my ideas without discussion	57 (10.88)
Taboo of death	40 (7.63)
Barriers to the DNR discussion with your family member with advanced disease	
Worry that they cannot handle the topic	307 (58.59)
Do not know when the appropriate timing is	216 (41.22)
Do not know how to discuss it with them	192 (36.64)
Do not know the progress of the disease	188 (35.88)
Should let the medical staff discuss it	153 (29.20)
Worry that they might refuse/reject treatment	136 (25.95)
Worry about the taboo of death	122 (23.28)
Worry about others' gossip (e.g., property)	96 (18.32)

CPR Cardiopulmonary resuscitation, *DNR* Do Not Resuscitate

Discussion

The study used scenarios to explore the factors related to a DNR decision. It was found that the participants were more willing to accept a DNR decision when the title referred to AND, when there was comprehensive information, and when there were worse outcomes. The participants took into account current physical conditions and future care plans, and they considered the consequences of DNR and the patient's willingness. More than 70% of participants agreed that DNR could reduce the patient's suffering and family's burden. However, family's worries, uncertainty about the physical conditions, and lack of skills were barriers to the DNR communication.

Similar to a previous study of medical staff [18], the results supported that the general population also prefer the title with AND rather than DNR. The document with "do not" in the title may hint at giving up and the medical jargon may be difficult to understand [14]. In addition, following the promotion of education about life and death and hospice palliative care by the government and hospice-related organizations, the general population can accept that death is natural and face the DNR issue.

The information contents may influence the decision. When the participants had comprehensive information, they had a higher willingness to sign the DNR order. Comprehensive information could include the prognosis of the disease, the goal of DNR, and the success rate and side effects of CPR. The outcome of CPR was one of important considerations [29]. People can evaluate whether the effect of CPR would match their goal and the patient's best interest. It might decrease the probability of CPR when the participants understand the survival rate of CPR for the dying patient [20]. In addition, they evaluated the level of functional impairment and dependence. If the patient had severe functional impairment and had to depend on others' care, they then tended to sign the DNR order.

Worse physical conditions and no curative treatment would make people choose DNR, as well as the suffering when receiving CPR. The reason was that if there was no chance to prolong life, then they would not increase the patient's suffering. If the patients were too old, they also would not want to increase the burden and suffering. In addition, future symptoms and the CPR procedure were regarded as important information about the level of suffering, and they may accept a DNR order if there was too much suffering.

People needed several information for making a DNR decision. The most important information needed for decision-making was "remaining life period," as has been found for patients with advanced lung cancer [30]. DNR was viewed as a death-related decision, and how much time the patients have was regarded as important information. They also needed information about the disease characteristics of diagnosis and prognosis, which can be used to determine if the patients were in the end-of-life stage. Expectancy about prolonging life was an important foundation of the DNR decision [31].

Patients' willingness was another important consideration. If the patients had expressed their opinions about DNR and end-of-life medical treatments, people could follow the patients' willingness. However, if there was no expression, they could make decisions based on only the current information they had, including the physicians' suggestions, previous understanding of the patient's values, and the best interest of the patient.

The participants considered that DNR can reduce suffering and the medical care can be arranged as the patients wish. It also decreases the family's burden, not only in terms of medical care but also the psychological burden, and they did not have to make the decision for the patient.

In spite of the benefits, there were still barriers to the discussion. Discussion of the DNR and end-of-life issues involve various skills. A lack of skill was one of the main barrier to discussion for the families with advanced disease [29]. They worried that they could not handle the topic, and did not know how to open and continue the discussion. In addition, the participants did not want to discuss their own DNR as it could contribute to the families' worries. The dialogue nature of the DNR discussion is related to death [32], and they were afraid of increasing the families' worries. On the other hand, they may not understand certain aspects of the physical changes and prognosis, and they did not have enough information about the symptoms and the dying process. Due to the uncertainty, it may be difficult to discuss it and to make a decision. The relevant medical information was also an obstruction that they would like to let the physicians take responsibility for in the discussion.

In the clinical situation, the health-care providers can address the concept of natural death and peaceful dying, and deliver comprehensive information about the goal, likelihood of success of CPR, potential harm, and outcomes. The health-care providers should help people to detect the benefits but also to overcome the barriers in terms of information and discussion skills.

Some limitations of this study should be acknowledged. First, this study used a scenario but there may be a difference between behaviors in real situations and choices in scenarios. Second, the participants had heard about DNR and were willing to participate in the DNR discussion; however, the results may not apply to participants who are not familiar with DNR. Third, the title and information were part of the communication, and other factors, such as the relationships between the families and patients, and between the physicians and patients, were not included in this study. Fourth, convenience sampling was used that the participants who were willing to join the study may have positive attitude about DNR and hospice care, and the results may not be generalizable beyond Taiwan. In future studies, an experimental design with a different title and different information could be conducted in clinical practice to exam whether the patients receiving AND tend to accept the order or have higher satisfaction.

Conclusion

Discussion about DNR is a process of communication, and the title that includes AND, comprehensive information about terminal illness, the goal of DNR, and the success rate and harm of CPR, and the worse outcomes of CPR with severe functional impairment and dependency may increase the DNR decision. The healthy adults needed information about the remaining life period, the prognosis of the disease, and future symptoms, the consequence of the CPR procedure and suffering when receiving CPR, and the patients' willingness. The barriers arising from the families' worries, uncertainty about future physical changes, and lack of skills may disrupt the DNR discussion.

Abbreviations

AND: Allow natural death; CPR: Cardiopulmonary resuscitation; DNR: Do not resuscitate

Acknowledgements

The authors would like to thank Miss Hsuan-An Chen and Chia-Ying Lin for data collection.

Funding

This work was supported by the National Science Council [grant numbers NSC 102–2410-H-006-123-].

Authors' contributions

SYF and YWW were involved in study conceptualisation and design and data collection. SYF and IML completed initial data analysis. SYF, YWW and IML contributed to manuscript preparation and approved the final manuscript.

Competing interests

The authors declare that they have no competing interests.

Author details

[1]Institute of Gerontology, College of Medicine, National Cheng Kung University, Tainan, Taiwan. [2]Department of Family Medicine, Buddhist Tzu Chi General Hospital, Hualien, Taiwan. [3]Department of Psychology, College of Humanities and Social Sciences, Kaohsiung Medical University, Kaohsiung, Taiwan.

References

1. Hazinski MF, Field JM. 2010 American Heart Association guidelines for cardiopulmonary resuscitation and emergency cardiovascular care science. Circulation. 2010;122:S639–946.
2. Bishop JP, Brothers KB, Perry JE, Ahmad A. Reviving the conversation around CPR/DNR. Am J Bioeth. 2010;10:61–7.
3. Cotter PE, Simon M, Quinn C, O'keeffe ST. Changing attitudes to cardiopulmonary resuscitation in older people: a 15-year follow-up study. Age Ageing. 2009;38:200–5.
4. Robinson C, Kolesar S, Boyko M, Berkowitz J, Calam B, Collins M. Awareness of do-not-resuscitate orders: what do patients know and want? Can Fam Physician. 2012;58:e229–33.
5. Kim DY, Lee KE, Nam EM, et al. Do-not-resuscitate orders for terminal patients with cancer in teaching hospitals of Korea. J Palliat Med. 2007;10: 1153–8.
6. Huang CH, Hu WY, Chiu TY, Chen CY. The practicalities of terminally ill patients signing their own DNR orders - a study in Taiwan. J Med Ethics. 2008;34:336–40.
7. Huang YC, Huang SJ, Ko WJ. Survey of do-not-resuscitate orders in surgical intensive care units. J Formos Med Assoc. 2010;109:201–8.
8. Lo YT, Wang JJ, Liu LF, Wang CN. Prevalence and related factors of do-not-resuscitate directives among nursing home residents in Taiwan. J Am Med Dir Assoc. 2010;11:436–42.
9. Lu CY, Johantgen M. Factors associated with treatment restriction orders and hospice in older nursing home residents. J Clin Nurs. 2011;20:377–87.
10. Covinsky KE, Fuller JD, Yaffe K, et al. Communication and decision-making in seriously ill patients: findings of the SUPPORT project. The study to understand prognoses and preferences for outcomes and risks of treatments. J Am Geriatr Soc. 2000;48:S187–93.
11. Liu JM, Lin WC, Chen YM, et al. The status of the do-not-resuscitate order in Chinese clinical trial patients in a cancer Centre. J Med Ethics. 1999;25:309–14.
12. Murphy DJ, Burrows D, Santilli S, et al. The influence of the probability of survival on patients' preferences regarding cardiopulmonary resuscitation. N Engl J Med. 1994;330:545–9.
13. Ebell MH, Smith MA, Seifert G, Polsinelli K. The do-not-resuscitate order: outpatient experience and decision-making preferences. J Fam Pract. 1990; 31:630–4.
14. Morrison RS, Meier DE. High rates of advance care planning in new York City's elderly population. Arch Intern Med. 2004;164:2421–6.
15. Morrison RS, Zayas LH, Mulvihill M, Baskin SA, Meier DE. Barriers to completion of health care proxies: an examination of ethnic differences. Arch Intern Med. 1998;158:2493–7.
16. Chen YY, Youngner SJ. "allow natural death" is not equivalent to " do not resuscitate": a response. J Med Ethics. 2008;34:887–8.
17. Knox C, Vereb JA. Allow natural death: a more humane approach to discussing end-of-life directives. J Emerg Nurs. 2005;31:560–1.
18. Venneman SS, Narnor-Harris P, Perish M, Hamilton M. "allow natural death" versus "do not resuscitate": three words that can change a life. J Med Ethics. 2008;34:2–6.
19. Wittmann-Price R, Celia LM. Exploring perceptions of "do not resuscitate" and "allowing natural death" among physicians and nurses. Holist Nurs Pract. 2010;24:333–7.
20. Schonwetter RS, Walker RM, Kramer DR, Robinson BE. Resuscitation decision making in the elderly: the value of outcome data. J Gen Intern Med. 1993;8: 295–300.
21. Thorevska N, Tilluckdharry L, Tickoo S, Havasi A, Amoateng-Adjepong Y, Manthous CA. Patients' understanding of advance directives and cardiopulmonary resuscitation. J Crit Care. 2005;20:26–34.
22. Cherlin E, Fried T, Prigerson HG, Schulman-Green D, Johnson-Hurzeler R, Bradley EH. Communication between physicians and family caregivers about care at the end of life: when do discussions occur and what is said? J Palliat Med. 2005;8:1176–85.
23. Malloy TR, Wigton RS, Meeske J, Tape TG. The influence of treatment descriptions on advance medical directive decisions. J Am Geriatr Soc. 1992; 40:1255–60.
24. High DM. Why are elderly people not using advance directives? J Aging Health. 1993;5:497–515.
25. Curtis JR, Patrick DL, Caldwell E, Greenlee H, Collier AC. The quality of patient-doctor communication about end-of-life care: a study of patients with advanced AIDS and their primary care clinicians. AIDS. 1999;13:1123–31.
26. Yuen JK, Reid MC, Fetters MD. Hospital do-not-resuscitate orders: why they have failed and how to fix them. J Gen Intern Med. 2011;26:791–7.
27. Curtis JR, Patrick DL, Caldwell ES, Collier AC. Why don't patients and physicians talk about end-of-life care?: barriers to communication for patients with acquired immunodeficiency syndrome and their primary care clinicians. Arch Intern Med. 2000;160:1690–6.
28. Wang SC, Chang CJ, Fan SY, Wang YW, Chang SC, Sung HC. Development of an advance care planning booklet in Taiwan. Tzu Chi Medical Journal. 2015;27:170–4.
29. Mockford C, Fritz Z, George R, et al. Do not attempt cardiopulmonary resuscitation (DNACPR) orders: a systematic review of the barriers and facilitators of decision-making and implementation. Resuscitation. 2015;88: 99–113.
30. Pardon K, Deschepper R, Vander Stichele R, et al. Are patients' preferences for information and participation in medical decision-making being met? Interview study with lung cancer patients. Palliat Med. 2011;25:62–70.
31. Olver I, Eliott JA. The perceptions of do-not-resuscitate policies of dying patients with cancer. Psycho-Oncology. 2008;17:347–53.
32. Anselm AH, Palda V, Guest CB, et al. Barriers to communication regarding end-of-life care: perspectives of care providers. J Crit Care. 2005;20:214–23.

First year experiences with a palliative out-patients structure for patients with COPD: a qualitative study of health professionals' expectations and experiences

Dorthe Gaby Bove[1,2*], Marie Lavesen[2], Maria Omel Jellington[2], Kristoffer Bastrup-Madsen Marsaa[3] and Suzanne Forsyth Herling[4]

Abstract

Background: To improve the care of patients with advanced COPD and be able to address their palliative needs a new outpatient organization (CAPTAIN) was developed and implemented. CAPTAIN was inspired by best practice and existing guidelines and changed the traditional organization of an outpatient structure including the roles of nurses and doctors. Only sparse knowledge exists of the health professionals' expectations and experiences to organizational changes in an outpatient setting. This insight is necessary as health professionals are key stakeholders in implementing new structures and successfully transforming knowledge into practice. The aim of this study was to explore the health professionals' expectations and experiences of a new palliative out-patients structure for patients with advanced COPD.

Methods: The design was interpretive description as described by Thorne. Focus groups and individual interviews were conducted with pulmonary nurses, pulmonary doctors and municipality nurses from 2014 to 2016.

Results: The overall theme was dualism. Both nurses and doctors were pending between aspiration and concern in their expectations to the new structure, meanwhile their actual experiences were pending between perceived gain and improvements versus consequences with the new structure. Nurses' and doctors' existing practice was altered and the new structure required new ways for them to cooperate and ways in which skills from each profession were most efficiently utilized.

Conclusion: Nurses and doctors considered the new structure as a quality boost and it fulfilled their hope of improving the quality of care offered to patients with advanced COPD, however with increased work-related stress as a derived consequence.

Keywords: Interpretive description, Dualism, Non-malignant palliative care, Multidisciplinarity, Organizational changes, Resource utilization, Qualitative research

Background

Chronic Obstructive Pulmonary Disease (COPD) is a progressive and incurable disease with a global prevalence of more than 6 million people and COPD represents 5% of all deaths worldwide [1]. In Denmark the prevalence of COPD is estimated to 320.000 people, whereas 50.000 of these are categorized as having advanced COPD [2]. When the patients have reached the stage of advanced COPD, they have a high symptom burden, low functional capacity, frequent hospital admissions, and impaired quality of life. The need of palliative care for patients with advanced COPD is comparable with the needs of patients with advanced pulmonary cancer [3]. However, in Denmark more than 96% of patients referred to hospices or palliative teams are patients with cancer [4], and as a result patients with

* Correspondence: dorthe.gaby.bove.01@regionh.dk
[1]Emergency Department, Copenhagen University Hospital, Nordsjælland, Dyrehavevej 29, 3400 Hillerød, Denmark
[2]Department of Pulmonary & Infectious Diseases, Copenhagen University Hospital, Nordsjælland, Dyrehavevej 29, 3400 Hillerød, Denmark
Full list of author information is available at the end of the article

advanced COPD live their last year of life with unmet palliative needs and low quality of life [5].

COPD is characterized by an unpredictable illness trajectory with numerous exacerbations, each potentially life threatening. During the last past years there has been an increasing focus on the palliative needs of patients with COPD [6] and key guidelines recommend that patients with advanced COPD are offered an early integrated patient-centred care [6–9]. However, how an early patient-centred and integrated palliative care is organized and operationalized is unknown and further knowledge is warranted [4, 10–12].

By tradition in Denmark, the outpatient treatment of patients with COPD has been organized as an annual routine check by a pulmonary specialist accompanied by a pulmonary nurse. As outpatient visits were planned far in advance the visits had no link to the patients' present needs or the progression of the disease. In case of acute exacerbations or symptom progression the patients were referred to their general practitioner (GP), municipal nurse, or an acute hospital admission. This traditional way of organizing an outpatient clinic failed to meet the individual and complex needs of patients with COPD and as a consequence the Department of Pulmonary Diseases at Nordsjællands Hospital designed and implemented a new palliative outpatient structure.

The Department of Pulmonary Diseases had a catchment area of 310.000 citizens in the Capital Region of Denmark, with a total of 650 patients affiliated the outpatient clinic. In average 240 patients died every year and 240 new patients were referred to the outpatient clinic. The new structure 'Comprehensive And Prospective Treatment And Individual Nursing' (CAPTAIN) was developed and implemented with a run-in-period of 2 years, and approximately 900 patients were enrolled in CAPTAIN during this period. The organisation is described in detail elsewhere [13]. The cornerstones of the new CAPTAIN structure was i) a multidisciplinary team-based approach, ii) nurses taking the responsibility of being case managers and iii) advanced care planning (ACP) [14]. The CAPTAIN-structure had an increased patient-centered approach compared to the current and traditional organisation [15]. The CAPTAIN structure was developed in collaboration between departmental management, a doctor and a nurse from the traditional pulmonary outpatient setting. The new structure was inspired by at that time limited existing knowledge and recommendations about COPD and palliation [4, 14, 16, 17].

The new structure required that both doctors and nurses changed their existing practices. The CAPTAIN-nurse had to take on the responsibility for establishing and maintaining an individualized patient and informal caregiver contact. In addition, the new structure required that both nurses and doctors altered their existing practice and found new ways to cooperate and ways to use skills from each profession in the best and most efficiently way.

To the best of our knowledge this way of organising a patient-centred outpatient structure for patients with advanced COPD is new, thus an unexplored research area with unknown perspectives and reactions of the involved health professionals. Nurses and doctors in the pulmonary outpatient clinic were introduced to the new structure by the chief physician and head nurse approximately 6 months before planned kick-off as their involvement was of paramount importance.

Several studies revealed that health professionals experienced barriers in providing palliative care for people with COPD [17–22]. Health professionals are key stakeholders in implementing new structures, and responsible of success of translating evidence into practice [23]. Insight in the involved health professionals' perspective can provide awareness for leaders and other stakeholders and derived possibility to address barriers and enhance facilitators in the process of planning and implementation of new structures.

This study is the first of two, and will be followed by a study with the aim of exploring the patients' perspective on the CAPTAIN-structure.

Methods

Aim

This study aimed to explore the health professionals' expectations and experiences of a new palliative out-patients structure for patients with advanced COPD.

Design

The methodology was interpretive description (ID) as described by Thorne [24]. ID is an inductive approach that focuses on meaning and how generated knowledge apply to clinical practice.

Setting and participants

We conducted a purposive sampling with a strategic identification based on the experiences and perspectives of key stakeholders in CAPTAIN. We defined the stakeholders of the CAPTAIN as pulmonary nurses, pulmonary doctors and primary nurses. In the following section the inclusion criteria for each stakeholder group are described. The concepts of pre and post CAPTAIN refer to the planning phase before implementing the new structure (pre) and the period after the CAPTAIN was introduced (post) (Fig. 1).

Pulmonary nurses

All nurses employed at the Department of Pulmonary Disease, Nordsjællands Hospital and affiliated to CAPTAIN ($n = 6$) participated in a focus group pre-CAPTAIN kick off and again 1 year after ($n = 7$). All the CAPTAIN nurses

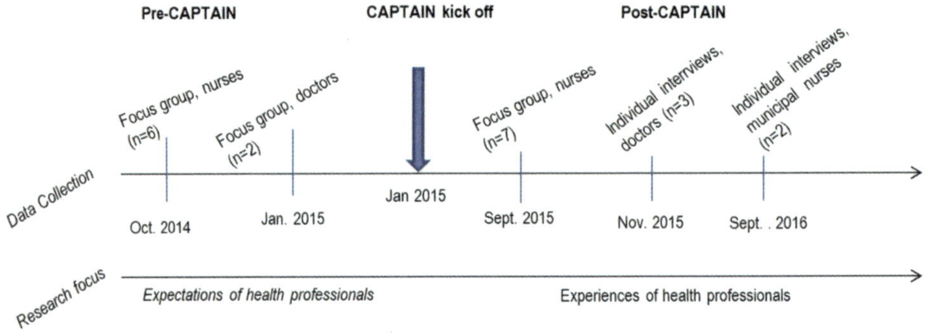

Fig. 1 Data collection phase and related perspectives over time

had a minimum of 5 years' experience caring for patients with COPD and were considered as specialist pulmonary nurses. Four nurses from the focus group pre-CAPTAIN also participated in the focus group post-CAPTAIN. All nurses were female.

Pulmonary doctors

All three doctors employed at the Department of Pulmonary Disease, Nordsjællands Hospital and affiliated to CAPTAIN were invited to a focus group pre-CAPTAIN ($n = 2$) and to semi-structured interviews ($n = 3$) post-CAPTAIN. All doctors had more than 10 years' experience as pulmonary consultants. One doctor was female.

Municipal nurses

Primary nurses from municipalities with patients affiliated to CAPTAIN participated in semi-structured interviews ($n = 2$). The municipalities were geographically located in the vicinity of North Zealand and the nurses had experience caring for patients with COPD affiliated CAPTAIN. The two municipal nurses were clinical specialists with several years of experience and dedicated caring for patients with COPD in their home environment. At the present time, the two municipal nurses represented at 100% of municipal nurses dedicated and highly experienced with caring for patients with COPD. All municipal nurses were female.

Data collection

Focus group and semi-structured interviews were used to generate data. Nurses and doctors were all familiar with each other, and we found that focus groups were an effective and suitable strategy to collect multiple perspectives and diverse experiences. Our aim with the focus groups was to facilitate a synergetic discussion among the informants about expectations and experiences with CAPTAIN. If we had knowledge about a small number of informants, individual interviews were chosen over focus groups. Individual interviews gave us the opportunity to ask more in-depth questions and clarify insights generated through the focus groups. The data was collected from 2014 to 2016 (Fig. 1).

Data collection was conducted by two nurse-researchers with experiences in mediating focus groups and conducting interviews. Immediately after the focus groups or individual interviews the interviewer wrote a memo, describing the immediate experience of the interview and the initial analysis. By choice the interviewer was uninvolved in CAPTAIN and unfamiliar with the study participants prior to the focus group or individual interviews. Data collection and data analysis was performed simultaneously as an iterative process where the preliminary analysis gave direction to further data collection. The opening question for all interviews was: *"Please tell me about your expectations or experience with CAPTAIN".*

Data analysis

All interviews were transcribed verbatim by a medical secretary or the interviewer and lasted in average for focus group and semi-structured interviews, respectively 94 min (range 90–97 min) and 38 min (range 32–42). All transcripts were organized in QSR NVivo 11 © software (QSR International Pty ltd, Cardigan, UK).

In the first step of the analysis all transcriptions were read and reread in an attempt to immerse and become familiar with data. In the next step we started sorting and organizing data into broad-based and generic codes. First each focus group or interview was considered to be one unit of analysis. Later in the process data was divided into pre and post CAPTAIN, and the units of analysis was all data regardless of profession (nurse, municipal nurse or doctor) or data collection method (interview or focus group). Next, we searched for intuitive meaning units in the participants' statements and the first themes and subthemes were identified. The themes and subthemes were explored by describing and discussing the content and meaning of each theme. In the next and final phase of the analysis we constructed multiple iterations of the themes by adding, re-organizing and merging several themes. As a final step in the analysis the first author (DB) read the original transcripts and the notes to ensure consistency among the themes and the informants' descriptions.

Rigour

To enhance credibility all steps in the research processes from the design of the study to the discussions of the themes have been conducted in discussion between two or more of the co-authors in accordance with the methodology ID [24]. All authors of this study are highly experienced in the field of COPD which has qualified the research process, the questions asked, the analysis and subsequent interpretation of the findings. This researcher triangulating has presumable reduced the risk of preconception and prejudices affecting the data collection and findings, and has contributed to keep focus on relevance of the findings for the clinical practice. The use of NVivo 11 was a valuable tool in strengthening dependability and the software contributed to transparency in the analysis process. Quotes underpinning the themes are presented in a concentrated and edited form to increase readability.

Results

The overall theme describing both the expectations and experience pre- and post-CAPTAIN was dualism, with the subtheme aspiration versus concern pre-CAPTAIN, and gain & improvement versus consequences post-CAPTAIN. The theme, subthemes and some of the underlying categories are illustrated in Figs. 2 and 3. The two figures are not an exhaustive illustration of the overall themes of the analysis, but merely an illustration of the nurses' perspective.

Aspiration and concern in the pre-CAPTAIN phase

Both nurses and doctors were characterized by dualism and pending between aspiration and concern in relation to what they expected the organizational changes would have of impact on both themselves and the patients.

> *I am overwhelmed by the thought that everything will be broken down and changed, and that we as nurses must stand for it all. It is both a cool initiative but also overwhelming if suddenly it is expected that you could handle and know everything about it all. It was my first thought that one would have to know it all (Nurse, pre-CAPTAIN)*

Because the focus of the interviews was on expectations to the future it required that the informants were able to create abstractions. In response the nurses spoke of uncertainties of the new structure and listed several new questions they were preoccupied with (Fig. 2).

The doctors' main concern was if they possessed the necessary communication skills to facilitate an advanced care planning (ACP) dialogue with the patient and their informal caregivers.

> *I think it is important that we quickly establish the training of both doctors and nurses in the process of conducting ACP dialogues. What does the ACP contain, what is our role as doctors and how should we prepare to facilitate these dialogues? (pre-CAPTAIN, doctor)*

The doctors hoped that the new organizational structure would result in better utilization of their knowledge and skills and increase and strengthen the teamwork between doctors and nurses. By excusing doctors from routine visits of patients in a stable phase of COPD, they hoped to be able to focus on the complex cases and overall increase the quality of palliative care to patients with advanced COPD.

> *Specifically, I see that we (doctors) see patients less often to routine visits than before and we give nurses more responsibility to establish and maintain contact with the patients. However, we also have more shared responsibility, doctors and nurses, in terms of communication. We have a shared responsibility to communicate and collaborate successfully, because if*

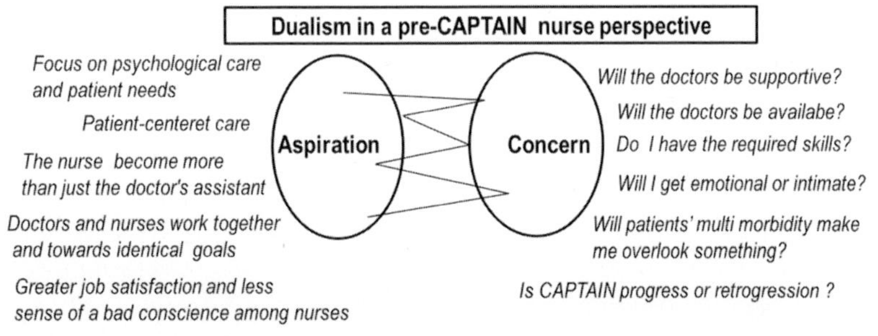

Fig. 2 Theme and subthemes supported by categories originated from nurses' perspectives pre-CAPTAIN

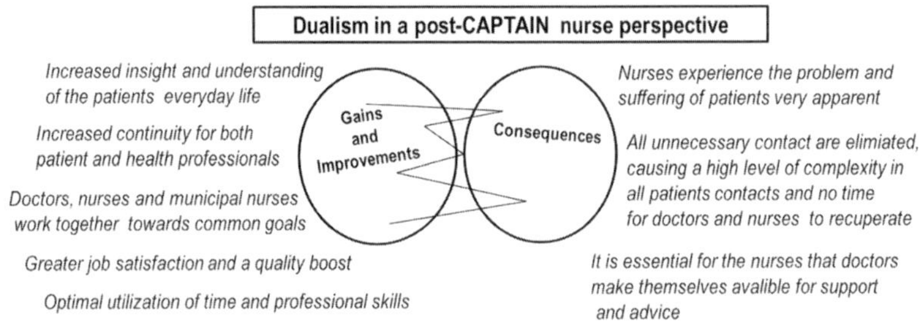

Fig. 3 Theme and subthemes supported by categories originated from nurses' perspectives post-CAPTAIN

we do not, this project will not succeed. This project requires a great deal of teamwork and communication between all involved, including the general practitioners (GP) (pre-CAPTAIN, doctor).

The nurses' main concern was whether they possessed the adequate competences. A few nurses described a concern as to whether they were able to maintain professionalism in their interaction with the patients when they became better acquainted. They worried if they could deal with the intimate nature of the contact with severe ill patients and their relatives, and especially if they could keep patients out of their private sphere. Another concern was related to the teamwork with doctors. Nurses felt that multidisciplinary collaboration was essential for them in order to take on the increased responsibility and fulfill the role as a CAPTAIN-nurse. Nurses expressed it was imperative that doctors supported them and made themselves available for coaching as well as counseling.

Gains and improvements and derived consequences in the post-CAPTAIN phase

The experiences of the health professionals are continuously characterized by a dualism, now pending between seeing the new structure as a quality boost and a positive change for patients but with the derived consequences triggering new concerns, predominantly among nurses. The new structure fulfilled aspirations and wishes described pre-captain by the health professionals. Although, the described concerns pre-CAPTAIN did not surface some of the concerns persisted in a vague or moderated form post-CAPTAIN (Fig. 3).

Gains and improvements but also concerns about derived consequences

Both nurses and doctors describe that the new CAPTAIN structure provide continuity and a better understanding of the patient's everyday life and perceived values and preferences. However, this increased insight in the patients' life and the awareness of suffering causes nurses to worry. Nurses realize that time does not permit them to render all the support patients are seeking or addressing all the problems patients are articulating.

Patients can be clear about end of life wishes or not, some patients want to talk about death and others prefer not to. It's not hard to talk to patients about death, what's hard is the suffering. The suffering in their life; now and here. I cannot take the suffering away, but it's hard to witness and not being able to accommodate the patient's wish for me to do something to relieve their suffering, just something. It is the frustration of the chronic progressive disease, and we meet it all along. Sometimes the patients are at the bottom of the pit, where their life is so full of suffering, it can be difficult to witness. I wish I could pull a rabbit out of the hat and fix it (post-CAPTAIN, nurse).

Nurses described how they together with the patient are forced to prioritize the current and the most important problem and decide what issues can be postponed to the next visit. This prioritizing highlights concern of quality and fear of overlooking anything important. The doctors, on the other hand, did not express this concern, neither on behalf of the nurses nor on their own behalf.

Increased insight and understanding of the patient struggles in everyday life was the result of caring for the same patient more continuously. More insight to the complexity of the patients' problems combined with the available time and resources made nurses realize that to provide the best care nurses had to strengthen patients' self-management capacity.

The CAPTAIN-structure redefines the role as a pulmonary doctor and nurse

Doctors described a change in their role as doctor. The new role was moving from being highly specialized toward a general pulmonologist more similar to a GP, as one doctor put it. Due to patient's increased influence on the agenda in the meeting with the health professionals, the existing and traditional doctor/nurse/patient relationship was changed toward a more patient-centered and holistic approach. The nurses described how patients with COPD did not distinguish between pulmonary, cardiological, social, or psychological problems. Patients had problems that overall affected their life with COPD and therefore they seeked help to solve or alleviate the problem. Opposed to the health professionals patients did not consider organizational structures or divisions in anatomy and specialties. As a consequence the health professionals could not ignore or avoid "non-pulmonary medicine" issues.

The CAPTAIN-structure support cross-sectoral collaboration

Both nurses and doctors described that success in supporting the patients' self-management capacity required an increased cross-sectoral collaboration, where the GP, municipal nurses and home care services were essential partners. This point of views was echoed by the municipal nurses. Municipal nurses described how CAPTAIN positively influence the quality of care delivered in the home due to the accessibility of the CAPTAIN-nurses, who provided them with an increased opportunity for seeking information about overall plans, treatment strategies, advice or support. The accessibility improved continuity for both patients and municipal nurses, and provided synergy as all health professionals across sectors were working towards identical goals.

> *There is no doubt that the patient is very pleased to find that we work together [hospital and home care]. My experience is that we are a group working together in a kind of team setting and that one hand knows what the other is doing. I think that because we can communicate about everything patients get an increased feeling of safety (post-CAPTAIN municipality nurse).*

The municipality nurses described feeling convinced that the CAPTAIN-structure prevented unnecessary hospital admissions.

> *I think CAPTAIN give us the opportunity to be more pro-active and preventive and thereby avoid the condition deteriorates and patient's situation getting worse (post-CAPTAIN, municipality nurse).*

Enhancement of utilization of professional skills of each profession

Nurses, municipal nurses and doctors described how their competences and time was better used post-CAPTAIN compared to pre- CAPTAIN. However, this optimization of resources also had disadvantages. Especially doctors described how all contact with patients had a more clear purpose being either exacerbations or ACP. All unnecessary consultations were eliminated, resulting in high complexity in every patient contact. This high level of complexity was perceived by both nurses and doctors as demanding and at times mentally exhausting. Pre-CAPTAIN, the shift between complex and routine consultations gave the health professionals an opportunity "to breathe" and recuperate.

> *Talking about death ... It's not a problem for me to be the patient's companion on the road to death. I'm not crying because somebody dies, but I think afterwards I might need to take a breather. I really think I may need to have a break and find myself again (post-CAPTAIN, nurse).*

Multidisciplinarity was key

The ACP-dialogues was perceived as cornerstone of CAPTAIN by the doctors, whereas the nurses described the continuity and increased accessibility for both nurses and other collaborator as most important. The ACP was perceived as somewhat unpredictable as it could be very diverse and take different directions according to the agenda of the patients and their relatives. ACP was described by both doctors and nurses as much more than a dialogue about types and intensity of treatment. Doctors played a leading role facilitating the ACP-dialogue, although they did not consider themselves experts. The doctors described how they practiced and slowly improved over time. Both doctors and nurses considered the multidisciplinary teamwork as a strength in ACP, and highlighted that quality in ACP demanded continuous supervision to develop and maintain necessary skills.

> *What patients express immediately after an ACP is that it was the best dialogue that have had with their doctor for years because the focus was not on lung function. Focus was on their anxiety and fear of being resuscitated by an emergency hospitalization (post-CAPTAIN nurse).*

Before CAPTAIN, nurses spoke of concerns about support and accessibility to the doctors, however this was un called for. Post CAPTAIN, nurses expressed seeing cooperation with doctors prerequisite for being able to fulfill the role as CAPTAIN-nurses. Doctors gave advice, guidance and support which still was considered essential for nurses in order to resume responsibility for establishing and maintaining contact with the patients throughout the disease trajectory. Being part of a multidisciplinary team and experiencing the support of doctors was described by nurses as of great importance to job satisfaction and provided motivation to take even more responsibility on. The nurses' concerns pre-CAPTAIN about making mistakes or lacking the required skills were persistent post-CAPTAIN, although none of the nurses spoke of specific experiences to this point.*I think it [the new role] is a huge challenge, it is great that we work very independently, but also a huge challenge because it is lurking at all time; have I overlooked something. (post-CAPTAIN, nurse)*

The doctors did not at any point substantiate this concern; in contrast they stated that nurses were considered highly competent and fully capable of solving the problems and ready to manage the increased responsibility.

Discussion

To the best of our knowledge this study is the first to offer insight into the health professionals' perspective on a new palliative outpatient structure aimed at improving treatment and care for patients with advanced COPD. This study does not explore the perceived value in a patient perspective, but exclusively focuses on the perspective of the health professionals, although it can be difficult to separate the two perspectives as they interact.

Our findings revealed that the health professionals' expectations to the new CAPTAIN-structure were both hope and concern, and their actual experience were achieved gains versus derived consequences. It is well known that changes causes concern and an attitudinal reaction to changes can be driven by feelings of uncertainty, loss of control and fear of failure engendered by the changing event [23]. Although that all informants in our study were highly experience and we assumed that they had every reason to be confident about own skills, they still expressed fear of failure, albeit most pronounced among nurses. It was notable how the nurses repeatedly articulated concerns about their own skills. The doctors did not question own skills and expressed a great confidence in the nurses' skills. The nurses were unaware of the doctors' confidence in them and the doctors' dedication to the multidisciplinary team and their intention to support them and make CAPTAIN a success. In general, it is considered unrealistic to eliminate all uncertainty in an initial phase of changing an existing structure; however it can be assumed that it would be beneficial to match expectations among nurses and doctors including discussion of present concerns in multidisciplinary meetings and supervision sessions.

A difference were also found in the description of what was required for respectively nurses and doctors to fulfill the role as CAPTAIN nurses or doctor. The doctors expressed a clear defined need for education and training in how to facilitate ACP dialogues, whereas the majority of nurses articulated a broader need for support and supervision related to complex cases and situations. This knowledge could be useful planning training- and education programs prior implementation of future organizational changes. Our findings indicate that it could be beneficial to combine formal education and training with sessions of supervision and scheduled time for interdisciplinary support.

According to Meleis' theory of transition [25, 26], transition always includes a form of change and take place over time. The process of transition is diverse, complex, multi-dimensional and do always have a direction (purpose). It can be facilitated or inhibited by factors like perceived meaning, realistic expectations level of knowledge/skill, environment, level of planning, emotional and physical well-being. In our study, the health professionals described experiences that can be interpreted as both inhibitors and facilitators. Facilitators of the transition could have been supported by focusing and clarifying the meaning with the new structure, expectations to the health professionals including expectations and frame for the interdisciplinary collaboration. By doing so we might have reduced the level of concern, especially among nurses.

After the implementation of CAPTAN, the experience was that the new structure was a quality boost, but not without derived consequences. Especially the nurses described how they experienced a transition from being the doctor's assistant to now having their own practice. Although, several nurses described a concern about becoming too emotional involved in the patients, none of them described episodes or experiences where this had actually happened or had caused a problem for them. However, the new structure exposed nurses to the patients suffering in a much greater extent than the traditional organization. Witnessing this suffering was described by nurses as hard and sometimes frustrating, but at the same time also seen as a consequence of the increased insight and understanding of the patient's life which was perceived as something positive. The nurses' fear of becoming too emotionally involved in the patient's life were associated with the new role as a CAPTAIN-nurse. To be a CAPTAIN-nurse required more from the nurses than just objective measurements like lung function and inhalation techniques. In CAPTAIN there were a focus on forming human relationship beyond the pulmonary disease and that required a broader professionalism from the nurses. The doctors did not have these considerations which can be explained with the fact the roles of the doctors did not changes as fundamentally as the nurses.

Another important finding was that although all health professionals experienced a better utilization of their professional resources and competences due to elimination of uncomplicated patient contact it also had a negative impact on their ability to restitute and prepare for the next patient. Both doctor and nurses described episodes of being mentally extinguished and the experience of having an increased level of stress. Exposure to suffering and caring for complex patients and families are recognized stressors associated with increased risk of work-related stress [27]. It is therefore highly recommended that leaders and other stakeholders consider how to give the health professionals the opportunity to restitute and self-care and thereby lowering their level of stress. In our opinion it makes no sense or is feasible to implement a new structure that on one hand improve patientcare but on the other hand increases the health professionals' level of stress and their derived risk of becoming ill.

This study is exploring the health professionals' perspectives and will be followed by another qualitative study with the aim of exploring the patients' perspectives. However, further research is needed to investigate the effectiveness of interventions like CAPTAIN and generate quantitative data about the impact on patients' quality of life, hospitals admissions, length of stay and mortality. Future studies should also examine how cross-sectoral cooperation is best organized without demanding extra resources both from an organizational and a patient perspective, besides evaluating the impact of the altered organization on the health professionals' workload and stress level.

As this paper very clearly illustrates, changing clinical practice is difficult and associated with an increased risk of stress among the health professionals, even though changes were well prepared in a group of experienced and collaborating nurses and physicians. At present, CAPTAIN is implemented as standard care for patients with severe COPD affiliated the pulmonary outpatient clinic. However, we do not consider the CAPTAIN structure as static, but rather it is under continuously development with the objective to reduce the perceived level of stress among the health professionals without lowering the quality for COPD patients or changing the fundamental framework of the CAPTAIN concept.

Limitations

The health professional perspective was only explored through nurse or doctor perspective, and it could have contributed further knowledge if the mixed professional perspective had been explored. The nurses' perspective was only explored through focus groups, and although focus groups contributes to multiple and diverse perspectives, the method do not allow for a deeper understanding of the participants experiences. It had to be noted the doctor focus group only consisted of two participants ($n = 2$), and that the municipality nurses' perspective only was explored post-CAPTAIN.

All nurses were female, and two of three doctors male, raising the question if gender had influence on the prevalence of experienced concerns. The nurses in our study articulate in general more concerns than doctors and especially regarding their level of both personal and professional competences. The literature illustrates, although somewhat inconsistent, that women respond with higher level of stress to work-related stressors, which implementation of a new structure is considered to be [28].

Conclusions

This study illustrates how it is possible, although challenging, to change the structure and roles of nurses and doctors in a pulmonary outpatient clinic for patients with advanced COPD. Both doctors and nurses experienced the new structure as a quality boost and it fulfilled the hope of improving the quality of care offered to patients with advanced COPD. The insight gained through this study highlight the need for addressing concerns continuously during both the planning and implementation phase, and in a multidisciplinary forum.

Especially, the nurses were insecure about possessing the required skills and wandered if the doctors would support them to the extent they needed.

Both doctors and nurses expressed that the new structure optimized the utilization of their professional resources, although with the consequence that all uncomplicated patient-contacts were eliminated. This meant that there was no opportunity to restitute between patient contacts, which increased the experience of work-related stress and in some cases led to feeling of being mentally exhausted.

Our findings may guide leaders and other stakeholders considering or standing before changing an existing organizational outpatient-structure to improve or implement palliative care to patients with COPD. We recommend that both leaders, nurses and doctors are aware and discuss pros and cons prior to implementing a new palliative structure. In a structure like CAPTAIN, the increased awareness of the patients' high symptom burden and suffering means that far more patients will be recognized as complex. The multidisciplinary team must have the time required to address this complexity, otherwise there is an increased risk of stress and dissatisfaction within the multidisciplinary team. However, we find it possible that by planning ongoing supervision and multidisciplinary dialogues this stress can be prevented or reduced. Although, this study is conducted in the context of a pulmonary outpatient clinic, our findings may be transferrable to other in-hospital settings and groups of patients with non-malign diseases with less tradition for palliative care as dementia and heart failure. This assumption is based on the health professionals' experience that the support the patients demanded was about management of life with a severe disease rather on specific pulmonary issues.

Abbreviations

ACP: Advanced Care Planning; CAPTAIN: Comprehensive and Prospective Treatment and Individual Nursing; COPD: Chronic Obstructive Pulmonary Disease; GP: General Practioner; ID: Interpretive Description

Acknowledgements

The authors would like to thank pulmonary consultant FinnVejlø Rasmussen for his dedication in all phases of the project. We would also like to thank the team of leaders affiliated the Department of Pulmonary Medicine and Infectious Diseases, who made the study possible: Britt Holmgaard, Puk Vad Vestergaard, and Thyge Lynghøj Nielsen and all the CAPTAIN nurses and doctors. Special thanks go to the CAPTAIN advisory board: Kirsten Lomborg, Helle Timm, Inge Vestbo and Jørgen Vestbo.

Funding

This research did not receive any specific grant from funding agency in the public, commercial, or not-for-profit sectors.

Authors' contributions

All authors contributed to the study design, analysis of the data and the manuscript. The focus groups were conducted by DGB and a colleague researcher (GK), the individual interviews with the doctors were conducted by GK and the interviews with the municipality nurses by MOJ. DGB and SFH led on the manuscript preparation. All authors have read and commented on drafts and approved the final version of the manuscript.

Competing interests

No conflict of interest has been declared by the authors DGB, MOJ, ML and SFH. K.M has received honoraria from Almirall, AstraZeneca, Boehringer Ingelheim, GlaxoSmithKline, Norpharma, Novartis, Intermune, and Roche for presenting at meetings and symposia and honoraria for participation in advisory board for AstraZeneca and Novartis.

Author details

[1]Emergency Department, Copenhagen University Hospital, Nordsjælland, Dyrehavevej 29, 3400 Hillerød, Denmark. [2]Department of Pulmonary & Infectious Diseases, Copenhagen University Hospital, Nordsjælland, Dyrehavevej 29, 3400 Hillerød, Denmark. [3]Department of Palliative Medicine, Copenhagen University Hospital, Herlev and Gentofte Hospital, Herlev Ringvej 75, 2730 Herlev, Denmark. [4]Neuroscience Centre, Copenhagen University Hospital, Rigshospitalet, Section 2091, Inge Lehmanns Vej 7, 2100 Copenhagen Ø, Denmark.

References

1. The World Health Organization (WHO): Chronic Respiratory Diseases. Burden of COPD. 2017, (05/08). www.lunge.dk/viden-noegletal-om-lungesygdomme.
2. Lungeforeningen: Nøgletal om lunger [key figures on lungs]. 2017, 2017(may 9). www.who.int.respiratory/copd/burden/en/.
3. Habraken JM, ter Riet G, Gore JM, Greenstone MA, Weersink EJ, Bindels PJ, Willems DL. Health-related quality of life in end-stage COPD and lung cancer patients. J Pain Symptom Manag. 2009;37(6):973–81.
4. Danmarks Lungeforening og Palliativt Videnscenter. Palliativ indsats til KOL-patienter [Palliative Care for COPD patients]. In: En deskriptiv undersøgelse af danske KOL-patienters sygdomsforløb og behov for palliativ indsats; 2013.
5. Harrington SE, Rogers E, Davis M. Palliative care and chronic obstructive pulmonary disease: where the lines meet. Curr Opin Pulm Med. 2017; 23(2):154–60.
6. Siouta N, van Beek K, Preston N, Hasselaar J, Hughes S, Payne S, Garralda E, Centeno C, van der Eerden M, Groot M, Hodiamont F, Radbruch L, Busa C, Csikos A, Menten J. Towards integration of palliative care in patients with chronic heart failure and chronic obstructive pulmonary disease: a systematic literature review of European guidelines and pathways. BMC Palliat Care. 2016;15(1):18 -016-0089-4.
7. Marså K, Knudsen T, Gundestrup S, Thorsen M, Larsen H, Kirkegaard N, Løkke A, Shaker S, Wilcke T, Lange P, Bendstrup E. Dansk Lungemedicinsk Selskab (Danish Society of Respiratory Medicine): Klarinigsrapport om palliation til voksne med kronisk fremadskridende non-malign lungesygdom. In: DLS klaringsrapport om palliation; 2015.
8. Celli BR, Decramer M, Wedzicha JA, Wilson KC, Agusti AA, Criner GJ, MacNee W, Make BJ, Rennard SI, Stockley RA, Vogelmeier C, Anzueto A, Au DH, Barnes PJ, Burgel PR, Calverley PM, Casanova C, Clini EM, Cooper CB, Coxson HO, Dusser DJ, Fabbri LM, Fahy B, Ferguson GT, Fisher A, Fletcher MJ, Hayot M, Hurst JR, Jones PW, Mahler DA, Maltais F, Mannino DM, Martinez FJ, Miravitlles M, Meek PM, Papi A, Rabe KF, Roche N, Sciurba FC, Sethi S, Siafakas N, Sin DD, Soriano JB, Stoller JK, Tashkin DP, Troosters T, Verleden GM, Verschakelen J, Vestbo J, Walsh JW, Washko GR, Wise RA, Wouters EF, ZuWallack RL. ATS/ERS task force for COPD research: an official American Thoracic Society/European Respiratory Society statement: research questions in COPD. Eur Respir Rev. 2015;24(136):159–72.
9. Global Initiative for Chronic Obstructive Lung Disease: Global strategy for the diagnosis, management, and prevention of chronic obstructive pulmonary disease (GOLD 2017). Avaible from http://goldcopd.org/. 2017, 2017 report:
10. Bergenholtz H, Holge-Hazelton B, Jarlbaek L. Organization and evaluation of generalist palliative care in a Danish hospital. BMC Palliat Care. 2015;14. https://doi.org/10.1186/s12904-015-0022-2.
11. Dalgaard KM, Bergenholtz H, Nielsen ME, Timm H. Early integration of palliative care in hospitals: a systematic review on methods, barriers, and outcome. Palliat Support Care. 2014;12(6):495–513.
12. Thuesen J, Mikkelsen T, Timm H. Koordinering af rehabilitering og palliation til mennesker med livstruende sygdom. In: REHPA - Videnscenter for rehabilitering og Palliation. 1.udgave ed; 2016.
13. Lavesen M, Marsa KB, Bove DG. A new way of organising palliative care for patients with severe chronic obstructive pulmonary disease. Int J Palliat Nurs. 2018;24(2):64–8.
14. Patel K, Janssen DJ, Curtis JR. Advance care planning in COPD. Respirology. 2012;17(1):72–8.
15. Ahmad A, Krelle E, Lawrie M. Person-centred care: from ideas to action. Bringing together the evidence on shared decision making and self-management support. In: The Health Foundation; 2014.
16. Crawford GB, Brooksbank MA, Brown M, Burgess TA, Young M. Unmet needs of people with end-stage chronic obstructive pulmonary disease: recommendations for change in Australia. Intern Med J. 2013;43(2):183–90.
17. Disler RT, Currow DC, Phillips JL, Smith T, Johnson MJ, Davidson PM. Interventions to support a palliative care approach in patients with chronic obstructive pulmonary disease: an integrative review. Int J Nurs Stud. 2012;49(11):1443–58.
18. Pinnock H, Kendall M, Murray SA, Worth A, Levack P, Porter M, MacNee W, Sheikh A. Living and dying with severe chronic obstructive pulmonary disease: multi-perspective longitudinal qualitative study. BMJ. 2011;342:d142.
19. Pastrana T, Junger S, Ostgathe C, Elsner F, Radbruch L. A matter of definition--key elements identified in a discourse analysis of definitions of palliative care. Palliat Med. 2008;22(3):222–32.

20. Gott M, Gardiner C, Small N, Payne S, Seamark D, Barnes S, Halpin D, Ruse C. Barriers to advance care planning in chronic obstructive pulmonary disease. Palliat Med. 2009;23(7):642–8.
21. Veigh CM, Reid J, Larkin P, Porter S, Hudson P. The provision of generalist and specialist palliative care for patients with non-malignant respiratory disease in the north and Republic of Ireland: a qualitative study. BMC Palliat Care. 2017;17(1). https://doi.org/10.1186/s12904-017-0220-1.
22. Mousing CA, Timm H, Lomborg K, Kirkevold M. Barriers to palliative care in people with chronic obstructive pulmonary disease in home care: a qualitative study of the perspective of professional caregivers. J Clin Nurs. 2018;27(3-4): 650–60.
23. Fedor D, Caldwell S, Herold DM. The effects of organizational changes om employee commitment: a multilevel investigation. Pers Psychol. 2006;59:1–29.
24. Thorne S. Interpretive Description. In: Qualitative research for applied practive. 2nd ed. New York: Routledge; 2016.
25. Meleis AI, Sawyer LM, Im EO, Hilfinger Messias DK, Schumacher K. Experiencing transitions: an emerging middle-range theory. ANS Adv Nurs Sci. 2000;23(1):12–28.
26. Schumacher KL, Meleis AI. Transitions: a central concept in nursing. Image J Nurs Sch. 1994;26(2):119–27.
27. Sinclair S, Raffin-Bouchal S, Venturato L, Mijovic-Kondejewski J, Smith-MacDonald L. Compassion fatigue: a meta-narrative review of the healthcare literature. Int J Nurs Stud. 2017;69:9–24.
28. Gyllensten K, Palmer S. The role of gender in workplace stress: a critical literature review. Health Educ J. 2005;64(3):271–88.

21

The experience of caring for patients at the end-of-life stage in non-palliative care settings

Xiao Bin Lai[1*], Frances Kam Yuet Wong[2] and Shirley Siu Yin Ching[2]

Abstract

Background: More patients are dying in non-palliative care settings than in palliative care settings. How health care providers care for adult patients at the end-of-life stage in non-palliative care settings has not been adequately explored. The aim of this study was to explore the experiences of health care providers in caring for patients at the end-of-life stage in non-palliative care settings.

Methods: This is a qualitative study. Twenty-six health care providers from eight health care institutions which are based in Shanghai were interviewed individually between August 2016 and February 2017. Three levels of health care, i.e., acute care, sub-acute care, or primary care, was provided in the health care institutions. The interviews were analyzed using qualitative content analysis.

Results: Three themes emerged from the interviews: (i) Definition of the end-of-life stage: This is mainly defined based on a change in treatment. (ii) Health care at the end-of-life stage: Most patients spent their last weeks in tertiary/secondary hospitals, transferring from one location to another and receiving disease- and symptom-focused treatment. Family-dominated decision making was common when discussing treatment options. Nurses instinctively provided extra care attention to patients, but nursing care is still task-oriented. (iii) Challenges, difficulties, and the future. From the interviews, it was found that pressure from families was the main challenge faced by health care providers. Three urgent tasks before the end-of-life care can become widely available in the future were identified from the interviews, including educating the public on death, extending government support, and creating better health care environment.

Conclusion: The end-of-life care system of the future should involve health care institutions at all levels, with established mechanisms of collaboration between institutions. Care should be delivered to patients with various life-threatening diseases in both palliative and non-palliative care settings. But first, it is necessary to address the obstacles to the development of end-of-life care, which involve health care providers, patients and their families, and the health care system as a whole.

Keywords: End-of-life care, Health care delivery, Qualitative research, Life-threatening diseases

Background

End-of-life care is that part of palliative care that focuses on patients who have life-threatening diseases and a life expectancy of 6 to 12 months [1, 2]. It helps patients to die in peace, comfort, and dignity [1]. Globally, the estimated number of people in need of end-of-life care is 20.4 million [1]. By 2040, an estimated 75% to 88% of patients at the end-of-life stage could benefit from palliative care [3]. All countries should take heed of the increasing need for end-of-life care [4].

Patients with life-threatening diseases at the end-of-life stage suffer multiple physical discomforts [5, 6], as well as a range of psychosocial and spiritual concerns [7–12]. With the progression of their diseases, the utilization of health services by patients increases at the end-of-life stage [13–19]. As a result, worldwide, a significantly large number of patients with chronic diseases (20–78%) die in acute care hospitals [20–22]. Yet acute care hospitals may not have specialized palliative care or hospice care wards.

* Correspondence: xblai@fudan.edu.cn
[1]School of Nursing, Fudan University, Shanghai, China
Full list of author information is available at the end of the article

With the huge number of patients at the end-of-life stage, more patients are dying in non- palliative care settings than in specialized hospice care wards in hospitals or hospice facilities [23, 24]. A nation-wide survey conducted in the United Kingdom (UK) reported that only 6% of those who passed away died in hospice facilities [25].

The situation in China is consistent with the international trend. The health care system in China has been undergoing reform for years. During the previous reform period (from the early 1980s to the 2000s), China dismantled the country's effective health care and public health system, which caused much turmoil years later [26]. One of the negative outcomes of this move has been the decentralization of the public health system, which has led to great disparities between rural and urban health care service [26]. Patients tend to bypass local health care institutions to seek care in the larger acute care hospitals in urban areas, even for relatively minor problems. As of the year 2017, there were 989,000 health care institutions in China, of which 30,000 were hospitals and 934,000 were primary health care institutions [27]. That same year, there were a total of 660 million health care visits in China, of which, 280 million were to hospitals, 360 million to primary health care institutions [28]. The hospitals have been overused for years.

Patients with chronic diseases usually go to large acute care hospitals to seek help. When their condition deteriorates, patients will stay in a hospital until they passed away. Previous studies found that more than half of patients at the end-of-life stage in Beijing, Shanghai, and Guangdong died in an acute care hospital [29–31]. Hospice care in China has developed rapidly since the announcement of several national policies on end-of-life care in 2015 [32–34]. Yet the care provided to dying patients is far from satisfaction. According to the 2015 Quality of Death Index report, mainland China ranked 71st out 80 countries and areas in its quality of death [35]. Before the wide introduction of the concept of hospice care, only 1% of patients at the end-of-life stage in China received hospice care [36]. The rate of utilizations of hospice care services is currently still low. In Shanghai, for example, a community-based hospice service was established with a great deal of support from the government, and the utilization of hospice beds was 43.8% [37]. However, only 11.8% of patients at the end-of-life stage died in hospice wards in the community [37].

In the face of the increasing need for palliative care, the World Health Organization and the Worldwide Palliative Care Alliance proposed that palliative care be delivered at all levels of care: (i) by all health care providers through a "palliative care approach"; (ii) by primary health care providers and those treating patients with life-threatening diseases, who would provide "general palliative care" and; (iii) by specialized teams treating patients with complex problems, who would provide "specialist palliative care" [1]. Palliative care should be provided wherever a person's care takes place [1]. Hence, as part of palliative care, it is necessary to develop and improve end-of-life care in non-palliative care settings.

Patients at the end of their life and living in non-palliative care settings may not be receiving care appropriate for their stage of illness [38, 39]. A review article found that the management of symptoms for dying patients was not adequate in many hospitals [39]. In the UK, nearly one-third (31%) of the bereaved families were not satisfied with the care that was provided in the hospital where a family member was a patient during the last 3 months of his/her life [25]. By comparison, the proportion of bereaved families who were dissatisfied with the care provided in hospice facilities, in their own home, and in care homes was 21%, 21%, and 18%, respectively [25]. Studies conducted in the United States (US), the UK, and the Netherlands found that the quality of dying and death in hospitals is not satisfactory [25, 40, 41]. Thus, how to enhance the end-of-life care in various clinical settings is a challenge faced by health care professionals.

Identifying gaps in service is a prerequisite to developing end-of-life care in non-palliative care settings. It is essential to know how patients at the end-of-life stage are cared for in hospitals from the perspectives of both health care providers and health care recipients. In the study by McIlvennan et al., the families felt that the hospice care provided to patients with a left ventricular assistance device was fragmented [42]. Peacock et al. reported that the family caregivers of dementia patients thought that physicians specializing in treating dementia patients did not seem like the idea of end-of-life care [43]. A recent review article suggested that a holistic approach be taken to providing end-of-life care to patients [44].

Patients at the end-of-life stage and their family caregivers have unmet needs in multiple domains. Mathews and Johnston identified the unmet needs of people with chronic obstructive pulmonary disease (COPD) and their caregivers as being in the physical, psychosocial and spiritual domains [45]. Of particular importance are appropriate and timely conversations to identify the personal preferences of patients at the end of their life and to provide relevant information on COPD [45]. The need for better communication with health care providers was also reported in another study [46]. Spending time and discussing important issues with patients have also been identified as family's needs [8, 47]. Clark et al. [8] found that family members with a relative who had died in an acute medical ward wished that they had been able to spend more time with the patient and address issues before he/she passed away. Mossin and Landmark's study [47] also found that families wanted to spend time with patients. The necessity of communicating with patients about death and important issues is echoed in another study on family members [48]. Family members also need more information and good support from health care providers, and good symptom management for patients [8].

Compared with the research that has been conducted on family caregivers, how health care providers care for adult patients at the end-of-life stage, especially in non-palliative care settings, has not been adequately explored. Garner et al. [49] found that, from the perspective of nurse executives, inadequate communication, lack of education, and hospital system constraints were three major barriers to providing end-of-life care in hospital settings. Another study found that, nurses considered it a challenge to provide end-of-life care in the complex and difficult environment of the medical units [50]. In their study, Gardiner et al. discovered that attitudinal differences to the care, a focus on curative treatments, and a lack of resources were the main barriers to providing palliative care for older people in acute care hospitals [51]. These studies explored the experiences of nurses in caring for patients at the end-of-life stage. Few studies have presented a comprehensive picture of how patients at the end-of-life stage are cared for in hospitals from the perspective of both physicians and nurses. Therefore, in this study the following research question was put forward: What have been the experiences of health care providers in caring for patients at the end-of-life stage in non-palliative care settings?

Methods

Aims

The aim of the study was to explore the experiences of health care providers in caring for patients at the end-of-life stage in non-palliative care settings.

Design

The experiences being examined in this study came from the health care providers' engagement in the health care system and their social interactions with patients and their families. The answer to the research question emerged through the dialogues that took place between the researcher and the participants. Hence, we aligned ourselves with an interpretivist perspective. Data were collected through interviews and analyzed using qualitative content analysis.

Participants

The criteria for the inclusion of participants were: (a) being a physician or a nurse working in a health care institution in Shanghai, where in a tertiary hospital (i.e., an acute care hospital), a secondary hospital (i.e., a sub-acute care hospital), or community health care center; (b) working in an internal medicine ward, intensive care unit (ICU), or acute and emergency department (AED); and (c) having cared for adult patients at the end-of-life stage during the past two years. The patients were those with cancer or a non-cancer chronic disease. Physicians or nurses who worked in palliative care units were excluded.

Purposive sampling was adopted to ensure that participants working in various wards could be interviewed. An advertisement was sent out via WeChat, the biggest social media application in China [52], with 963 million users in the country [53]. The advertisement of this project was sent to people on WeChat who were acquaintances of the first author (X.B.L.). It was estimated that more than 300 people saw the advertisement. Eligible health care providers were introduced to the first author (X.B.L.) by friends and colleagues if they expressed an interest in the research topic. X.B.L. then sent the information sheet to the eligible health care providers at least one week before the interviews. Any concerns were answered immediately. The interviews were confirmed after the health care providers agreed to participate. The consent form was signed on the day of the interview after the participant was given a face-to-face introduction to the study.

Data collection

The data were collected between August 2016 and February 2017. Semi-structured individual interviews were conducted by X.B.L. using an interview guide (see Table 1) in quiet rooms in the wards. Each participant was interviewed once. A minor revision was made to the interview guide after it was pilot tested in two interviews that were not included in the data analysis. The interviewer is an academic staff member with a PhD, who has a great deal of experience in conducting interviews. All of the interviews were audio taped and averaged 41 min in length. Participant recruitment was stopped when data saturation was achieved [54]. Data saturation was determined using the criterion of "informational redundancy" proposed by Grady and Sandelowski [55, 56]. When the researcher began to hear the same comments again and again in the interviews, data saturation was reached.

Ethical considerations

Ethical approval was obtained from the ethics committee of the university in which the first author works before the study began (Reference number: IRB#2017-10-1). The informants were assured that their participation was voluntary and confidential. Each participant was identified by a research number. All of the participants signed the consent form before the interviews were conducted.

Table 1 Interview Guide

Interview questions
1. Please enlighten me on the trajectory of disease(s) in your specialty. From your point of view, how would you define the end-of-life stage of the disease?
2. What kinds of treatment/care have you provided to patients at this stage?
3. What challenges/difficulties have you experienced when caring for such patients?
4. From your point of view, how should these patients be cared for?

Data analyses

The interviews were transcribed verbatim in Mandarin. A transcript was sent to one participant to check against with the audio record for accuracy. The transcripts were then imported into NVivo software [57] and analyzed using qualitative content analysis [58]. The analytic steps included: (a) thoroughly reading the transcripts; (b) dividing the interviews into *content areas* according to the interview questions; (c) extracting and condensing *meaning units*; (d) abstracting and labeling a *code*; (e) sorting the codes into *categories*; and (f) creating *sub-themes/themes* [58]. The data were mainly coded by the first author and reviewed by the other two authors. The analytic results were discussed by all three authors.

Rigor

The rigor of a study refers to its credibility, transferability, dependability, and conformability [59]. Health care providers in different specialties at several institutions were interviewed as a way of triangulating sources of data [60]. In each ward, one physician and one nurse were interviewed. Triangulation through multiple analyses was also performed [60]. The three researchers, all academic staff members, reviewed the data set independently, held group discussions on the findings, addressed the differences in their views, and finally arrived at a consensus. One participant reviewed the findings as another approach to analytical triangulation [60]. Verbatim quotations were provided to boost the transferability and credibility of the study [59]. A personal journal was kept to record the researcher's thoughts, including the frustrations, challenges, and highlights that were encountered while conducting the study [61].

Results

Twenty-six health care providers from eight institutions were approached. All agreed to participate. Their demographic characteristics are listed in Table 2. Three themes emerged from the interviews: (i) Definition of the end-of-life stage; (ii) Health care at the end-of-life stage; (iii) Challenges, difficulties, and the future. An illustration of the coding process has been included as Additional file 1.

Definition of the end-of-life stage

The participants defined the end-of-life stage of a person who has a chronic disease mainly in terms of a change in treatment.

> "A patient could be described as being at the end-of-life stage if he/she needs intravenous drugs to maintain (his/her physical status)." (Physician 15, cardiology)

Some few criteria for the end-of-life stage of those with specific diseases were also mentioned, including

Table 2 Demographics of the Participants

	Physician ($N = 13$)	Nurse ($N = 13$)
Age (Mean [*SD*])	39.00 (9.28)	37.15 (4.34)
Gender (n [%])		
Female	5 (38.5)	13 (100)
Education (n [%])		
Tertiary school	5 (38.5)	12 (92.3)
Master's degree	5 (38.5)	1 (7.7)
Doctoral degree	3 (23.0)	0 (0)
Religion (n [%])		
Buddhist	3 (23.0)	1 (7.7)
None	10 (76.9)	12 (92.3)
Marital status (n [%])		
Married	12 (92.3)	12 (92.3)
Divorced	1 (7.7)	0 (0)
Single	0 (0)	1 (7.7)
Working since graduation (year) (Median [range])	10 (5–37)	17 (4–25)
Working in this specialty (year) (Median [range])	10 (0.2–19)	11 (1–16)
Level of health care institution (n [%])		
Tertiary hospital	7 (53.8)	6 (46.2)
Secondary hospital	4 (30.8)	5 (38.5)
Community health care center	2 (15.4)	2 (15.4)
Specialty (n [%])		
AED	4 (30.8)	3 (23.1)
ICU	1 (7.7)	1 (7.7)
Cardiology department	2 (15.4)	2 (15.4)
Pulmonary department	0 (0)	2 (15.4)
Gastroenterology department	1 (7.7)	0 (0)
Hepatology department	1 (7.7)	1 (7.7)
Nephrology department	2 (15.4)	2 (15.4)
General practice	2 (15.4)	2 (15.4)
Diagnoses of patients cared for by the participants (n [%])	Total ($n = 26$)	
Cancer	22 (84.6)	
Cardiovascular disease	22 (84.6)	
Diabetes	11 (42.3)	
Chronic obstructive pulmonary disease	12 (46.2)	
Renal failure	16 (61.5)	
Cirrhosis	11 (42.3)	
Dementia	5 (19.2)	
Parkinson's disease	7 (16.9)	
Multiple sclerosis	2 (7.7)	

increased hospital admissions (Nurse 8, pulmonary), being bed-bound all day (Nurse 10, cardiology), and having a Creatinine level over 400 (Physician 16, nephrology). They stated that the duration of the end-of-life stage varies from days to months, and is unpredictable.

Health care at the end-of-life stage

Hospitalization: Drifting in the health care system

The need for hospitalization increases at the end-of-life stage. Some patients were directly admitted to a ward. More patients stayed in the AED of a tertiary/secondary hospital. From there, some patients were then transferred to a ward. The others remained in the AED until the end.

"If a patient does not die soon, we will try to transfer him/her to a ward for further treatment." (Physician 2, AED)

Local medical insurance policies allow patients to stay in a tertiary hospital for 7 days, or in a secondary hospital for 21 days. This amount of time is insufficient for patients at this stage, so they are transferred from one location to another. The transfers can be arranged to take place within the same hospital or among hospitals.

"After a patient stays in a ward for three weeks, we can arrange a self-financed re-admission. This means that the patient continues to stay in the ward, but pay all expenses by themselves for one week. After they can use their medical insurance again, we discharge and re-admit the patient again. All of the administrative procedures are done in the hospital information system. The patient stays in our ward throughout this period." (Nurse 3, pulmonary)

Regardless of which of the above arrangement is made, such transfers brought suffering to patients and their families.

"The patients had to keep moving. It was really painful for the patients and their families." (Physician 1, hepatology)

In the end, apart from a small number of patients who died in community health care centers or at home, most patients died in tertiary/secondary hospitals, especially in AEDs. However AEDs were not a good place in which to die.

"Eight to nine hundred patients died in our AED each year, the majority was patients with a chronic disease. We usually have more than 100 patients stay in the AED hall. Most are dying. They lie on trolleys. There are no curtains between the trolleys. They spend their last days in a place like a refugee camp." (Physician 12, AED)

Spending one's last days in a hospital was common, but it was not a good way to die. The patients usually underwent worthless treatments. In a way, it was a waste of health care resources, because other patients who truly needed high-level treatment and highly technical facilities could not be admitted, due to the presence of these patients.

"For the patients, it was worthless." (Physician 8, cardiology)

"For the tertiary hospitals, it was a waste of health care resources." (Physician 1, hepatology)

Physiologically focused and excessive treatment

Treatment at the end-of-life stage may continue to focus on the primary disease. As the disease progresses, attention turns to the symptoms and complications of the disease, is described as "conservative" or "symptom-focused" treatment. Both kinds of treatments may continue until the end.

"We usually provide symptom-focused treatment, which is the main treatment in the last few days." (Physician 12, AED)

Another change in treatment occurs after the patient is judged to be dying. Several treatments are used during the dying phase. In some wards, many drugs, including life-sustaining drugs, nutrition supplements, antibiotics, and even organ protective drugs, are used. Oxygen therapy and vital sign monitoring also continued to be delivered too. Only two participants mentioned the application of minimal treatment.

"I can only control the pain and prescribe oxygen therapy. Other treatments (i.e., life-sustaining drugs, antibiotics, resuscitation equipment, etc.) are unavailable here." (Physician 10, community)

The physicians acknowledged the patients' psychological needs, but could not do more.

"It is difficult to address this (psychological) area because of China's health care system, or the doctors' energy." (Physician 8, cardiology)

Roles of patients and families in making treatment decisions

Few participants had heard about advanced directives. After judging a patient's prognosis to be poor, the physician would initiate a conversation with the family to discuss future treatment. The essence of the conversation was to decide on whether to use invasive treatments and procedures. It was assumed that other treatments would continue to be delivered, but that they could be changed if the family proposed a change.

> "Others, such as intravenous medications or nutritional support, would usually not be discussed, unless the family proposed it." (Physician 5, nephrology)

In most cases, the family made the decisions without the patient's participation. The family's decision was influenced by many factors, such as the financial burden of the treatment, the perception of the patient's clinical condition, age, societal norms, and so on.

> "Some families continued treatment under the pressure of social judgment. They did not want to be blamed." (Physician 14, ICU)

Only in a few special cases did the patients make their own decisions.

> "We had (such a case) before. It was a young patient with cancer, who was able to communicate and had some medical knowledge. Only with such a patient could we have such a discussion (about the treatment)." (Physician 3, AED)

The physicians seldom discussed the patient's treatment and prognosis with the patients themselves. Although patients sometimes spoke of giving up (i.e., terminating treatment), it was the decisions of their family that was finally followed. Under the circumstance of family-dominated decision making, a patient's real wish could hardly be known.

> "Definitely the doctors discuss it [treatment] with the families. We are not sure whether the families previously discuss it with the patients." (Nurse 1, hepatology)

More than half of the families decided to terminate active treatment, while others chose resuscitation.

> "Most gave up at last." (Physician 15, cardiology)

Efforts to keep the patient alive occurred when the family had not yet decided what to do or when the family insisted on resuscitation. In a few cases, the patient was kept alive to give all members of the family time to arrive to "see the patient for one last time." Such resuscitation only brought suffering to the patient, and consumed resources unnecessarily.

> "We encountered such a situation. The family decided to give up. Then, the patient's condition worsened at night. We used drugs and carried out cardiopulmonary resuscitation (CPR) to keep the patient alive in order to wait for all family members to come." (Physician 10, community)

Instinctively enhanced nursing care

Although nurses were seldom involved in judging the end-of-life stage or dying phase, they instinctively provided more care to patients at the end-of-life stage.

> "I can only try my best. If the environment in the room is not good, I try to keep the room clean and tidy, and more comfortable, and to keep extraneous people out of the room." (Nurse 13, AED)

They made necessary adjustments on administration, caring for patients at a higher level of nursing care. For example, one nurse said, "We would pay extra attention to their basic nursing care" (Nurse 1, hepatology). Another nurse said, "We would have more intensive surveillance on them" (Nurse 3, pulmonary). Meanwhile, they tried to provide psychological support.

> "I would hold the patient's hand if the patient was conscious. I think it was a comfort for him/her." (Nurse 8, pulmonary)

Only one community nurse claimed that some basic nursing care procedures were no longer followed when the patient was dying, in order to minimize disturbance to the patient. Nursing care after death was quite procedure-related. None of the participants mentioned the provision of bereavement support.

Challenges, difficulties, and the future

Great pressure from families

The greatest challenge came from the families of the patients. Some families did not accept their loved one's condition.

> "The biggest challenge is the unwillingness of the family to accept the patient's condition. Some people had quarreled with us. At that time, my work became very difficult." (Physician 5, nephrology)

Sometimes, the physicians had to repeatedly explain a patient's condition to his/her family. Some families contacted physicians with their personal interests in mind. The physicians had to deal carefully with these complicated families.

> "Some families were involved in their own interests when discussing the treatment plan. For example, they wanted to inherit the patient's apartment. These

kinds of families were very difficult to communicate with." (Physician 14, ICU)

Meanwhile, the nurses' work became difficult because many families expressed mistrust, showed poor cooperation and a lack of understanding, and made unreasonable demands.

> "The biggest challenge was the poor cooperation of the family. Last time, there was an elderly patient. We suggested that the family spend more time with the patient. But the family said,'You should take care of him since he is in the hospital'. Then they left." (Nurse 10, cardiology)

Despite the participants' efforts, some families insisted on aggressive treatment. Worse, conflict and violence sometimes occurred after the patients died.

> "There was a patient who died suddenly. The family thought the treatment was delayed because of us. They could not accept this and smashed things in the ward everywhere." (Nurse 2, AED)

Practical difficulties in the delivery of care

Several difficulties in the delivery of care were also mentioned. A common difficulty was how to transfer patients out of a tertiary/secondary hospital after stabilization. Due to the lack of an effective referral system among health care institutions, physicians did not know where to place the patients.

> "We don't collaborate with nearby hospitals at lower levels. Therefore, it is difficult for us to transfer our patients out." (Physician 2, AED)

The physicians also felt that it was a challenge to comfort patients who did not know their real condition.

> "The family usually requests us to not tell the patient the truth. So it becomes very difficult to comfort the patient when his/her condition is deteriorating." (Physician 1, hepatology)

For the nurses, the difficulties included an increased workload, great stress during the night shift, skill-related difficulties, and feeling powerless to solve family conflicts. A lack of effective interventions to manage symptoms or problems was another difficulty faced by the participants.

> "The biggest difficulty was that some of their suffering could not be solved with my ability and skills" (Nurse 13, AED)

Urgent tasks in the future

The participants believed that some essential tasks need to be completed before local end-of-life care is developed in the future. The most important and repeatedly mentioned task, was educating the public on death, so that they would have the proper attitude towards it.

> "I think it is the attitude towards death. The society holds an attitude of avoidance towards death. Many Chinese cancer patients did not know their diagnosis until they died. They did not have the chance to realize their wishes." (Physician 14, ICU)

Meanwhile, the participants thought that government support was ultimately essential to develop local end-of-life care. Creating a better health care environment was another important but challenging task.

> "There are too many conflicts between patients and health care providers. We become exceptionally self-protective and careful when caring for dying patients. It causes great stress. I hope the environment can improve." (Nurse 16, nephrology)

End-of-life care model in the future

In terms of how patients at the end-of-life stage would best be cared for in the future, some participants stated that patients would be better cared for in non-palliative care settings, and that end-of-life care should be integrated into routine work.

> "I think patients in tertiary hospitals still need this service. We may have one or two health care providers in each ward to deliver the care after training." (Physician 1, hepatology)

Others thought that patients should be cared for in specialized end-of-life units in health care institutions at all levels. A few suggested that patients should be cared for at home. Regardless of the car model, there is a long road ahead in developing local end-of-life care service.

Discussion

This study describes how health care providers in non-palliative care settings care for patients with life-threatening diseases at the end-of-life stage. The findings indicate a lack of general end-of-life care in non-palliative care settings in Shanghai. Although symptom management is practiced to certain extent, aggressive disease management, the overuse of medication in the last 48 h, and visits to emergency rooms are common, especially among patients with non-cancer chronic diseases [62–65]. The nursing care in this study has mainly physical and task-oriented, similar to the nursing care provided in other settings [66–68]. The participants in this study thought that the quality of death was unsatisfactory. However, since there have been few studies in China on the quality of death of patients, great effort is needed in the future to develop a localized scale to evaluate the quality of death and examine the level of satisfaction of the patients and their families.

Having conversations about a patient's poor prognosis and final treatment plan is a difficult task for physicians, and such conversations are usually initiated at a very late stage in the study. This is similar to the practice of British physicians [69]. Having been trained in an atmosphere of active treatment for years, some doctors still think that patients should be actively treated until the end [69]. Others want to avoid deeper concerns [69], which they may not feel confident about discussing with patients and their families. Despite the similarities to other areas in the world, dying in a family-oriented society is more complicated. Traditional Chinese cultural values, i.e., filial piety and the power of the family, exert a deep influence on decision making at the end-of-life stage [70]. Chinese people feel "culturally obliged to provide every possible means to keep a patient alive" [71]. Accordingly, over-treatment at this stage is common. It is also common for family members to make medical decisions on behalf of the patient, even when the patient is conscious [72]. In the future, how to involve patients in end-of-life care, and to allow them to voice their wishes will be a great challenge in China.

The nurses interviewed in this study meet a number of patients at the end-of-life stage in their work. This suggests that end-of-life care is an area of practice for nurses working in general wards [73], but they are seldom involved in judging the end-of-life stage or the dying phase. Bloomer et al. [65] also found that nurses took a passive role in recognizing dying. The nursing care that was described in this study is still physical and task-oriented, although a certain amount of comfort care is given both physical and psychological. This is similar to the nursing care provided in other settings [67, 68]. High-quality end-of-life nursing care in non-palliative care settings is lacking.

Several challenges must be addressed before general end-of-life care can be developed in local settings. Fridh (2014) suggested that education about the end-of-life stage and a supportive environment are essential for providing end-of-life care [74]. These are exactly what are needed in Shanghai. A major obstacle to providing end-of-life care is that health care providers lack a clear idea of what end-of-life care means, as well as the relevant competencies. Relevant training is necessary to bring about change. With regard to patients and their families, the lack of a proper attitude towards death is a considerable obstacle in initiating end-of-life care in China. Chinese people usually hold a negative attitude towards death, even when the patient is dying [75]. Meanwhile, many Chinese people mistakenly believe that health care services are part of the general service industry [76]. They believe that health care providers must fix the patient's problem as they requested, since they are paying for it. These factors also contribute to delayed discussions of final treatment plans and to the constant seeking of medical support in acute care hospitals. This places a great burden on hospitals and wastes valuable health care resources.

Much work needs to be done at the system level in Shanghai. A care pathway or special insurance policy should be considered, as this would allow patients to remain in one location without drifting among institutions. An end-of-life care network linking health care institutions at all levels should be considered as well. In recent years, new measures have been implemented to optimize health care services in China. For instance, medical treatment partnerships and community-based end-of-life care have been developed [77, 78]. These measures facilitate the management of chronic diseases and provide more beds for cancer patients at the end-of-life stage. However, end-of-life care should be considered in various settings. Additionally, the health care environment in China needs to be ameliorated. The tension between patients and the health care system over the years has had a significant impact on the work of health care providers, causing them great stress and even danger. It has made them particularly self-protective, which may ultimately compromise the quality of care provided to patients.

Limitations

This study reveals the service gaps in local end-of-life care and identifies future directions for research. The participants were not invited from hospitals in each division, which would have provided a comprehensive representation of views. Using WeChat was a more efficient way to recruit participants, but, it may have compromised the representativeness of the study population. In addition, due to limited time and human resources, this study was conducted in one city. The experiences of health care providers in other areas and countries may differ.

Conclusions

General end-of-life care is underdeveloped in China. As health care institutions in China, and around the world, are faced with increasing numbers of patients at the end-of-life stage with longer life expectancies, it is time to bring this topic to the forefront of health care service reform. An end-of-life service network that could benefit patients with life-threatening diseases, and that could be set up in institutions at all three levels, should be developed. The obstacles impeding the development of end-of-life care should be resolved before a comprehensive end-of-life care system is established. Training programs for health care providers and death education programs for the public should also be developed. In the future, more studies should be conducted to provide empirical evidence for designing localized end-of-life care programs, since patients with different diagnoses and from social backgrounds may have different preferences for end-of-life care.

Abbreviations

AED`: Acute and emergency department; COPD: Chronic obstructive pulmonary disease; CPR: Cardiopulmonary resuscitation; ICU: Intensive care unit; UK: The United Kingdom; US: The United States

Acknowledgments

The authors would like to thank all of the participants and all of the colleagues and friends who helped to approach eligible health care providers.

Funding

This work was supported by the New Staff Funding program of Fudan University [Grant number JIF400104].

Authors' contributions

The authors of the manuscript are XBL, FKYW, and SSYC. All of the three authors were involved in the study. The study was designed by XBL and finalized after discussions with FKYW and SSYC. The data were collected and mainly analyzed by XBL. The results of the analysis were discussed by all three authors. XBL drafted the manuscript. FKYW and SSYC reviewed the manuscript, gave comments, approved the final manuscript, and agreed to be accountable for all aspects of the work. All authors read and approved the final manuscript.

Competing interests

The authors declare that they have no competing interests.

Author details

[1]School of Nursing, Fudan University, Shanghai, China. [2]School of Nursing, The Hong Kong Polytechnic University, Hung Hom, Hong Kong.

References

1. Worldwide Palliative Care Alliance: Global atlas of palliative care at the end of life. http://www.who.int/nmh/Global_Atlas_of_Palliative_Care.pdf (2014). Accessed 30 May 2018.
2. The Gold Standards Framework: The GSF Prognostic indicator guidance. http://www.goldstandardsframework.org.uk/cd-content/uploads/files/General%20Files/Prognostic%20Indicator%20Guidance%20October%202011.pdf (2011). Accessed 10 Sep 2018.
3. Etkind SN, Bone AE, Gomes B, Lovell N, Evans CJ, Higginson IJ, et al. How many people will need palliative care in 2040? Past trends, future projections and implications for services. BMC Med. 2017;15(1):102.
4. Mitchell G. Rapidly increasing end-of-life care needs: a timely warning. BMC Med. 2017;15(1):126.
5. Button E, Chan R, Chambers S, Butler J, Yates P. Signs, symptoms, and characteristics associated with end of life in people with a hematologic malignancy: a review of the literature. Oncol Nurs Forum. 2016;43(5):E178–87.
6. Ekstrã MM, Allingham SF, Eagar K, Yates P, Johnson C, Currow DC. Breathlessness during the last week of life in palliative care: an Australian prospective, longitudinal study. J Pain Symptom Manag. 2016;51(5):816–23.
7. Ben Natan M, Garfinkel D, Shachar I. End-of-life needs as perceived by terminally ill older adult patients, family and staff. Eur J Oncol Nurs. 2010; 14(4):299–303.
8. Clark K, Cain J, Campbell L, Byfieldt N. Caring for people dying in acute hospitals: a mixed-methods study to examine relative's perceptions of care. Palliat Support Care. 2015;13(2):335–43.
9. Egan R, MacLeod R, Jaye C, McGee R, Baxter J, Herbison P, et al. Spiritual beliefs, practices, and needs at the end of life: results from a New Zealand national hospice study. Palliat Support Care. 2017;15(2):223–30.
10. Perrar KM, Schmidt H, Eisenmann Y, Cremer B, Voltz R. Needs of people with severe dementia at the end-of-life: a systematic review. J Alzheimers Dis. 2015;43(2):397–413.
11. Saleem TZ, Higginson IJ, Chaudhuri KR, Martin A, Burman R, Leigh PN. Symptom prevalence, severity and palliative care needs assessment using the palliative outcome scale: a cross-sectional study of patients with Parkinson's disease and related neurological conditions. Palliat Med. 2013; 27(8):722–31.
12. Virdun C, Luckett T, Lorenz K, Davidson PM, Phillips J. Dying in the hospital setting: a meta-synthesis identifying the elements of end-of-life care that patients and their families describe as being important. Palliat Med. 2017; 31(7):587–601.
13. Abarshi E, Echteld M, Van Den Block L, Donker G, Deliens L, Onwuteaka-Philipsen B. Transitions between care settings at the end of life in the Netherlands: results from a nationwide study. Palliat Med. 2010;24(2):166–74.
14. Green E, Ward S, Brierley W, Riley B, Sattar H, Harris T. They shouldn't be coming to the ED, should they? A qualitative study of why patients with palliative care needs present to the emergency department. Am J Hosp Palliat Care. 2017;34(10):984–90.
15. Houttekier D, Vandervoort A, Van Den Block L, van der Steen JT, Vander Stichele R, Deliens L. Hospitalizations of nursing home residents with dementia in the last month of life: results from a nationwide survey. Palliat Med. 2014;28(9):1110–7.
16. Kim SJ, Han KT, Kim TH, Park EC. Does hospital need more hospice beds? Hospital charges and length of stays by lung cancer inpatients at their end of life: a retrospective cohort design of 2002-2012. Palliat Med. 2015;29(9):808–16.
17. Reyniers T, Deliens L, Pasman HR, Vander Stichele R, Sijnave B, Cohen J, et al. Reasons for end-of-life hospital admissions: results of a survey among family physicians. J Pain Symptom Manag. 2016;52(4):498–506.
18. Rosenwax LK, McNamara BA, Murray K, McCabe RJ, Aoun SM, Currow DC. Hospital and emergency department use in the last year of life: a baseline for future modifications to end-of-life care. Med J Aust. 2011;11(194):570–3.
19. Teno JM, Gozalo PL, Bynum JP, Leland NE, Miller SC, Morden NE, et al. Change in end-of-life care for Medicare beneficiaries: site of death, place of care, and health care transitions in 2000, 2005, and 2009. JAMA. 2013;309(5): 470–7.
20. Bekelman JE, Halpern SD, Blankart CR, Bynum JP, Cohen J, Fowler R, et al. Comparison of site of death, health care utilization, and hospital expenditures for patients dying with cancer in 7 developed countries. JAMA. 2016;315(3):272–83.

21. Broad JB, Gott M, Kim H, Boyd M, Chen H, Connolly MJ. Where do people die? An international comparison of the percentage of deaths occurring in hospital and residential aged care settings in 45 populations, using published and available statistics. Int J Public Health. 2013;58(2):257–67.
22. Cohen J, Bilsen J, Addington-hall J, Löfmark R, Miccinesi G, Kaasa S, et al. Population-based study of dying in hospital in six European countries. Palliat Med. 2008;22(6):702–10.
23. Department of Health. More care less pathway: A review of the Liverpool Care Pathway. https://www.gov.uk/government/uploads/system/uploads/attachment_data/file/212450/Liverpool_Care_Pathway.pdf (2013). Accessed 30 May 2018.
24. William L. Non-palliative care staff need to deliver generalist end of life care. BMJ. 2014;348:3426.
25. Office for National Statistics. National survey of bereaved people (VOICES): England. https://www.ons.gov.uk/peoplepopulationandcommunity/healthandsocialcare/healthcaresystem/bulletins/nationalsurveyofbereavedpeoplevoices/england2015#preferences-and-choice-at-the-end-of-life (2015). Accessed 30 May 2018.
26. Blumenthal D, Hsiao W. Privatization and its discontents—the evolving Chinese health care system. N Engl J Med. 2005;353(11):1165–71.
27. National Health Commission of the People's Republic of China. [The total number of health care institutions in China till Oct 2017]. http://www.moh.gov.cn/mohwsbwstjxxzx/s7967/201712/cb133528a46d4e98af757e6a657bdb9c.shtml (2017). Accessed 10 Sep 2018. Chinese.
28. National Health Commission of the People's Republic of China. [The health care utilization in 2017]. http://www.nhfpc.gov.cn/mohwsbwstjxxzx/s7967/201706/6044508d72144fc8b343adc2f024f9d1.shtml (2017). Accessed 10 Sep 2018. Chinese.
29. Han M, Jin WZ, Qian NS, Cai RS, Wang CF. characteristics analysis on death among elderly people aged 60 years and above in Shanghai in 2014. Shanghai J. Prev. Med. 2015;27(9):523–7 Chinese.
30. Han S, Zhou Y, Wang LJ, He Y. factors influencing the place of death in Beijing dongcheng south district patients with Cancer, 2007-2012. J Med Res. 2015;44(5):57–61 Chinese.
31. Liu ZH, He MF, Zhang YJ, Chen JL, Tang Q. study on distribution of hospital death. Chin Gen Prac. 2010;13(32):3635–8 Chinese.
32. Xinhua Net. [The plan of Health China 2030 is published]. http://news.xinhuanet.com/health/2016-10/25/c_1119786029.htm (2016). Accessed 30 may 2018. Chinese.
33. National Health Commission of the People's Republic of China. The standards of hospice care center and management guideline. Chin Nurs Manag. 2017;17(3):289–90 Chinese.
34. The State Council of the People's Republic of China. [The notification of the publication of hospice care practice guideline]. http://www.moh.gov.cn/yzygj/s3593/201702/83797c0261a94781b158dbd76666b717.shtml (2017). Accessed 10 Sep 2018. Chinese.
35. The Economist Intelligence Unit. The 2015 quality of death index: Ranking palliative care across the world. https://www.eiuperspectives.economist.com/sites/default/files/2015%20EIU%20Quality%20of%20Death%20Index%20Oct%2029%20FINAL.pdf (2015). Accessed 10 Sep 2018.
36. Liu XM. to reduce the pain of the dying—developing hospice care was suggested on the biweekly CPPCC meeting. Chinese People's political consultative conference news. 2016;4(22):01 Chinese.
37. Wang HP, Shi YX, Zhou JQ. the service status of hospice care pilot settings in Shanghai. Chin gen prac. 2015;18(34):4244–7 Chinese.
38. Reyniers T, Houttekier D, Cohen J, Pasman HR, Deliens L. The acute hospital setting as a place of death and final care: a qualitative study on perspectives of family physicians, nurses and family carers. Health Place. 2014;27(3):77–83.
39. Wilkie DJ, Ezenwa MO. Pain and symptom management in palliative care and at end of life. Nurs Outlook. 2012;60(6):357–64.
40. Walling AM, Asch SM, Lorenz KA, Roth CP, Barry T, Kahn KL, et al. The quality of care provided to hospitalized patients at the end of life. Arch Intern Med. 2010;170(12):1057–63.
41. Witkamp FE, Van Zuylen L, Borsboom G, van der Rijt CCD, van der Heide A. Dying in the hospital: what happens and what matters, according to bereaved relatives. J Pain Symptom Manag. 2015;49(2):203–13.
42. Mcllvennan CK, Jones J, Allen LA, Swetz KM, Nowels C, Matlock DD. Bereaved caregiver perspectives on the end-of-life experience of patients with a left ventricular assist device. JAMA Intern Med. 2016;176(4):534–9.
43. Peacock S, Duggleby W, Koop P. The lived experience of family caregivers who provided end-of-life care to persons with advanced dementia. Palliat Support Care. 2014;12(2):117–26.
44. Broady TR, Saich F, Hinton T. Caring for a family member or friend with dementia at the end of life: a scoping review and implications for palliative care practice. Palliat Med. 2018;32(3):643–56.
45. Mathews G, Johnston B. Palliative and end-of-life care for adults with advanced chronic obstructive pulmonary disease: a rapid review focusing on patient and family caregiver perspectives. Curr Opin Support Palliat Care. 2017;11(4):315–27.
46. Dose AM, Carey EC, Rhudy LM, Chiu Y, Frimannsdottir K, Ottenberg AL, et al. Dying in the hospital: perspectives of family members. J Palliat Care. 2015; 31(1):13–20.
47. Mossin H, Landmark BT. Being present in hospital when the patient is dying - a grounded theory study of spouses experiences. Eur J Oncol Nurs. 2011; 15(5):382–9.
48. Mori M, Yoshida S, Shiozaki M, Baba M, Morita T, Aoyama M, et al. Talking about death with terminally-ill cancer patients: what contributes to the regret of bereaved family members? J Pain Symptom Manag. 2017;54(6): 853–60.
49. Garner KK, Goodwin JA, McSweeney JC, Kirchner JE. Nurse executives' perceptions of end-of-life care provided in hospitals. J Pain Symptom Manag. 2013;45(2):235–43.
50. Oliveira I, Fothergill-Bourbonnais F, Mcpherson C, Vanderspank-Wright B. Battling a tangled web: the lived experience of nurses providing end-of-life care on an acute medical unit. Res Theory Nurs Pract. 2016;30(4):353–78.
51. Gardiner C, Cobb M, Gott M, Ingleton C. Barriers to providing palliative care for older people in acute hospitals. Age Ageing. 2011;40(2):233–8.
52. Tencen Ltd. WeChat. Shenzhen. China: Tencent Ltd; 2017.
53. Hexun Net. [The user of WeChat in China has been reached the peak]. http://tech.hexun.com/2017-09-05/190730980.html (2017). Accessed 10 Sep 2018. Chinese.
54. Saumure K, Given LM. Data saturation. In: Given LM, editor. The SAGE encyclopedia of qualitative research methods. Thousand Oaks: SAGA Publications; 2008. https://doi.org/10.4135/9781412963909.n99.
55. Grady MP. Qualitative and action research: a practitioner handbook. Bloomington: Phi Delta Kappa Intl Inc; 1998. p. 26.
56. Sandelowski M. Theoretical saturation. In: Given LM, editor. The SAGE encyclopedia of qualitative research methods. Thousand Oaks: SAGA Publications; 2008. https://doi.org/10.4135/9781412963909.n99.
57. QSR International Pty Ltd. NVivo 11. Victoria: QSR International Pty Ltd; 2017.
58. Graneheim UH, Lundman B. Qualitative content analysis in nursing research: concepts, procedures and measures to achieve trustworthiness. Nurse Educ Today. 2004;24(2):105–12.
59. Lincoln YS. Trustworthiness criteria. In: Lewis-Beck MS, Bryman A, Liao TF, editors. The SAGE encyclopedia of social science research methods. Thousand Oaks: SAGA Publications; 2008. https://doi.org/10.4135/9781412950589.n1035.
60. Patton MQ. Enhancing the quality and credibility of qualitative analysis. Health Serv Res. 1999;34(5):1189–208.
61. Mayan MJ. Essentials of qualitative inquiry. London: Routledge; 2016.
62. Brown C, Drosdowsky A, Krishnasamy M. An exploration of medical emergency team intervention at the end of life for people with advanced cancer. Eur J Oncol Nurs. 2017;31:77–83.
63. Garrison CM, Overcash J, Mcmillan SC. Predictors of quality of life in elderly hospice patients with cancer. J Hosp Palliat Nurs. 2011;13(5):288–97.
64. Van Den Noortgate NJ, Verhofstede R, Cohen J, Piers RD, Deliens L, Smets T. Prescription and deprescription of medication during the last 48 hours of life: multicenter study in 23 acute geriatric wards in Flanders, Belgium. J Pain Symptom Manag. 2016;51(6):1020–6.
65. Bloomer MJ, Endacott R, O'Connor M, Cross W. The 'dis-ease' of dying: challenges in nursing care of the dying in the acute hospital setting. A qualitative observational study. Palliat Med. 2013;27(8):757–64.
66. Wachterman MW, Lipsitz SR, Lorenz KA, Marcantonio ER, Li Z, Keating NL. End-of-life experience of older adults dying of end-stage renal disease: a comparison with cancer. J Pain Symptom Manag. 2017;54(6): 789–97.
67. Ong KK, Ting KC, Chow YL. The trajectory of experience of critical care nurses in providing end-of-life care: a qualitative descriptive study. J Clin Nurs. 2018;27(1–2):257–68.
68. Sekse RJT, Hunskår I, Ellingsen S. The nurse's role in palliative care: a qualitative meta-synthesis. J Clin Nurs. 2018;27(1–2):e21–38.

69. Horn R. 'I don't need my patients' opinion to withdraw treatment': patient preferences at the end-of-life and physician attitudes towards advance directives in England and France. Med Health Care Philos. 2014;17(3):425–35.
70. Chen X, Fan R. The family and harmonious medical decision making: cherishing an appropriate Confucian moral balance. J Med Philos. 2010; 35(5):573–86.
71. Lee I. Filial duty as the moral foundation of caring for the elderly: its possibility and limitations. In: Fan RP, editor. Family-oriented informed consent: east Asian and American perspectives. London: Springer International Publishing; 2015. p. 137–47.
72. Yang Y. A family-oriented Confucian approach to advance directives in end-of-life decision making for incompetent elderly patients. In: Fan RP, editor. Family-oriented informed consent: east Asian and American perspectives. London: Springer International Publishing; 2015. p. 257–70.
73. Croxon L, Deravin L, Anderson J. Dealing with end of life-new graduated nurse experiences. J Clin Nurs. 2017;27(1–2):337–44.
74. Fridh I. Caring for the dying patient in the ICU - the past, the present and the future. Intensive Crit Care Nurs. 2014;30(6):306–11.
75. Hsu C, O'Connor M, Lee S. Understandings of death and dying for people of Chinese origin. Death Stud. 2009;33(2):153–74.
76. Chen SM. [the rise, harm and solution of medical consumerism]. [Medicine & Philosophy]. 2015;36(2A):62-6. Chinese.
77. Eastday. [The 5th meeting of the 13th People's Congress of Shanghai was held this morning]. http://sh.eastday.com/qtmt/lh2012/u1a953218.html (2012). Accessed 30 may 2018. Chinese.
78. The State Council of the People's Republic of China. [The state council promotes medical treatment partnerships]. http://www.gov.cn/zhengce/content/2017-04/26/content_5189071.htm (2017). Accessed 23 Apr 2018. Chinese.

Intranasal fentanyl for respiratory distress in children and adolescents with life-limiting conditions

Lucas Pieper[1], Julia Wager[1,2] and Boris Zernikow[1,2*]

Abstract

Background: Respiratory distress is one of the most common and frightening symptoms of children with life-limiting conditions. Because treatment of the underlying cause is frequently impossible or insufficient, in many children, symptomatic treatment is warranted. The purpose of this study was to describe the circumstances of the use of intranasal fentanyl in an acute attack of respiratory distress (AARD) in children receiving palliative care, as well as to describe outcomes and adverse events after its use.

Methods: Children and adolescents treated in a pediatric palliative unit or attended by a specialized home care team between 2010 and 2016 were included in this study. A retrospective chart review was conducted of those who were treated with intranasal fentanyl for an AARD.

Results: During the study period 16 children (0.5–18.6 years) with various life-limiting conditions were treated with intranasal fentanyl for AARD. In total, 70 AARDs were analyzed. In 74% of all AARDs, a single dose of intranasal fentanyl was used. Frequent causes for an AARD were excessive secretions and acute respiratory infection. The median starting dose of intranasal fentanyl was 1.5 μg/kg body weight. Labored breathing (96%), tachypnea (79%) and related suffering (97%) improved after treatment. An adverse event occurred in one child.

Conclusions: Intranasal fentanyl may be a safe and effective medication for the treatment of acute attacks of respiratory distress in children with life-limiting conditions. However, prospective studies with larger sample sizes and a control group are needed to validate these findings.

Keywords: Dyspnea, Fentanyl, Intranasal application, Palliative, Pediatric

Background

Respiratory distress (RD) is a concerning symptom with high prevalence in children with life-limiting conditions (LLCs) [1–15]. RD is frequently reported in cancer, advanced heart or pulmonary disease, neurological disorders and many other rare LLCs [1–8, 10–12, 14]. The management of RD is therefore an important part of pediatric palliative care.

In children and adolescents of all ages, RD can occur with a wide range of physical signs and unpleasant perceptions [16]. The latter are often described as dyspnea, "a subjective experience of breathing discomfort that consists of qualitatively distinct sensations that vary in intensity" [17]. The multidimensional concept of dyspnea describes the complex pathophysiology of this symptom with interacting biological, psychological, social and environmental factors. Numerous chemo- and mechanoreceptors as well as neural pathways are involved in this condition [17–19]. RD can also be caused by increased respiratory drive, mechanical impedance, respiratory muscle failure, wasted ventilation and psychological stress [19] causing sensations such as air hunger, a sense of increased work of breathing, labored breathing and chest tightness [20, 21].

The most effective treatment of RD is the identification and therapy of underlying causes. However, this approach is frequently limited when no specific cause is apparent or

* Correspondence: B.Zernikow@kinderklinik-datteln.de
[1]Department of Children's Pain Therapy and Paediatric Palliative Care, Witten/Herdecke University, Faculty of Health – School of Medicine, Witten, Germany
[2]Paediatric Palliative Care Centre, Children's and Adolescents' Hospital Datteln, Dr.-Friedrich-Steiner-Str.5, 45711 Datteln, Germany

no effective treatment at hand [22]. In this situation, symptomatic treatment is warranted. Non-pharmacological approaches include physiotherapy, management of secretions, fans to blow in the face, psychological and behavioral therapy and (noninvasive) positive pressure ventilation [1, 22, 23]. Pharmacological treatment mainly consists of opioids and anxiolytics [1, 22, 24]. In the pharmacological treatment of RD in adults, opioids are used frequently with good evidence for the oral and parenteral route [24, 25].

One treatment approach is intranasal fentanyl (INF); it is used to treat dyspnea in adults with chronic obstructive pulmonary disease, chronic heart failure and lung cancer [26, 27]. Fentanyl is a lipophilic opioid and can therefore easily traverse the highly vascularized and permeable nasal mucosa [28]. Intranasal drug delivery is described as an effective and non-invasive approach for systemic administration [28]. In pain treatment, the onset of action occurs within 5 min after the application of INF [29]. This is very short, compared to the long onset of action of 15–30 min when short acting morphine is given orally [30]. INF also avoids the hepatic first pass effect [28]. In one study, INF treatment led to significantly higher fentanyl plasma levels and had a higher bioavailability than the oral-transmucosal administration of fentanyl [31].

In pediatric pain management INF is a rather new treatment approach; it has been used with good evidence postoperatively and in acute pain due to burns or fractures [32–34]. Although evidence for the effectiveness of INF administration for RD is scant [35, 36], clinical experience indicates a safe reduction of symptom intensity and related suffering [26, 37, 38]. A case series with 11 newborns and infants describes the good effectiveness and tolerability of INF for the palliation of RD, without the occurrence of apnea or chest wall rigidity [37]. Nonetheless, the use of INF for the palliation of RD in children requires further exploration, specifically the use in various age groups and for various underlying diseases. Solid knowledge regarding the circumstances of administration, dosage, outcomes, safety and adverse effects needs to be generated.

The primary purpose of this study is to report the application of INF for RD treatment in a sample of palliative attended children and adolescents with various LLCs based on data from a retrospective chart analysis. First, the symptoms and conditions leading to the administration of INF are described. Second, the extent and frequency in which INF has been used during acute attacks of RD are presented. Third, the therapeutic response and potential adverse events are analyzed.

Methods

Study design and sample

We performed a retrospective chart review of pediatric in- and outpatients, who were either treated in a pediatric palliative ward or by a specialized pediatric palliative home care team. From June 2010 to July 2016, 402 patients with LLC were treated inpatient, and 198 patients were treated by the home care team. All children received palliative care in various phases of their illness trajectory. A prior study showed that approximately 30% of inpatients suffer from RD [14].

Patients were considered eligible for the study if they were treated with INF for RD. Those treated with INF were detected via the controlled drugs register ($n = 28$). In 57% of the patients ($n = 16$), INF was used for the palliation of RD. In the remaining 43% of the patients ($n = 12$), the drug was administered for breakthrough pain control.

Data collection

A retrospective chart review was conducted for the 16 eligible patients. Both, electronic and handwritten medical charts, pharmacy data and doctor's letters were screened for this research. The documentation did not change over time. At all time points, electronic and handwritten charts were used in parallel for the documentation of different aspects. All documents were screened for indicators of an acute attack of respiratory distress (AARD). For this purpose, descriptions and acronyms of RD and associated conditions such as suffering and restlessness were searched in the documents (Table 1). A mean of 2 and a maximum of 5 different verbal descriptions of RD were documented during an AARD.

For each AARD, symptoms and conditions leading to the administration of INF were extracted. Additionally, the continuous medication and adjunctive therapies for RD were documented.

To measure the therapeutic response of the INF application, any reported improvement of RD, RD-associated symptoms, suffering and restlessness were ranked on a 4-point scale (0 = no, 1 = slight, 2 = moderate, and 3 = complete resolution). For that purpose, the researchers collected typifying terms of the different levels of improvement (no/ slight/ moderate/ complete resolution) in the medical charts. The assignment of these terms to the 4-point scale was carried out in an interdisciplinary

Table 1 Indicators for dyspnea: searched terms for symptoms and general conditions

symptoms/condition	descriptions in the documents
respiratory distress	"labored breathing" incl. "chest wall retractions", "use of accessory muscles", "nasal flaring", "heavy breathing", "difficult breathing"
	"tachypnea"
	"dyspnea"[b]
	"wheezing"
	"cyanosis"
suffering	"suffering", "sorrow", "crying"
restlessness	"is restless"
exhaustion	"is weak", "is exhausted"

palliative care team consisting of physicians, psychologists and nurses. Following, a researcher (LP) assessed any reported improvement of RD in an AARD guided by the collections of typifying terms. The ranking could only be applied if the same symptom was reported prior to the INF application and after treatment. A symptom was considered resolved if it was reported prior to the INF application and not reported afterward. Vital signs such as heart rate, oxygen saturation, respiratory rate and blood pressure before and after the administration were collected. However, vital signs were not documented in all AARDs; they are regarded with rather low importance in pediatric palliative care (PPC). Due to the small number of usable findings, they are not reported in this manuscript.

We recorded the circumstances of every single INF application, number of doses of INF applied per AARD, the cumulative dosage and the length of intervals between 2 INF doses. The end of an AARD was defined as the absence of signs of RD occurring for at least 1.5 h. The adverse effects occurring in association with INF application were documented.

Statistical analysis

Analyses were conducted with the SPSS 24 statistical software program. The results of the descriptive statistics are reported as the total number (n) and percentages (%), as well as the median and the range of values or mean and standard deviation (SD). A comparison regarding the initial dose of INF between opioid naïve children and non-naïve children was calculated with a Mann-Whitney U-Test. A significance level of $p < .05$ is considered significant.

Results are reported separately for 1) the first dose of INF ($n = 70$), 2) the second dose of INF ($n = 18$) and 3) the last dose of INF ($n = 70$). The section "last dose of INF" deals with the final dose of all reviewed AARD (n = 70, 100%) and also includes all AARD treated with only one dose of INF. For the first dose, circumstances prior to administration, details of treatment and treatment success are reported. For the second dose, only details on treatment are presented, while for the last dose, only the treatment success is reported.

Results

Patient characteristics

The characteristics of all 16 patients included in this study are summarized in Table 2. Nine patients were male and seven were female. The age of patients ranged from 0.5 to 18.6 years. The median patient age was 5.9 years. All patients had different diagnoses, except for three children who suffered from spinal muscular atrophy type I and two patients from hypoxic-ischemic encephalopathy. Thirteen children (81%) were unable to self-report RD or related suffering due to young age or cognitive impairment.

Table 2 Sample characteristics

N = 16	*n*	%
sex		
male	9	56
female	7	44
setting		
outpatient	5	31
inpatient	10	63
inpatient+ outpatient	1	6
underlying condition		
acute lymphoblastic leukemia	1	
alveolar rhabdomyosarcoma	1	
chronic granulomatous disease, Graft-versus-host disease	1	
Cockayne syndrome	1	
global developmental delay of unknown origin	1	
hypoxic-ischemic encephalopathy	2	
Menkes disease, prematurity	1	
neurodegenerative disease of unknown origin	1	
neuronal ceroid lipofuscinosis type 3	1	
Prune belly syndrome, periventricular leukomalacia	1	
spinal muscular atrophy type 1	3	
Tetralogy of Fallot, hypoxic ischaemic encephalopathy	1	
Trisomy 13	1	

Note: percentages are rounded and may therefore add up to more than 100%

General description of intranasal fentanyl application

In the 16 patients, 70 AARDs (100%) were treated with 122 INF applications. In total, 38 (54%) of the AARDs occurred in opioid naïve children, and 32 (46%) occurred in children already receiving opioids via various administration routes on a daily basis. The median daily oral morphine equivalent dose of the continuous opioid application was 0.72 mg/kg body weight (bw) (range 0.1–12.24 mg/kg bw/day).

The mean number of administered doses in a single AARD was 1.74 (SD = 1.98). One child with infectious hypoxic encephalopathy received 12 doses in a single AARD during his terminal phase, but the majority ($n = 52$, 74%) of attacks were treated with a single dose of INF (Fig. 1). The used drugs were either 1) nebulized intravenous fentanyl (50 μg/ml) for lower doses or 2) Instanyl (500-2000 μg/ml) for higher doses.

First dose of INF

Circumstances prior to administration

Various potential reasons for RD were recorded (Table 3). Excessive secretion was documented in 70% of all AARDs. Furthermore, in 67% of AARDs, an acute respiratory infection was documented when the first dose of INF was administered. Other, less frequently described pathophysiologies were anxiety, pain, pleural effusion, atelectasis and hepatosplenomegaly.

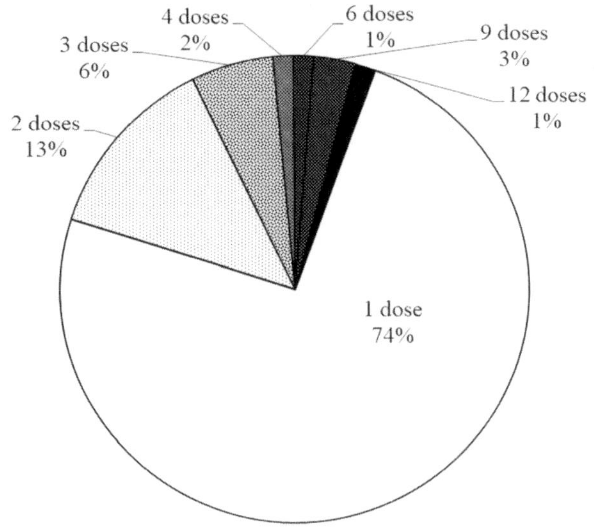

Fig. 1 Number of INF doses in a single acute attack of respiratory distress. Note: percentages are rounded and add up to less than 100%

Table 3 Documented circumstances prior to the first administration of intranasal fentanyl ($n = 70$)

Circumstances prior to administration	number of AARDs	
	n	%
underlying pathophysiology		
excessive secretion	49	70
respiratory infection	47	67
muscular hypotonia	19	27
limited ability to cough	14	20
lower airway obstruction	14	20
upper airway obstruction	4	6
others[a]	14	20
general condition		
suffering	34	49
restlessness	29	41
exhaustion	13	19
sleepiness	12	17
description of respiratory distress		
labored breathing	47	67
tachypnea	41	59
dyspnea	27	39
wheezing	7	10
cyanosis	6	9

Note: percentages are rounded; multiple responses possible
[a]others includes: atelectasis, pleural effusion, anxiety

The initial usage of INF was connected in timely fashion to the occurrence of various descriptions of RD and the impairment of the general condition (Table 3). In the majority of AARDs, several signs of RD appeared simultaneously. The most prevalent descriptions prior to the first administration of INF was labored breathing (67%), followed by tachypnea (59%). "Dyspnea" as a descriptor was documented in 39% of all AARDs. General suffering was reported in nearly half of all AARDs. In 41% of the children, restlessness was reported.

Treatment of an AARD

The median starting dose of INF was 40 μg (range 10–100 μg), which equals 1.5 μg/kg bw (range 0.4 μg–5.1 μg/kg bw). Opioid-naïve children were initially treated with a median dose of 0.97 μg/kg bw (range 0.42–1.5 μg/kg bw), while children already receiving opioid treatment started with a significantly higher dose of 1.7 μg/kg bw (range 0.54–5.1 μg/kg bw) ($p < .001$; U-Test).

In addition to INF application, various approaches of adjunctive therapy were used to improve the patient's respiratory situation (Table 4). Continuous medication for RD palliation was applied in 67 AARDs (96%). Most common were inhaled salbutamol (74%) and ipratropium bromide (39%). Other continuous medications for RD were inhalations with NaCl 0.9%, salmeterol and budesonide or treatment with opioids, glucocorticoids, furosemide and xylometazoline. In 81% of all AARDs, oxygen was applied initially with a range from 2 to 15 l and a median of 4.5 l. Additional on-demand medication was used in 4 AARDs (6%).

Treatment success

Figure 2 displays the effects of INF application for the various symptoms and conditions. The administration of the first INF dose in an AARD had the greatest effect on "labored breathing" (improved in 89%) and "tachypnea" (improved in 73%). When the term "dyspnea" was documented, it improved in more than half of all AARDs after the first INF application (59%). With regard to the general condition of the patient, "suffering" and "restlessness" were reduced in 85% and 76% of all AARDs after the first INF dose, respectively.

Adverse events

In just one case, an adverse event was documented after the first INF dose. The affected child had Trisomy 13, with body weight of 55 kg. The child was treated with a starting dose of 50 μg (0.9 μg/kg bw) of INF during "labored breathing", "suffering" and "restlessness". After the INF administration, Cheyne-Stokes respiration occurred, and a decrease in the oxygen saturation was documented. The only continuous drugs admitted at the time were furosemide and ipratropium bromide inhalation.

Table 4 Adjunctive therapy administered when the first dose of intranasal Fentanyl was given ($n = 70$)

adjunctive therapies	number of AARDs	
	n	%
continuous medication		
Budesonide, inhalation	12	17
Furosemide, orally/intravenously	13	19
Glucocorticoids, orally/intravenously	15	21
Ipratropium bromide, inhalation	27	39
Levamethadone, orally	4	6
Morphine, patient controlled analgesia	7	10
Morphine, continual intravenous infusion	2	3
Morphine, slow release, orally	19	27
NaCl 0.9%, inhalation	25	36
Salbutamol, inhalation	52	74
Salmeterol/Fluticasone, inhalation	20	29
Xylometazoline, intranasally	8	11
Other medications	3	4
on demand medication		
Ipratropium bromide, inhalation	3	4
Salbutamol, inhalation	1	1
Oxygen	57	81
non-pharmacological treatments		
mechanical suction of secretion	38	54
physiotherapy	11	16
others	4	6

Note: Percentages add up to more than 100% because multiple responses are possible

After the administration of oxygen (10 l/min) the oxygen saturation improved. The Cheyne-Stokes respiration disappeared shortly afterward. In this child, four administrations of similar INF doses in the days prior and six applications after this event occurred without any recorded side effects. The described adverse effect was not noted with other doses of INF. Further adverse effects like chest wall rigidity did not occur.

Second dose of INF

In 18 (26%) AARDs, a second dose of INF was administered. The time interval between the first and second dose ranged from 15 to 80 min, with a median interval of 30 min. For all patients, the amount of the second INF dose was the same as that of the first dose. The median dose was 1.3 µg/kg bw (range 0.67–4.08 µg/kg bw).

Last dose of INF

The cumulative INF dose in one AARD (median 50 µg) ranged from 10 µg in two toddlers to 500 µg in a 19-year-old with neuronal ceroid lipofuscinosis type 3 in the terminal phase. The highest rate of improvement was achieved when "labored breathing" (96%) and "tachypnea" (79%) occurred before the last administration of INF (Fig. 3). When the term "dyspnea" was documented just prior to the last INF application, it improved in 72% of the AARDs after the last dose of INF and was completely resolved in 48% of the AARDs. "Cyanosis" was completely resolved in all children after the last dose of INF. An improvement of "suffering" was achieved in 97% of all attacks. There was only one documented AARD in which the child's suffering did not improve at all, although previous attacks that day were treated successfully.

Adverse events

No additional adverse events were documented after the last dose of INF.

Discussion

Beside the previous report of INF in eleven infants and newborns [37], this is the first study that describes the usage of INF for the treatment of RD in children with LLC receiving palliative care. The results show that in many children of various ages and with varying diagnosis, symptoms improve after the first INF application;

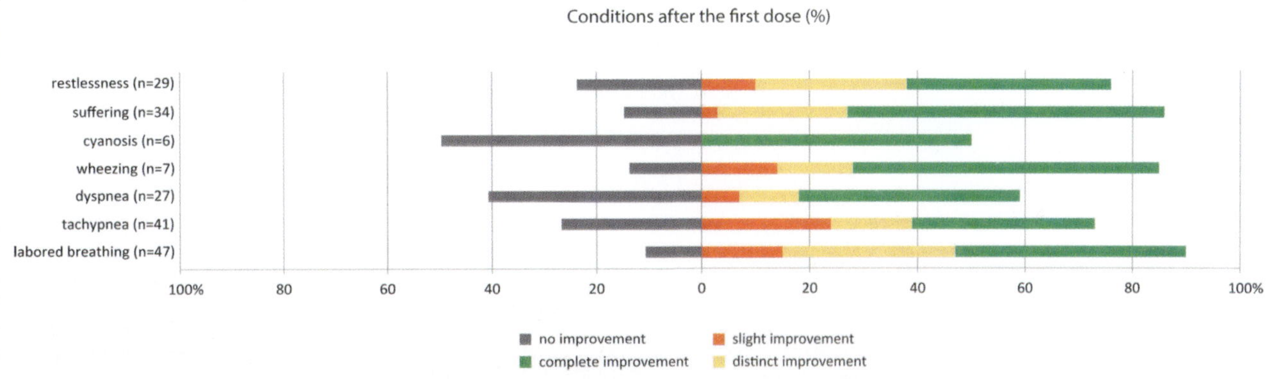

Fig. 2 Conditions after the first intranasal fentanyl dose. Note: rounded percentages

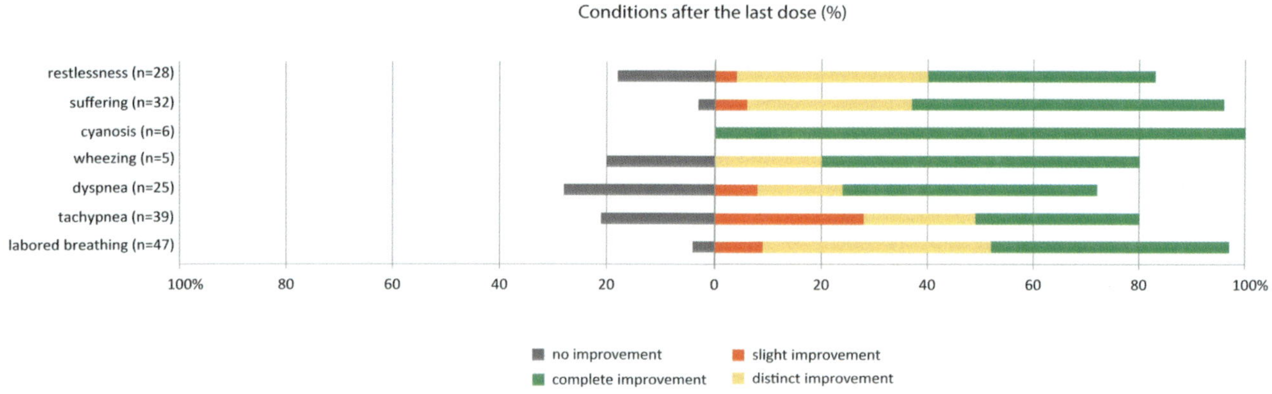

Fig. 3 Conditions after the last dose of intranasal fentanyl dose. Note: rounded percentages

only a small number of patients require a second or more doses. Furthermore, this study indicates that adverse events after INF application are rare. Taken together, this study offers preliminary evidence that INF is a safe and effective medication for the treatment of RD in children with LLC.

In PPC settings, the assessment of RD is often hindered by patients being unable to self-report. The majority of patients have severe psycho-motor impairments and are not able to report dyspnea [14, 16]. Our results underline the complexity of RD. Various descriptions of RD and related suffering are used to paraphrase the patient's respiratory condition in the chart. This fact impedes comparability. For future research and for clinical communication, it may be of great help to generate a reliable and valid assessment tool for the measurement of RD in children unable to self-report. Furthermore, the small number of self-assessment tools for communication-competent children needs to be extended and adapted to younger ages and validated for a wide range of underlying diseases [16].

During the retrospective chart review, we also noticed that vital signs are not recorded routinely during AARD. Only in approximately 50% of all AARDs, vital signs were documented prior to the administration of INF. The documentation after INF treatment was even more incomplete. This finding suggests that the clinical assessment of a patient may be more relevant in palliative care than the evaluation of vital signs. However, for research purposes, the documentation of AARD in standard care needs to be improved. An assessment tool for RD could therefore be supplemented by documentation of vital signs optionally, if the situation allows the measurement. The patient's conditions and quality of life should not be affected by the measurement.

This study supports the notion that underlying conditions leading to RD in children with LLC differ from those in adults, who often suffer from chronic obstructive pulmonary disease, heart failure or pulmonary cancer [39–42]. The children in our study suffer from a wide variety of underlying conditions. Diverse biological and psychological pathophysiologies can be found. Excessive and thick secretions and airway infections are the most frequently reported causes of the AARDs, but pain and anxiety may also contribute to the children's RD. These findings support the multidimensional concept of dyspnea [17, 18, 43].

Similar to previous research in adults [26, 27] and infants [37], this study highlights the suitability of INF treatment for RD. One dose of INF seems frequently adequate to clinically improve RD. In an AARD, the intranasal route has advantages over the oral or oral-transmucosal administration of fentanyl. The rather quick effect of INF is important for the treatment. An AARD is an emergency situation that requires prompt relief. Because the effect of INF becomes apparent very quickly, it also becomes obvious very quickly if an additional dose is required. In our sample, a median time of 30 min passed until the next dose. The minimum interval between first and second dose was 15 min.

The initial median INF dose of 1.5 μg/kg bw for the treatment of an AARD in children reported in this study corresponds to doses used in pediatric pain management. In pediatric pain management, effective analgesia is reported at a dose of 1–2 μg/kg bw of INF [29, 44–51]. In adults, the use of INF for treatment of dyspnea is reported in a few case reports only. In these case reports, the initial INF dose ranged from 50 to 100 μg in opioid-naïve patients. In patients already on continuous opioids, a four-hour equivalent INF dose leads to relief of RD [26, 27]. The only study available describing the palliation of RD in infants and newborns reports initial doses of 0.2–3.8 μg/kg bw of INF, of which more than one half of the children were treated with 1–2 μg/kg bw of INF [37]. The results of our study show that the doses applied are safe and appeared to be rather effective in RD.

The low number of adverse effects is remarkable and supports the assumption of former studies of INF being a good treatment option for RD [26, 27, 37]. The good safety profile, the ease of use, and the effectiveness of INF [26, 27, 32, 37] enable the application in the in- and outpatient setting. However, this study showed that opioids should be used carefully, as adverse effects can occur even in children used to opioids.

The retrospective design of the study and the lack of standardized documentation and a validated assessment tool for the children's RD may have negatively affected the data collection. Furthermore, the small sample size of this study limits generalizability.

Limitations

The validity of the data on the efficacy of INF in an AARD may be affected as the ranking was conducted by one researcher. To prevent any bias in the assessment the 4-point scale was designed by an interdisciplinary palliative care team. It provided collections of typifying terms to guide the assessment-process and ensure consistency.

Conclusions

Our findings suggest that INF is one option to treat acute RD in children with diverse underlying life-limiting conditions and different ages. Good reasons for the INF treatment are the short onset of action, the low invasiveness, and the easy and safe application in a range of children. However, knowledge regarding the palliation of RD with INF needs to be extended. Prospective studies and a control-group-design would be desirable, though challenging. A standardized and validated tool to measure RD in children unable to self-report would help to measure treatment outcome and to identify a requirement for the pharmacological treatment of RD.

Abbreviations

AARD: Attack of respiratory distress; bw: Body weight; INF: Intranasal fentanyl; LLC: Life-limiting conditions; PPC: Pediatric palliative care; RD: Respiratory distress

Funding

This research did not receive any specific grant from funding agencies in the public, commercial, or not-for-profit sectors.

Authors' contributions

LP, JW and BZ made substantial contributions to the conception of the work; LP collected data, performed the statistical analysis and drafted the paper; JW and BZ added to the interpretation of data and revised the paper critically for important intellectual content. All of the authors gave their final approval of the version to be published.

Competing interests

The authors declare that they have no competing interests.

References

1. Craig F, Henderson EM, Bluebond-Langner M. Management of respiratory symptoms in paediatric palliative care. Curr. Opin. Support. Palliat. Care. 2015;9(3):217–26.
2. Blume ED, Balkin EM, Aiyagari R, Ziniel S, Beke DM, Thiagarajan R, Taylor L, Kulik T, Pituch K, Wolfe J. Parental perspectives on suffering and quality of life at end-of-life in children with advanced heart disease: an exploratory study*. Pediatr. Crit. Care Med. 2014;15(4):336–42.
3. von Lutzau P, Otto M, Hechler T, Metzing S, Wolfe J, Zernikow B. Children dying from cancer: parents' perspectives on symptoms, quality of life, characteristics of death, and end-of-life decisions. J Palliat Care 2012, 28(4):274–281.
4. Hechler T, Blankenburg M, Friedrichsdorf SJ, Garske D, Hubner B, Menke A, Wamsler C, Wolfe J, Zernikow B. Parents' perspective on symptoms, quality of life, characteristics of death and end-of-life decisions for children dying from cancer. Klinische Padiatrie. 2008;220(3):166–74.
5. Wolfe J, Hammel JF, Edwards KE, Duncan J, Comeau M, Breyer J, Aldridge SA, Grier HE, Berde C, Dussel V, et al. Easing of suffering in children with cancer at the end of life: is care changing? J. Clin. Oncol. Off. J. Am. Soc. Clin. Oncol. 2008;26(10):1717–23.
6. Wolfe J, Grier HE, Klar N, Levin SB, Ellenbogen JM, Salem-Schatz S, Emanuel EJ, Weeks JC. Symptoms and suffering at the end of life in children with cancer. N Engl J Med. 2000;342(5):326–33.
7. Theunissen JM, Hoogerbrugge PM, van Achterberg T, Prins JB, Vernooij-Dassen MJ, van den Ende CH. Symptoms in the palliative phase of children with cancer. Pediatr Blood Cancer. 2007;49(2):160–5.
8. Schindera C, Tomlinson D, Bartels U, Gillmeister B, Alli A, Sung L. Predictors of symptoms and site of death in pediatric palliative patients with cancer at end of life. Am. J. Hosp. Palliat. Care. 2013;31(5):548–52.
9. Gormley PK, Colreavy MP, Patil N, Woods AE. Congenital vascular anomalies and persistent respiratory symptoms in children. Int J Pediatr Otorhinolaryngol. 1999;51(1):23–31.
10. St-Laurent-Gagnon T. Paediatric palliative care in the home. Paediatr Child Health. 1998;3(3):165–8.
11. Hunt AM. A survey of signs, symptoms and symptom control in 30 terminally ill children. Dev Med Child Neurol. 1990;32(4):341–6.
12. Drake R, Frost J, Collins JJ. The symptoms of dying children. J Pain Symptom Manag. 2003;26(1):594–603.
13. Monnier P, Lang F, Savary M. Partial cricotracheal resection for pediatric subglottic stenosis: a single institution's experience in 60 cases. Eur. Arch. Otorhinolaryngol. 2003;260(6):295–7.
14. Garske D, Schmidt P, Hasan C, Wager J, Zernikow B. Palliativversorgung auf der pädiatrischen Palliativstation "Lichtblicke" – Eine retrospektive Studie. Zeitschrift für Palliativmedizin. 2016;17(06):302–7.
15. Collins JJ, Byrnes ME, Dunkel IJ, Lapin J, Nadel T, Thaler HT, Polyak T, Rapkin B, Portenoy RK. The measurement of symptoms in children with cancer. J Pain Symptom Manag. 2000;19(5):363–77.
16. Pieper L, Zernikow B, Drake R, Frosch M, Printz M, Wager J. Dyspnea in children with life-threatening and life-limiting complex chronic conditions. J Palliat Med. 2018;
17. American Thoracic Society. Dyspnea. Mechanisms, assessment, and management: a consensus statement. American Thoracic Society. Am J Respir Crit Care Med. 1999;159(1):321–40.
18. Manning HL, Schwartzstein RM. Pathophysiology of dyspnea. N Engl J Med. 1995;333(23):1547–53.
19. Leach RM. Palliative care in non-malignant, end-stage respiratory disease. In: Hanks G, Cherny NI, Christakis NA, Fallon M, Kaasa S, Portenoy RK, editors. Oxford textbook of palliative medicine. Edn. New York, NY: Oxford University Press; 2010. p. 1231–67.

20. Lansing RW, Gracely RH, Banzett RB. The multiple dimensions of dyspnea: review and hypotheses. Respir Physiol Neurobiol. 2009;167(1):53–60.
21. Parshall MB, Schwartzstein RM, Adams L, Banzett RB, Manning HL, Bourbeau J, Calverley PM, Gift AG, Harver A, Lareau SC, et al. An official American Thoracic Society statement: update on the mechanisms, assessment, and management of dyspnea. Am J Respir Crit Care Med. 2012;185(4):435–52.
22. Robinson WM. Palliation of dyspnea in pediatrics. Chronic respiratory disease. 2012;9(4):251–6.
23. Bausewein C, Booth S, Gysels M, Higginson I. Non-pharmacological interventions for breathlessness in advanced stages of malignant and non-malignant diseases. The Cochrane database of systematic reviews 2008(2): Cd005623.
24. Jennings AL, Davies AN, Higgins JP, Gibbs JS, Broadley KE. A systematic review of the use of opioids in the management of dyspnoea. Thorax. 2002; 57(11):939–44.
25. Abernethy AP, Currow DC, Frith P, Fazekas BS, McHugh A, Bui C. Randomised, double blind, placebo controlled crossover trial of sustained release morphine for the management of refractory dyspnoea. BMJ (Clinical research ed). 2003;327(7414):523–8.
26. Sitte T, Bausewein C. Intranasal fentanyl for episodic breathlessness. J Pain Symptom Manag. 2008;36(6):e3–6.
27. Sitte T. Nasal application of fentanyl citrate as symptom control against breathlessness in palliative care--overview and case report. Wien. Med. Wochenschr (1946). 2009;159(23–24):566–70.
28. Grassin-Delyle S, Buenestado A, Naline E, Faisy C, Blouquit-Laye S, Couderc LJ, Le Guen M, Fischler M, Devillier P. Intranasal drug delivery: an efficient and non-invasive route for systemic administration: focus on opioids. Pharmacol Ther 2012, 134(3):366–379.
29. Crellin D, Ling RX, Babl FE. Does the standard intravenous solution of fentanyl (50 microg/mL) administered intranasally have analgesic efficacy? Emerg. Med. Australas. : EMA. 2010;22(1):62–7.
30. Freye E, Levy JV, Braun D. Effervescent morphine results in faster relief of breakthrough pain in patients compared to immediate release morphine sulfate tablet. Pain practice : the official journal of World Institute of Pain. 2007;7(4):324–31.
31. Nave R, Schmitt H, Popper L. Faster absorption and higher systemic bioavailability of intranasal fentanyl spray compared to oral transmucosal fentanyl citrate in healthy subjects. Drug delivery. 2013;20(5):216–23.
32. Mudd S. Intranasal fentanyl for pain management in children: a systematic review of the literature. J. Pediatr. Health Care. 2011;25(5):316–22.
33. Murphy A, O'Sullivan R, Wakai A, Grant TS, Barrett MJ, Cronin J, McCoy SC, Hom J, Kandamany N. Intranasal fentanyl for the management of acute pain in children. The Cochrane database of systematic reviews 2014(10): Cd009942.
34. Davis MP. Fentanyl for breakthrough pain: a systematic review. Expert Rev Neurother. 2011;11(8):1197–216.
35. Simon ST, Koskeroglu P, Gaertner J, Voltz R. Fentanyl for the relief of refractory breathlessness: a systematic review. J Pain Symptom Manag. 2013; 46(6):874–86.
36. Bausewein C, Simon ST. Inhaled nebulized and intranasal opioids for the relief of breathlessness. Curr. Opin. Support. Palliat. Care. 2014;8(3):208–12.
37. Harlos MS, Stenekes S, Lambert D, Hohl C, Chochinov HM. Intranasal fentanyl in the palliative care of newborns and infants. J Pain Symptom Manag. 2013;46(2):265–74.
38. Graff GR, Stark JM, Grueber R. Nebulized fentanyl for palliation of dyspnea in a cystic fibrosis patient. Respiration; international review of thoracic diseases. 2004;71(6):646–9.
39. Bausewein C. Management of refractory breathlessness in patients with advanced disease. Internist. 2016;57(10):978–82.
40. Solano JP, Gomes B, Higginson IJ. A comparison of symptom prevalence in far advanced cancer, AIDS, heart disease, chronic obstructive pulmonary disease and renal disease. J Pain Symptom Manag. 2006;31(1):58–69.
41. Alt-Epping B, Staritz AE, Simon ST, Altfelder N, Hotz T, Lindena G, Nauck F. What is special about patients with lung cancer and pulmonary metastases in palliative care? Results from a nationwide survey. J Palliat Med. 2012;15(9): 971–7.
42. Reuben DB, Mor V. Dyspnea in terminally ill cancer patients. Chest. 1986; 89(2):234–6.
43. Kamal AH, Maguire JM, Wheeler JL, Currow DC, Abernethy AP. Dyspnea review for the palliative care professional: assessment, burdens, and etiologies. J Palliat Med. 2011;14(10):1167–72.
44. Borland ML, Jacobs I, Geelhoed G. Intranasal fentanyl reduces acute pain in children in the emergency department: a safety and efficacy study. Emergency medicine (Fremantle, WA). 2002;14(3):275–80.
45. Borland ML, Clark LJ, Esson A. Comparative review of the clinical use of intranasal fentanyl versus morphine in a paediatric emergency department. Emerg. Med. Australas. : EMA. 2008;20(6):515–20.
46. Borland M, Jacobs I, King B, O'Brien D. A randomized controlled trial comparing intranasal fentanyl to intravenous morphine for managing acute pain in children in the emergency department. Ann Emerg Med. 2007;49(3): 335–40.
47. Finkel JC, Cohen IT, Hannallah RS, Patel KM, Kim MS, Hummer KA, Choi SS, Pena M, Schreiber SB, Zalzal G. The effect of intranasal fentanyl on the emergence characteristics after sevoflurane anesthesia in children undergoing surgery for bilateral myringotomy tube placement. Anesth Analg. 2001;92(5):1164–8.
48. Galinkin JL, Fazi LM, Cuy RM, Chiavacci RM, Kurth CD, Shah UK, Jacobs IN, Watcha MF. Use of intranasal fentanyl in children undergoing myringotomy and tube placement during halothane and sevoflurane anesthesia. Anesthesiology. 2000;93(6):1378–83.
49. Holdgate A, Cao A, Lo KM. The implementation of intranasal fentanyl for children in a mixed adult and pediatric emergency department reduces time to analgesic administration. Acad Emerg Med Off J Soc Acad Emerg Med. 2010;17(2):214–7.
50. Manjushree R, Lahiri A, Ghosh BR, Laha A, Handa K. Intranasal fentanyl provides adequate postoperative analgesia in pediatric patients. Can. J. Anaesth. 2002;49(2):190–3.
51. Younge PA, Nicol MF, Kendall JM, Harrington AP. A prospective randomized pilot comparison of intranasal fentanyl and intramuscular morphine for analgesia in children presenting to the emergency department with clinical fractures. Emerg Med. 1999;11:90–4.

23

Addressing the needs of terminally-ill patients in Bosnia-Herzegovina: patients' perceptions and expectations

S. Aebischer Perone[1*], R. Nikolic[2], R. Lazic[2], E. Dropic[3], T. Vogel[4], B. Lab[4], S. Lachat[4], P. Hudelson[5], C. Matis[6], S. Pautex[6] and F. Chappuis[1]

Abstract

Background: Many terminally ill patients in Bosnia-Herzegovina (BiH) fail to receive needed medical attention and social support. In 2016 a primary healthcare centreer (PHCC) in Doboj (BiH) requested the methodological and technical support of a local partner (Fondacija fami) and the Geneva University Hospitals to address the needs of terminally ill patients living at home. In order to design acceptable, affordable and sustainable solutions, we involved patients and their families in exploring needs, barriers and available resources.

Methods: We conducted interviews with 62 purposely selected patients using a semi-structured interview guide designed to elicit patients' experiences, needs and expectations. Both qualitative and quantitative analyses were conducted, using an inductive thematic approach.

Results: While patients were aware that their illnesses were incurable, they were poorly informed about medical and social support resources available to them. Family members appeared to be patients' main source of support, and often suffered from exhaustion and financial strain. Patients expressed feelings of helplessness and lack of control over their health. They wanted more support from health professionals for pain and other symptom management, as well as for anxiety and depression. Patients who were bedridden or with reduced mobility expressed strong feelings of loneliness, social exclusion, and stigma from community members and – occasionally - from health workers.

Conclusions: Our findings suggest a wide gap between patients' end-of-life care needs and existing services. In order to address the medical, psychological and social needs of terminally ill patients, a multi-pronged approach is called for, including not only better symptom management through training of health professionals and improved access to medication and equipment, but also a coordinated inter-professional, inter-institutional and multi-stakeholder effort aimed at offering comprehensive medical, psycho-social, educational and spiritual support.

Keywords: Terminally ill patients, End of life care, Palliative care, Home care, Patients' perceptions, Transition countries, Low and middle income countries, Bosnia-Herzegovina

Background

At any time, over 40 million individuals live with incurable diseases in need of palliative care [1]. More than three quarters of them (78%) live in low and middle-income countries with poor access to palliative care. As put forward by Mitchell [2], the organisation and delivery of palliative and end-of-life care (EoLC) must be improved globally and the World Health Organisation states in one of its resolutions, that EoLC should be integrated into mainstream health care [1]:

> "To develop and strengthen, where appropriate, evidence-based guidelines on the integration of palliative care into national health systems, across disease groups and levels of care..."

EoLC includes medical treatment and support offered to patients with incurable, life-threatening, and/or chronic

* Correspondence: sigiriya.aebischerperone@hcuge.ch
[1]Division of Tropical and Humanitarian Medicine, Geneva University Hospitals, Rue Gabrielle-Perret-Gentil 6, 1205 Geneva, Switzerland
Full list of author information is available at the end of the article

progressive diseases when curative care is no longer a primary objective. The aim is to provide patients with the best possible quality of life before death, while also providing appropriate support to their relatives. End of life care aims at preventing suffering and complications and includes medical treatment and care as well as psychological, social and spiritual support [3, 4].

Our study took place in Bosnia and Herzegovina (BiH), a former Yugoslav republic situated at the heart of the Balkans. In the post conflict reconstruction and through the health system reform, strengthening primary health care, based on the family medicine (FM) model, has been set as a priority. Currently more than 80% of municipalities of BiH are served by FM teams. However, palliative care services are limited to services provided by community nurses and two hospices in Tuzla and Ljubuski (*Personal communication, Samir Husic, chief of Palliative Care Center of Tuzla*) and the palliative home care department of the PHCC "Centar Sarajevo" covering the population of Sarajevo (*Personal communication Fuad Husic, director of PHCC of Sarajevo Canton*). In hospitals no beds are allocated for palliative care patients [5]. There are no other outpatients' services organised in BIH for palliative care patients. Therefore, it appears that the range of services needs to be further extended to improve access to healthcare for elderly, patients with incurable conditions and terminally-ill patients who stay at home with little support or wait to be admitted in a hospital. Despite national laws stating that EoLC should be provided by primary care services [6–8] and hospital services [9], policies and resources are insufficient to guide the development of EoLC in BiH. EoLC are currently provided on an ad-hoc basis outside any existing system or community network.

The municipality of Doboj, northern BiH, covers a population of about 80´000 persons. Doboj has an above average need for EoLC, because its population has a relatively high proportion of people over 65 years of age (28%) [10], as compared to the EU (19.4%) [11]. High mortality from cardiovascular diseases (47%), cancer (22%) and metabolic and respiratory conditions (10%) [12] was recorded in all age groups in 2015.

Early 2016, the management of the municipal PHCC approached a local non-governmental organisation, the Fondacija fami, and the Geneva University Hospitals (HUG) with the intent to improve the type and level of services made available to terminally ill patients living at home. Indeed, research [13] demonstrated in rural communities a reduction in avoidable hospital admissions for patients at their end of life when cared by general practitioners.

Since little was known about the needs and perceptions of these patients in BiH, we undertook a qualitative study to investigate patients' perceptions, expectations and proposals for improvement. This paper presents the results from interviews with patients as a first step of an ongoing program to improve care and support offered to terminally-ill patients in Doboj municipality.

Methods

Study design

We conducted semi-structured interviews with a purposely selected sample of 62 terminally ill patients, in order to explore their perceptions, experiences and expectations regarding their health care and social support.

Setting and participants

The study was conducted in Doboj municipality between November and December 2016. To identify study participants, we used a 2-tier, purposive sampling strategy. We first asked 31 family medicine teams (FM teams) from Doboj PHCC (totalling 35 doctors and 68 nurses) to identify each up to 30 patients in need for EoLC. Inclusion criteria were: registered patients with incurable disease, over 18 years of age, and able to understand and answer the interview questions. Exclusion criteria were: patients unable to provide informed consent to participate in the study, or with any disability that impeded communication. A total of 900 patients were identified.

From each of the FM team's list of patients, we chose and invited 2 patients to participate in the study, for a total of 62 patients. Individuals were chosen to reflect the geographical and demographic characteristics of terminally-ill patients in Doboj municipality. All 62 selected patients (31 male, 31 female) accepted to be interviewed. Forty-six were interviewed alone, while 16 were interviewed with the assistance of a family member. All but one were interviewed in their home. Weekly supportive debriefing was offered to the interviewers.

Table 1 summarizes participants' characteristics.

Data collection

Based on preliminary exchanges and a review of relevant literature [14–17], we developed an interview guide consisting of 15 open-ended questions to explore patients' experiences and expectations, investigating the following dimensions as shown in Table 2.

In addition to the open-ended questions, we also asked patients to rate their current perceptions about each of the 15 dimensions using a 4-points severity scale (See interview guide in Additional file 1).

The interviews were jointly conducted by two investigators: the project coordinator from the Fondacija fami and an appointed PHCC health worker, who noted down answers on hard copy interview guides in the local language. All interviews lasted between 45 and 90 min.

Table 1 Characteristics of participants interviewed in Doboj municipality, Bosnia and Herzegovina ($n = 62$)

Gender	
Male	31
Female	31
Age (years)	
≤ 29	1
30–39	2
40–49	6
50–59	11
60–69	10
70–79	17
80–89	15
Place of interview	
Home	61
Field clinic	1
Education	
No formal education	5
Primary school	26
Secondary school	29
Higher education	2
Distance to health facility	
< 5 min	15
6–15 min	36
> 16 min	11

Data analysis

Interview notes were anonymised, translated into English and entered in Epi-Info 7 to facilitate analysis.

Respondents' answers to the open-ended questions were first grouped by interview question, and then themes within each question were identified by the interviewer from the Fondacija fami and a social scientist from the HUG. Descriptive codes were created to reflect emerging themes. Consensus about findings was reached over weekly conference calls and discussions among research team members from BiH and Switzerland.

Table 2 Dimensions explored in the interview guide

1. Information about the health condition, right / desire to know
2. Dignity, respect
3. Autonomy (physical and functional)
4. Depression, anxiety
5. Tiredness/drowsiness
6. Respiratory distress
7. Pain
8. Nutrition, appetite
9. Nausea/vomiting
10. Other digestive problems: constipation/diarrhoea
11. Distress, fear
12. Spiritual needs and believes
13. Financial issues
14. Administrative issues
15. Family and concern about their future

Ethics approval

The study was approved by the Geneva Canton Research Ethics Commission (CCER) (N°2016-01422) and the ethical board of the PHCC in Doboj. We required and obtained written consent from all patients prior to the interviews.

Results

Quantitative analyses

The quantitative analysis of the ratings given by the interviewed patients show – in decreasing order - the relative importance of: (i) lack of autonomy in daily activities, (ii) depression and loneliness, (iii) pain control and symptom management, (iv) burden on families, (v) deontology and professionalism and finally the (vi) lack of information. This analysis of the ratings confirmed the relative importance of the six identified themes as shown in the figures below (Figs. 1 and 2).

Qualitative analysis

We took the emerging themes forward to proceed with a qualitative analysis that would provide further ground for the needs assessment and (future) interventions.

Theme 1 – Lack of autonomy

The majority of study participants ($n = 50$; 81%) depended entirely on their families for care and support and most persons mentioned being exhausted ($n = 46$).

- *«I depend on my family, especially my wife. I can just turn myself in the bed. My wife feeds me, I cannot get up, I lose my mind, I often forget things and have difficulties to speak. » (P6Q3a, M, 60–69, urban setting, lives with his relative)*
- *«I cannot move, pain exhausts me. I have no strength. I did not get help. They do not know how to help me. » (P11Q5a, M, 70–79, urban setting, lives with his relative)*

Theme 2 – Loneliness, depression and social exclusion

A majority of patients ($n = 39$; 63%) declared to be depressed (24 most of the time and 15 very often), particularly because of isolation and loneliness. The more restrained in their mobility and dependent they were, the more depressed they felt. Facing the deterioration of their condition and their impending death as well as painful symptoms were also sources of depression.

- *« We are both not well. I am exhausted and we both do not enjoy our lives any more. I wish we both die together and I wish it happens soon. » (P25Q4a, F, 50–59, urban setting, lives with her relative)*

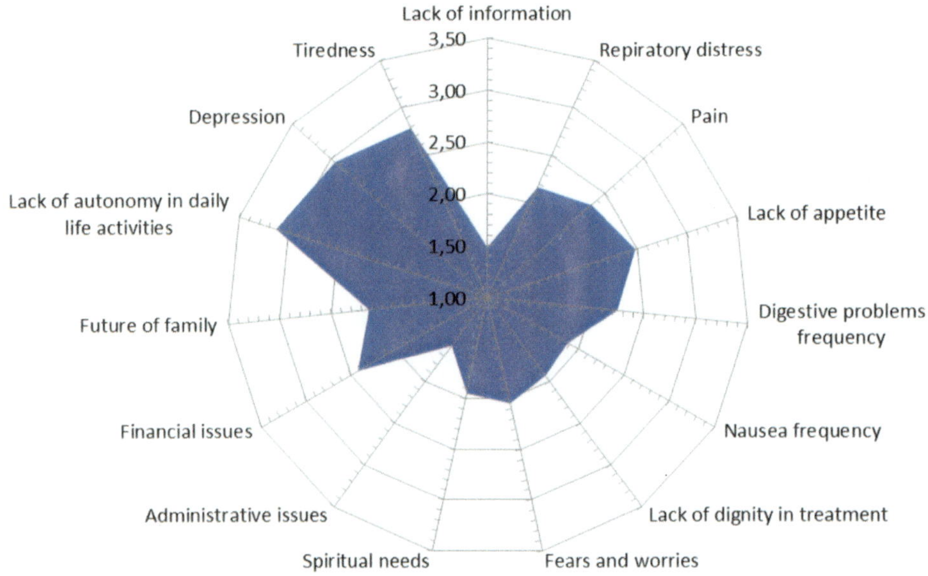

Fig. 1 Fifteen themes and their relative weight according to patients

- *« I cry, I lay down all the time in bed. This is no life any more. I do not enjoy my life at all. My husband as well. I wait for death and that is it. » (P28Q4a, F, 80–89, rural setting, lives with her relative)*

Some patients spontaneously stressed the need for psychological support and treatment against anxiety. Others explained that their ability to enjoy life could improve with increased social interaction, home visits by volunteers, peer support or even through technology-based interactions. Simply being able to go out from their bed or their home was also mentioned as a source of relief.

- *« We are isolated, people avoid us. Can people with this problem meet, or have volunteers to visit us and make us feel like human? » (P2Q4d, F, 80–89, urban setting, lives alone)*
- *« People know I am seriously ill and they either avoid me or feel sorry about me. I am not happy about it. It makes me forced to isolate myself from people. I am better off alone. » (P58Q2a, M, 60–69, rural setting, lives with his relative)*

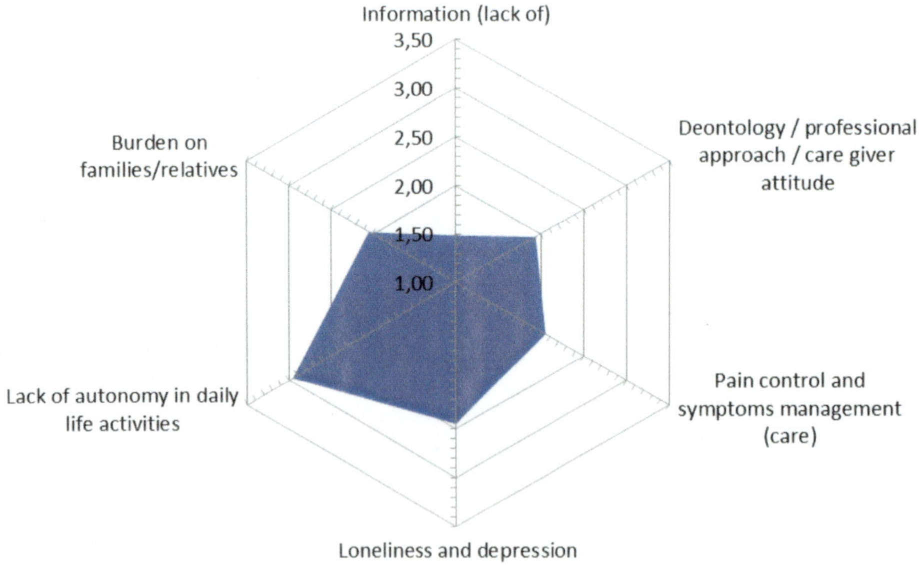

Fig. 2 Emerging themes (grouping)

Many patients ($n = 27$; 44%) found relief in faith, going to church, getting the communion and having the religious leaders visiting them.

- *« I believe in God and he helps me when I feel the worst. I have regular visits from the priest. » (P24Q12a, M, 30–39, urban setting, lives with his relative)*
- *« I did not solve those issues yet. Maybe I am angry at God because of all that has happened to me. I did not look for help. It is something I have to deal with myself. » (P18Q12a, M, 80–89, urban setting, lives with his relative)*

Theme 3 – Dissatisfaction with pain control and symptoms management

The majority of patients ($n = 51$; 82%) said they suffered from pain, and rated it from moderate ($n = 21$; 34%) to severe ($n = 29$; 47%) with one patient suffering from "the worst pain". Almost all patients were treated with pain killers - including opioids - but reported that "it doesn't help". Many patients wished for home visits, some wanted stronger pain killers, others wanted physiotherapy or simply advice from specialists. Many were self-medicating with additional pain.

- *« My pain is strong and I would like sometimes to jump out of the window. Patients with such pain should have proper therapy. » (P1Q7c, F, 70–79, urban setting, lives with her relative)*
- *« I have strong pain. I buy pain killers. My doctor prescribes medication, but they help only for a short while. I become immune to this medication. I buy some pain killers that help my friends too. » (P16Q7a, F, 70–79, urban, lives with her relative)*

Most of the patients ($n = 53$; 85%) reported breathing difficulties, loss of appetite and weight ($n = 53$; 85%), digestive problems ($n = 45$; 73%), severe nausea ($n = 15$; 24%) often related to medication side effects (e.g. chemotherapy) or pain. In some cases ($n = 3$; 5%) the consequences of skin irritation from diarrhoea were worse than the diarrhoea itself. Some patients confirmed they were receiving medical treatment to address these problems but most were coping through self-adaptation (body position, diet, etc.) or by simply accepting that nothing could be done to improve their situation. Finally, more than two thirds of patients reported being exhausted (n = 45; 73%) due to their underlying condition or treatment.

- *« I did not ask for help. My disease influences my breathing. These breathing problems cause many difficulties. I know this is the consequence of my diagnosis. » (P13Q6a, F, 40–49, urban, lives with her relative)*
- *« I need support for my wounds, not for the diarrhoea. I need advice about what to do. I suffer because of diarrhoea's consequences. » (P27Q10b, M, 50–59, urban setting, lives with his relative)*

Theme 4 -Burden on families

The majority of patients ($n = 41$; 66%) also worried about their family members and their future, and were afraid of becoming a burden on them. Most respondents ($n = 43$; 69%) expressed concern about the physical, social and financial strain on their family members as a result of their illness.

- *« My family worries more about me. I also worry about them. I am concerned on how they cope now and what will happen with them after I die. » (P27Q15a, M, 50–59, urban setting, lives with his relative)*
- *«I worry about my mum, she is exhausted. It is difficult to care for me. I worry about the financial situation of my family. I did not get sufficient support, just basic. » (P9Q15a, M, 40–49, rural setting, lives with his relative)*

Specifically, patients complained about the lack of access to paid caregivers, home based care, physiotherapy, wheelchairs or diapers.

- *« He could not even get a free wheelchair. He is neglected by the society. » (P14Q2a, M, 20–29, urban setting, lives with his relative)*
- *« Our families need better support, especially those who are all the time with us. My husband is exhausted. My daughter studies in Banja Luka and she comes from time to time. My husband takes care of everything. He works and earns for us. » (P13Q3b, F, 40–49, urban setting, lives with her relative)*

Only a few patients reported paying for full-time caregivers or nurses (day or night care) and some mentioned that in some circumstances the social services of Doboj paid for the caregivers. More than half of the patients ($n = 32$; 52%) mentioned financial difficulties when they needed to buy medicines, diapers or pay for caregivers. Only 14 (23%) did not have any financial issues. Most of the patients facing financial difficulties received support from their families and only few from social services and disability compensation.

Theme 5 – Deontology, professional approach and dignity of patients

One third of patients reported being mistreated, ($n = 20$; 32%), with five patients stating they had never been treated with dignity. Patients told of being refused care by emergency medical services "as they are dying anyway", and of being left on their own, abandoned by friends and neighbours. More home visits were particularly desired.

- *« I do not want to go to the hospital. I feel bad there. They treat me bad, they just give me medication and nobody cares about me there. » (P18Q1c, M, 80–89, urban setting, lives with his relative)*
- *« Help patients have dignity in the last days of their life. We need better home care. » (P3Q2c, M, 80–89, urban setting, lives with his relative)*

However respondents benefitting from family support, friends, and sometimes medical staff reported being better off ($n = 27$; 44%). This helped them to gain a sense of dignity in the face of terminal illness and loss of autonomy.

- *« I am satisfied. The nurse comes once a month, she brings the doctor sometimes. The nurse is our blessing, we would be lost without her. » (P55Q1d, M, 50–59, rural setting, lives with his relative)*
- *« Thank God I had support from my daughter. I think that support only comes from the family. I feel bad about the patients who do not have family or lack their support. Every patient should have human support and understanding. » (P35Q2b, F, 70–79, urban setting, lives alone)*

Theme 6 – Lack of information

Almost all patients ($n = 57$; 92%) stated they were quite a bit ($n = 19$; 30%) or completely (38; 61%) informed about the course of their condition. However, a majority complained that nobody explained to them how to cope with their condition, feeling lost and left alone with their condition. Like their caregivers, they were asking for more support by health services and other public services, which – according to them – often do not pay enough attention. A few patients were not informed about their diagnosis, although they suspected the severity of their disease. It is important to stress that in most of these cases, the family members knew the diagnosis but did not inform the patient. Patients who were aware of their condition seemed better off:

- *« I have some problems with my brain. I do not know what the problem is. Something appeared on my CT. » (P26Q1a, M,60–69, urban setting, lives with his relative)*
- *« We are all lost. He is not talking or moving. He is completely paralyzed. Nobody told us what to do. He was sent home to die. We ask ourselves what to do now. » (P10Q1e, M, 50–59, rural setting, lives with his relative)*

Many ($n = 19$; 31%) patients reported a lack of information about available services. They reported challenges to access social and financial support (e.g. for diapers, catheters, care givers or transport to the medical referral centre). They also claimed a need for more information about health insurance, succession procedures, patients' rights and general administrative procedures.

- *« It is difficult to have this disease. It is even more difficult to go through all procedures. This kind of patients are ill and still they have to organize everything themselves. » (P35Q1e, F, 70–79, urban setting, lives alone)*
- *« There should be a counselling service for cancer patients. Many people have cancer, it is like an epidemic. » (P36Q1f, M, 40–49, urban, lives with his relative)*

Discussion

Our results suggest that in the absence of adequate services and support for terminally ill patients, symptom management may be unsatisfactory, patients may feel abandoned, and the burden of care may fall on family members who are challenged in taking on such a role. This situation can accentuate patients' anxiety, and lead to financial and social problems for family members.

The exploration of patients' needs and perceptions at the end of their life in Doboj reveals four key areas of concern.

Firstly, and as described by Sand [18], restricted social interaction caused by either loss of autonomy or by being left alone without adequate support led to isolation and loneliness for most patients. Patients with no relatives to take care of them appeared worse off. Feelings of neglect and stigma from community - but also from some health services or the society as a whole - were common, reported both by patients and caregivers. Home visits and home based care were asked for frequently.

Secondly, management of symptoms, especially of pain, anxiety and depression may be insufficient. Regarding pain, many patients stated the need for adaptation of medication but also physiotherapy and general home based care. Other symptoms were often accepted, considered secondary to their underlying condition with no possibility for improvement. Physical symptoms had an important impact on the mood of patients, causing depression, increasing their dependency, leading to isolation and contributing to exhaustion of care givers. Anxiety was common among patients, which is also described in the literature as secondary to the uncertainties of living with their condition and approaching death [19]. In this regard, while only a few mentioned the need for specialised psychological support, perhaps due to cultural sensitivity, many found relief in faith and in the possibility to exchange their feelings, particularly with peers. Therefore, comprehensive symptom and pain management is essential to quality end of life care and support [20].

Thirdly, exhaustion of caregivers (essentially spouses or close relatives) emerged as significant, which has also been found elsewhere [21]. In addition, financial difficulties were recurrent and may put additional strain on caregivers [22]. While support to caregivers has been recognised as critical [23], their needs remain unmet. Patients and caregivers suggested home visits, both by volunteers, faith representatives and medical teams would reduce the burden and provide emotional support. Improving availability and affordability of consumables (e.g. diapers, urinary catheters) and equipment (e.g. wheelchairs) were also regularly mentioned in this regard. Our study highlighted how interlinked these factors are, stressing the importance of a comprehensive response that goes beyond medical palliative care.

Finally, information seems to be lacking about patient's condition, prognosis and availability of services. Lack of understanding of their condition may result in feelings of helplessness with impeded decision making and control over their lives. Many patients did not ask for additional medical care, considering that symptoms could not be adequately managed. Indeed, provision of adequate information is crucial, as stated by Fallowfield [24]: "although truth hurts, deceit may well hurt more". In addition, information about disease management is also needed in order for caregivers to support appropriately their sick family member [25].

Strengths and limitations

Although the importance of end of life care and support is well established in many countries, palliative care services remain scarce in BiH and care is essentially provided by general practitioners [26]. Little information exists on existing services [27]. Here we have focused on the patients' needs and perceptions to provide insights into the most adequate interventions [28]. The results of this study, in addition to further investigations about perceptions of care providers, social workers, volunteers and municipal authorities, will serve as the basis for developing acceptable, feasible and sustainable solutions, involving all stakeholders. Our participatory approach will help us to build a common understanding and a shared intervention strategy for quality patient centred end-of-life care and services in the municipality of Doboj. Based on the identification of needs and perceptions of both patients and providers to jointly design an intervention aimed at improving palliative care and support, our approach could be replicated successfully elsewhere to develop context specific strategies [29] and could help to reduce the significant burden carried by individuals, families and local communities [30]. Mobilisation of all actors and integration into the public health system is key to delivering sustainable services in settings with limited resources [31]. In addition, as stated by Gwyther [32], sharing of lessons learned from this initiative with policy makers at both the national and international level could trigger policy changes and promote integration of EoLC into BiH's health programmes, which is a priority for the European Association for Palliative Care Initiative in Eastern Europe [33].

We acknowledge as limitation the possibility of selection bias of participants, as the FM teams of Doboj municipality had to list all patients which would qualify for end of life care. There might be patients recently discharged from hospital or not registered with FM teams who have not been listed and therefore, not selected. Nevertheless, the probability that patients are discharged without information to FM teams is quite small and more than 90% of the population is registered with FM. Patients unable to provide informed consent to participate, or with any disability that impedes communication were also excluded. The small sample size of our study may limit generalisation and external validity of the findings. However, we used a 2-tier, purposive sampling strategy and chose individuals to reflect the geographical and demographic characteristics of terminally ill patients. Another limitation might be that an appointed PHCC worker interviewed the patients. Patients may have been reluctant to make negative statements about care provided at the primary care level. On the other hand, the presence of a PHCC professional facilitated identification of patients needing immediate attention and referral to appropriate services.

Conclusion

Our study, conducted in a resource limited setting where such issues are barely investigated, emphasised a wide gap between patients' expectations and currently available care and services. While there is a need to improve symptoms management through training of health professionals including capacity building of nurses [34], better medication and provision of adequate material and devices, this will only tackle the patients' most urgent concerns. Addressing the needs of patients at the end of their life, aiming at maintaining them with the best possible quality of life while providing appropriate support to their relatives, thus remains a much broader challenging task.

In order to ensure a comprehensive response to expressed needs, a coordinated inter-professional, inter-institutional and multi-stakeholder approach is required, including appropriate information to the patients and their caregivers about the disease, its stages and its management as well as adequate psychosocial, spiritual, administrative and financial support. The concept of nurse-led navigation / stewardship [35], that would provide patients with comprehensive services could be explored. A culture of anticipation should be adopted while providing end of life care and support.

Abbreviations
BiH: Bosnia-Herzegovina; DTHM: Division of Tropical and Humanitarian Medicine; EoLC: End of life care; FM : Family medicine; HUG: Hôpitaux Universitaires de Genève, Geneva University Hospitals; PHCC: Primary Health Care Centre; WHO: World Health Organisation

Acknowledgements
The authors wish to acknowledge the support of the HUG leadership as well as the funding that enabled this project to be developed. Special recognition is given to all the BiH partners of the DTHM for their Invaluable contributions and friendship in ensuring a successful project.

Funding
The research was funded by the Division of Tropical and Humanitarian Medicine (DTHM) of the Geneva University Hospitals (HUG).

Authors' contributions
All authors contributed to the concept of the study and the analysis. ED and RL conducted the interviews. SAP drafted the original manuscript with input from all other authors to finalise this manuscript. All authors read and approved the final manuscript.

Competing interests
The authors declare that they have no competing interests.

Author details
[1]Division of Tropical and Humanitarian Medicine, Geneva University Hospitals, Rue Gabrielle-Perret-Gentil 6, 1205 Geneva, Switzerland. [2]Primary Health Care Center, Dom zdravja Doboj, Nemanjina 18, 74000 Doboj, Bosnia and Herzegovina. [3]Fondacija fami, Kralja Aleksandra 52, 74000 Doboj, Bosnia and Herzegovina. [4]Division of Tropical and Humanitarian Medicine, Geneva University Hospitals, Avenue de Beau-Séjour 22, Geneva, Switzerland. [5]Transcultural consultation and interpretation, Geneva University Hospitals, Rue Gabrielle-Perret-Gentil 4, 1211 Geneva 14, Switzerland. [6]Geriatrics and community palliative care unit, Geneva University Hospitals, Avenue Cardinal-Mermillod 36, 1227 Carouge, Switzerland.

References
1. WHA67.19 - Strengthening of Palliative Care as a Component of Comprehensive Care Throughout the Life Course. WHA Resolution; Sixty-seventh World Health Assembly. 2014. http://apps.who.int/medicinedocs/documents/s21454en/s21454en.pdf
2. Mitchell S, Loew J, Millington-Sanders C, Dale J. Providing end-of-life care in general practice: findings of a national GP questionnaire survey. Br J Gen Pract. 2016;66:e647-653. PubMed PMID: 27381483.
3. World Health Organization. Palliative care. Fact sheet. 2017. [online] available from: http://www.who.int/mediacentre/factsheets/fs402/en/
4. Organisation faitière nationale du monde du travail Santé. Compétences des professionnels de la santé dans le donaine des soins palliatifs de base. Un projet d'OdASanté sur mandat du Secrétariat de l'Etat à la formation, à la recherche et à l'innovation (SERI). Rapport de projet du janvier 2015. Confédération Suisse. 2015. https://www.bag.admin.ch/.../competences-des-professionnels.pdf.
5. EAPC Task Force on the development of Palliative Care in Europe. Bosnia and Herzegovina. information correct as at 7th August 2006, no up-date available. https://www.eapcnet.eu/home
6. The Primary Health Care Strategy of the Republika Srpska, BiH http://www.vladars.net/sr-SP-Cyrl/Vlada/Ministarstva/MZSZ/Documents/Primarna%20zastita%20Brosura.pdf
7. The Primary Health Care Strategy of the Federation of Bosnia and Herzegovina. http://www.fmoh.gov.ba/images/federalno_ministarstvo_zdravstva/zakoni_i_strategije/strategije_i_politike/dokumenti/strategija_razvoja_PZZ.pdf
8. Law on health protection of the Republika Srpska, BiH, Article 36. http://www.vladars.net/sr-SP-Cyrl/Vlada/Ministarstva/MZSZ/Documents _106_09.pdf
9. Law on health protection of the Federation of Bosnia and Herzegovina, Article 93. http://www.fmoh.gov.ba/index.php/zakoni-i-strategije/zakoni/zakon-o-zdravstvenoj-zastiti
10. Census of population, households and dwellings in Bosnia and Herzegovina, 2013. Final results. Agency for Statistics of Bosnia and Herzegovina. 2016. http://www.popis2013.ba/popis2013/doc/Popis2013prvoIzdanje.pdf
11. Eurostat Population structure and ageing, Population age structure by major age groups, 2007 and 2017 (% of the total population). *Data extracted in May 2018.* https://ec.europa.eu/eurostat/statistics-explained/pdfscache/1271.pdf.
12. Statistical Yearbook 2015. Institute of Statistics of Republic of Srpska. 2016. http://www.rzs.rs.ba
13. Carson SS, Cox CE, Wallenstein S, Hanson LC, Danis M, Tulsky JA, Chai E, Nelson JE. Effect of palliative care–led meetings for families of patients with chronic critical illness. A randomized clinical trial. JAMA. 2016;316(1):51–62. https://doi.org/10.1001/jama.2016.8474 PMID: 27380343.
14. World Health Organisation. Palliative Care: symptom management and end of life care. Integrated management of adolescent and adult illness. Interim guidelines for first level facility health workers. 2004. http://apps.who.int/iris/bitstream/10665/68535/4/WHO_CDS_IMAI_2004.4.pdf
15. Matis C. Mission report Kirghizstan. Geneva: Geneva University Hospitals. 2015.
16. Zulian G., Pautex S. Aide-mémoire de soins palliatifs destiné aux soignants. Programme des soins palliatifs. Geneva University Hospitals. https://docplayer.fr/69977319-Soins-palliatifs-aide-memoire-destine-aux-soignants.html.
17. Pirnazarova G, Matis C, Loutan L, Heller O, Grivel A, Guisado H. Caring for palliative patients: the 9 symptoms booklet. Geneva: Geneva University Hospitals; 2015.
18. Sand L, Strang P. Existential loneliness in a palliative home care setting. J Palliat Med. 2006;9(6):1376–87. PMID:17187546. https://doi.org/10.1089/jpm.2006.9.1376.
19. Traeger L, Greer JA, Fernandez-Robles C, Temel JS, Pirl WF. Evidence-based treatment of anxiety in patients with cancer. J Clin Oncol. 2012;30(11):1197–205. https://doi.org/10.1200/JCO.2011.39.5632 Epub 2012 Mar 12. PMID: 22412135.
20. Wilkie DJ, Ezenwa MO. Pain and symptom management in palliative care and at end of life. Nurs Outlook. 2012;60(6):357–64. https://doi.org/10.1016/j.outlook.2012.08.002 Epub 2012 Sep 14.
21. Clark MM, Atherton PJ, Lapid MI, Rausch SM, Frost MH, Cheville AL, et al. Caregivers of patients with cancer fatigue: a high level of symptom burden. Am J Hosp Palliat Med. 2014;31(2):121–5. https://doi.org/10.1177/1049909113479153.

22. Götze H, Brähler E, Gansera L, Polze N, Köhler N. Psychological distress and quality of life of palliative cancer patients and their caring relatives during home care. Support Care Cancer. 2014;22(10):2775–82. https://doi.org/10.1007/s00520-014-2257-5 Epub 2014 May 9.
23. Simonič A, Furlan M, Ravnjak T, Dirkse D. Caring for caregivers: a right way to do it? Curr Opin Support Palliat Care. 2012;6(3):379–85. https://doi.org/10.1097/SPC.0b013e328356ab0c.
24. Fallowfield LJ, Jenkins VA, Beveridge HA. Truth may hurt but deceit hurts more: scommunication in palliative care. Palliat Med. 2002;16(4):297–303. PMID:12132542. https://doi.org/10.1191/0269216302pm575oa.
25. Wilkes L, White K, O'Riordan L. Empowerment through information: supporting rural families of oncology patients in palliative care. Aust J Rural Health. 2000;8(1):41–6 PMID:11040579.
26. Taché S, Chapuis V, Goehring C, Loutan L. Access to palliative care in Bosnia-Herzegovina: a primary care issue. J Gen Pract. 2004;10(1):31–2. https://doi.org/10.3109/13814780409094225.
27. Centeno C. et al. EAPC atlas of palliative care in Europe. European Association for Palliative Care 2007. ISBN 978-0-9758525-5-2.
28. Véron C, Pautex S, Weber C, Janssens JP, Cedraschi C. Recollection of participating in a trial: a qualitative study of patients with severe and very severe chronic obstructive pulmonary disease. PLoS One. 2018;13(9):e0204701.
29. Jünger S, Klose J, Brearley S, Hegedus K, Payne S, Radbruch L. Palliative care information needs in central and Eastern Europe and the commonwealth of independent states. J Palliat Care. 2015;31(2):109–17 PubMed PMID: 26201213.
30. Anderson RE, Grant L. What is the value of palliative care provision in low-resource settings? BMJ Global Health. 2017;2:e000139. https://doi.org/10.1136/bmjgh-2016-000139.
31. Logie DE, Harding R. An evaluation of a public health advocacy strategy to enhance palliative care provision in Zambia. BMJ Support Palliat Care. 2012; 2(3):264–9. https://doi.org/10.1136/bmjspcare-2012-000232.
32. Gwyther L, et al. Advancing palliative care as a human right. J Pain Symptom Manag. 2009;38(5):767. https://doi.org/10.1016/j.jpainsymman.2009.03.003.
33. Fürst CJ. The European Association for Palliative Care initiative in Eastern Europe. J Pain Symptom Manag. 2002;24(2):134–5 Review. PubMed PMID: 12231130.
34. Grimes C, Wanless RS, Damonti J. New models for elevating the practice and status of community-based nursing across the spectrum of cancer care in Central and Eastern Europe. Eur J Oncol Nurs. 2014;18(Suppl 2):S97–122. https://doi.org/10.1016/j.ejon.2014.07.008 Epub 2014 Aug 27. Erratum in: Eur J Oncol Nurs. 2014 Dec;18(6):649. PubMed PMID: 25174879.
35. Pesut B, et al. Nurse-led navigation to provide early palliative care in rural areas: a pilot study. BMC Palliat Care. 2017;16(1):37. https://doi.org/10.1186/s12904-017-0211-2.

Attitudes to specialist palliative care and advance care planning in people with COPD: a multi-national survey of palliative and respiratory medicine specialists

Natasha Smallwood[1,2*], David Currow[3], Sara Booth[4], Anna Spathis[5], Louis Irving[1] and Jennifer Philip[6,7]

Abstract

Background: Chronic obstructive pulmonary disease (COPD) guidelines recommend early access to palliative care together with optimal, disease-directed therapy for people with advanced disease, however, this occurs infrequently. This study explored the approaches of respiratory and palliative medicine specialists to palliative care and advance care planning (ACP) in advanced COPD.

Methods: An online survey was emailed to all specialists and trainees in respiratory medicine in Australia and New Zealand (ANZ), and to all palliative medicine specialists and trainees in ANZ and the United Kingdom.

Results: Five hundred seventy-seven (33.1%) responses were received, with 440 (25.2%) complete questionnaires included from 177 respiratory and 263 palliative medicine doctors. Most respiratory doctors (140, 80.9%) were very or quite comfortable providing a palliative approach themselves to people with COPD. 113 (63.8%) respiratory doctors recommended referring people with advanced COPD to specialist palliative care, mainly for access to: psychosocial and spiritual care (105, 59.3%), carer support (104, 58.5%), and end-of-life care (94, 53.1%). 432 (98.2%) participants recommended initiating ACP discussions. Palliative medicine doctors were more likely to recommend discussing: what palliative care is ($p < 0.0001$), what death and dying might be like ($p < 0.0001$) and prognosis ($p = 0.004$). Themes highlighted in open responses included: inadequate, fragmented models of care, with limited collaboration or support from palliative care services.

Conclusions: While both specialties recognised the significant palliative care and ACP needs of people with advanced COPD, in reality few patients access these elements of care. Formal collaboration and bi-directional support between respiratory and palliative medicine, are required to address these unmet needs.

Keywords: COPD, Survey, Health professionals, Palliative care, Attitudes, Advance care planning

Background

Chronic obstructive pulmonary disease (COPD) is characterised by airflow limitation, persistent symptoms and respiratory failure [1]. By 2020, COPD is projected to be the third leading cause of death worldwide [2]. Yet despite many people expressing a desire to die at home, seven out of ten people with COPD die in hospital in Australia and the United Kingdom (UK) [3, 4].

Many patients with severe COPD experience reduced quality of life due to severe, chronic breathlessness, which persists at rest or on minimal exertion despite optimal treatment of the underlying causes [5–7]. Disease progression is also reflected in reduced function, limiting basic activities of daily living and requiring additional support from informal and paid caregivers, often for long periods of time [8]. In addition to other physical symptoms such as cough, pain, anorexia and fatigue, many patients have significant psychological comorbidity, with all these factors contributing to

* Correspondence: Natasha.smallwood@mh.org.au
[1]Department of Respiratory and Sleep Medicine, The Royal Melbourne Hospital, Melbourne, VIC 3050, Australia
[2]Department of Medicine (Royal Melbourne Hospital), University of Melbourne, Melbourne, VIC 3050, Australia
Full list of author information is available at the end of the article

reduced quality of life and increasing social isolation for both patients and caregivers [9, 10].

Given the significant physical, psychosocial and communication needs of people with COPD [11], guidelines recommend that patients with advanced disease should receive early access to palliative care in conjunction with optimal, disease-directed therapy [1, 12]. Therefore all health professionals have a role in providing palliative care to their patients [12]. Indeed when palliative care is provided by the usual treating clinician (such as the general practitioner or a medical specialist), it is termed *generalist* palliative care or a *palliative approach* [13]. By contrast, *specialist* palliative care is provided by health professionals who have specialist qualifications and/or significant experience in palliative care. Specialist palliative care teams not only support the usual treating clinician to offer a palliative approach, but have an important role in caring for people with challenging symptoms or complex needs [12]. Thus a palliative approach and specialist palliative care are not separate entities, but may be complementary aspects of care for patients with advanced COPD.

Despite guidelines recommending palliative care for people with advanced COPD, referral to specialist palliative care service occurs infrequently [14–16]. Only 1.7% of patients with end-stage COPD in the USA were referred to specialist palliative care when admitted with an exacerbation [16]. Similarly, in the UK and Australia only 16.7–17.9% of COPD patients accessed any specialist palliative care in their last year of life [15, 17, 18]. Yet people with severe COPD have documented needs which are similar to those of people at the end-of-life, irrespective of the underlying life-limiting illness [19]. Advance care planning (ACP), which by definition should include discussion of each patient's palliative care wishes, also seldom occurs in routine practice [20–22].

Well-described barriers to accessing palliative care include difficulty prognosticating in COPD due to the variable disease trajectory [23, 24], clinicians lacking time to discuss palliative care or being fearful of taking away hope [25], and availability of specialist palliative care from services which are already overburdened [26, 27]. Given these issues, a survey was undertaken to explore physicians' knowledge and practices managing people with advanced COPD. This manuscript reports current beliefs and practices of respiratory and palliative medicine doctors regarding the role of specialist palliative care and advance care planning in patients with severe COPD.

Methods

The full methodology including the research questionnaire utilised for this study have been published elsewhere [28], therefore the methods are summarised here. A voluntary survey was designed for specialists and specialist trainees working in respiratory medicine in Australia and New Zealand (ANZ) and palliative medicine in ANZ and the United Kingdom (UK). The questionnaire included a case vignette describing an outpatient with severe COPD, receiving maximum disease modifying therapies and worsening, severe chronic breathlessness (modified Medical Research Council breathlessness score of 4). Survey participants were told the case patient did not have anxiety and was *not* in the terminal phase (last few days) of his illness. Respondents were asked to consider how they would manage the case patient or people with COPD similar to the case. All survey questions (including demographic information at the start of the survey) required an answer, before the respondent could proceed to the next question.

The link to the online survey (written in Survey Monkey) was distributed by the Thoracic Society of Australia and New Zealand, the Australian and New Zealand Society of Palliative Medicine, and the Association for Palliative Medicine of Great Britain and Ireland to their members. Each society member received two email invitations including the survey link, 2–4 weeks apart. The online survey was open to participants for six months from August 2015 to February 2016, with participants only able to submit one response from their IP address. Consent to participate was implied by completion of the survey questionnaire. Ethics approval was granted by the Melbourne Health Research Office (QA2014171). Separate ethics approvals from each specialist society were not required. Similarly health professional research studies that did not collect sensitive data, did not require ethics approval in the UK in 2015 [29].

Statistical analysis

Demographic data and responses are reported descriptively using frequencies and proportions. The Pearson Chi-Square test was used to identify associations between participants' responses and exposure variables measured as proportions (age, gender, country, specialty, position and location of practice); and Student's t test was used for exposures measured as continuous numerical values (mean years worked in specialty and mean number of patients with severe COPD seen per month). Statistical analyses were performed using IBM SPSS Statistics Version 24.0, with a p-value of less than 0.05 indicating statistical significance. Free text responses to open ended questions were analysed using thematic analysis.

Results

Five hundred and seventy-seven (33.0%) responses were received from 1047 doctors working in palliative medicine (323 in ANZ and 724 in the UK) and 702 working in respiratory medicine who were emailed the survey link. Responses were excluded from participants who: provided incomplete responses regarding patient management (94), were not respiratory or palliative medicine doctors (35), or were non-medical (8). Of the 440 (25.2%) responses included, 263 (25.1%) were palliative medicine doctors and 177 (25.2%) participants were respiratory doctors (Table 1). Results from Australia and New Zealand were combined, given the smaller workforce and thus limited number of participants from New Zealand (21 palliative medicine specialists and 25 respiratory physicians).

The majority of respiratory doctors (140, 80.9%) reported being very or quite comfortable providing a palliative approach to people with COPD. Only eight (4.6%) respiratory participants were quite or very uncomfortable offering this care, and the remainder were neutral. Respiratory doctors' demographic characteristics and experience (including age, gender, country, specialty, position and location of practice, mean years worked in specialty and mean number of patients with severe COPD seen per month) were not associated with level of comfort providing a palliative approach.

Almost two thirds of respiratory doctors (113, 63.8%) recommended referring the person in the case vignette to specialist palliative care, with 90 (50.8%) recommending referring for long-term specialist palliative care input and 23 (13.0%) for an opinion only. Thirteen (7.3%) participants were uncertain if they would refer and the remainder would not. Female respiratory doctors were twice as likely as their male colleagues to recommend referral to the specialist palliative care service (OR = 2.0, 95%CI = 1.0–3.9, $p = 0.048$). No other demographic characteristics or experience were associated with respiratory doctors recommending referral to specialist palliative care.

Respiratory doctors referred people with COPD for many reasons including for: psychosocial and spiritual care (105, 59.3%), carer support including future bereavement support (104, 58.5%), and end-of-life care (94, 53.1%) (Table 2). Of the 64 (36.2%) respiratory physicians who would not or were unsure if they would refer to specialist palliative care, 27 (15.3%) reported being able to provide a palliative approach themselves, 19 (10.7%) reported difficulty accessing palliative care in their location and 13 (7.3%) thought the person described in the case vignette was unlikely to die within the next 12 months.

Nearly all doctors working in both respiratory (172, 97.2%) and palliative medicine (260, 98.9%) reported that they would initiate a discussion with the person in the case vignette (or similar people) regarding prognosis and advance care planning. Only 4 doctors (all respiratory) reported that they would not initiate this discussion with the person in the case vignette (or similar patients), with 2 reporting lack of time as a barrier. Holding the belief that advance care planning should be undertaken was not associated with any of the participants' demographic characteristics or experience for each specialty.

Both specialist groups recommended discussing multiple topics during ACP conversations including: mechanical ventilation and/or intensive care unit admission in the future, the utility of cardiopulmonary resuscitation, and the nature and role of palliative care (Table 3).

Table 1 Participant demographics

	Palliative Medicine ($n = 263$)			Respiratory Medicine	Specialties Compared
	ANZ ($n = 129$)	UK ($n = 134$)	All (n = 263)	ANZ ($n = 177$)	
Female	80 (62.0%)	112 (83.6%)	192 (73.0%)	61 (34.4%)	$p < 0.0001$
Age					
25–35	25 (19.3%)	31 (23.1%)	56 (21.3%)	40 (22.6%)	$p = 0.953$
36–45	27 (20.9%)	50 (37.3%)	77 (29.3%)	57 (32.2%)	
46–55	31 (24.0%)	36 (26.9%)	67 (25.5%)	39 (22.0%)	
56–65	29 (22.5%)	15 (11.2%)	44 (16.7%)	27 (15.3%)	
> 65	11 (8.5%)	0	11 (4.2%)	8 (4.5%)	
Missing	6 (4.7%)	2 (1.5)	8 (3.0%)	6 (3.4%)	
Position					
Consultant	89 (69.0%)	107 (79.9%)	196 (74.5%)	145 (81.9%)	$p = 0.068$
Specialist trainee	40 (31.0%)	27 (20.1%)	67 (25.5%)	32 (18.1%)	
Mean years in specialty [a]	12.5 (9.1)	12.3 (7.3)	12.4 (8.2)	15.0 (10.8)	$p = 0.006$
Mean no. of COPD patients seen/month [a]	3.1 (3.1)	2.5 (3.4)	2.8 (3.3)	14.1 (12.0)	$p < 0.0001$

Data are represented as either frequencies or means (denoted by [a]), with either proportions or standard deviations in parentheses

Table 2 Respiratory doctors' referrals to specialist palliative care

Reasons for referring COPD patients to palliative care	$N = 113^a$
For holistic care including psychosocial and spiritual care	105 (59.3%)
For carer support including future bereavement support	104 (58.8%)
For future end-of-life care	94 (53.1%)
To access community palliative care	92 (52.0%)
To access respite care	78 (44.1%)
For management of symptoms including breathlessness	75 (42.4%)
For completion of advance care planning	63 (36.2%)
Reasons for not referring COPD patients to palliative care	$N = 64^b$
I am capable of providing generalist palliative care myself	27 (15.3%)
Palliative care services are difficult to access in my location	19 (10.7%)
I do not think the patient might die in the next 12 months	13 (7.3%)
I do not want the patient to feel abandoned by me	7 (4.0%)
The patient does not require specialist palliative care yet	6 (3.4%)
I do not want to take away the patient's hope	4 (2.3%)
Previously have not found palliative care teams helpful for COPD patients	3 (1.7%)

Data are represented as frequencies with proportions of the total group (n = 177) in parentheses
[a]Only participants who said they would refer to palliative care were directed to answer this question
[b] Only participants who said they would NOT/were unsure regarding referral to palliative care were directed to answer

Palliative medicine doctors were significantly more likely to recommend discussing: what palliative care is and whether indicated ($p < 0.0001$), what death and dying might be like from COPD ($p < 0.0001$), the likely prognosis ($p = 0.004$) and changing treatment goals to aim for palliation ($p = 0.028$).

Many themes were identified in the extensive free text comments participants wrote, including that specialists believed current palliative care arrangements for people with advanced COPD are inadequate and fragmented:

> *"(This is a) difficult and big problem, and an area that clearly requires greater investment into formal palliative care services for this patient group, and greater formal systems of collaboration between respiratory physicians, palliative care teams, and community health providers."* [Respiratory Medicine Specialist number 13, ANZ]

Fear of palliative care by both clinicians and patients was also noted as an issue:

> *"Of our palliative care patients I think they have the greatest number of unmet needs, but often they or their clinicians are fearful of what palliative care entails."* [Palliative Medicine Specialist number 39, ANZ]

There was also concern that both people with COPD and their caregivers experience issues such as anxiety:

> *"COPD is hard to palliate. Patients find the exacerbations distressing and panic inducing. This also contributes to carer anxiety."* [Palliative Medicine Specialist number 62, UK]

Additionally, limited available support from palliative care services currently was highlighted as an issue.

> *"Unfortunately our local palliative care service is under-resourced to support similar patients to this due to the frequent longevity of their needs. This is likely to be a growing problem in the future."* [Respiratory Medicine Specialist number 71, ANZ]

Finally, both respiratory and palliative medicine physicians raised concerns regarding each other's knowledge and practices.

> *"Palliative care physicians manage this (COPD patients) very poorly."* [Respiratory Medicine Specialist number 4, ANZ]

> *"It's end organ disease - we need to enable respiratory physicians to manage their patients in all phases of the illness, and use consultative services when necessary, rather than 'handing over' care to palliative care when goals of care are palliative."* [Palliative Medicine Specialist number 57, UK]

Discussion

Recent international surveys of respiratory doctors have examined referral practices to specialist palliative care in the context of organisation of current service models, availability and local health policies [21, 30, 31]. In this large, multi-national study spanning three countries, in addition to examining recognised barriers to referring to specialist palliative care, we also uniquely identified that the majority of respiratory doctors are comfortable providing a palliative approach, but also recognise the role of specialist palliative care for people with advanced COPD. Additionally, both respiratory and palliative

Table 3 Recommended ACP discussion topics

	Resp Med	Pall Med
ACP topics		
The utility of CPR in the future	159 (89.8%)	249 (94.7%)
Mechanical ventilation and/or ICU admission in the future	164 (92.7%)	241 (91.6%)
What palliative care is and if this is indicated	139 (78.5%)	246 (93.5%)
What death and dying might be like from COPD	97 (54.8%)	200 (76.0%)
The likely prognosis in months and years	100 (56.5%)	191 (72.6%)
Changing treatment goals to be palliative	111 (62.7%)	191 (72.6%)
Appointing a medical power of attorney or substitute decision maker	123 (69.5%)	185 (70.3%)
Other treatment limitations	4 (2.3%)	20 (7.6%)
Other suggested topics		
Desired place of future care (home/hospital/hospice)	0	39 (14.8%)
Desired place of death	0	37 (14.1%)
The patient's goals, values, wishes, hopes & fears	2 (1.1%)	27 (10.3%)
Ascertain the patient's understanding and knowledge first	3 (1.7%)	4 (1.5%)
Patient led discussion	0	22 (8.4%)
Future wishes regarding antibiotics	3 (1.7%)	10 (3.8%)
Future wishes regarding NIV	3 (1.7%)	9 (3.4%)
Advance treatment directives	0	12 (4.6%)
Making a will or arranging affairs	1 (0.6%	7 (2.7%)

Data are represented as frequencies with proportions of the total group (n = 177) in parentheses
CPR Cardiopulmonary resuscitation, *ICU* Intensive Care Unit, *NIV* Non-invasive ventilation

medicine doctors acknowledge the importance of ACP discussions and identify similar key topics to discuss. However, current working models are considered inadequate with insufficient communication and collaboration between the many health professionals often involved in caring for people with advanced COPD.

Attitudes to palliative care

The vast majority of respiratory doctors from Australia and New Zealand, including doctors in specialist training, reported being very or quite comfortable providing a palliative approach to people with COPD. This finding is novel and may partly explain why people with COPD are infrequently referred to specialist palliative care services in Australia [15, 17]. Interestingly few participants in this study reported poor access to specialist palliative care services as an obstacle to referring COPD patients. By contrast respiratory physicians in the UK, Netherlands, and Sweden have cited lack of access to specialist palliative care services as an important barrier for people with COPD [32]. Instead, in this study participants highlighted that whilst specialist palliative care services were available, these services did not have the capacity or experience to manage advanced COPD patients, and importantly established relationships between respiratory and palliative medicine were absent.

Senior doctors' attitudes to specialist palliative care have been described as a barrier to referring people with cancer to these services [33]. However, the majority of respiratory doctors in our study recognised the benefits of referring people with advanced COPD to specialist palliative care. However, some respiratory doctors focussed on the prognosis and limited survival, as opposed to patients' needs when considering referral to specialist palliative care. Notably female doctors were considerably more likely to recommend referral to specialist palliative care. Likewise, when Australian junior doctors within their first five years of qualifying were surveyed (using this same questionnaire) regarding their knowledge and experiences managing people with advanced COPD, female trainees were approximately three times more likely to suggest referring to palliative care than male trainees [34]. This consistent finding requires further investigation to understand the reasons behind this difference in female doctors' reported practices.

The principle reasons for referring to specialist palliative care in this survey were for access to psychosocial and spiritual care, carer support including bereavement support, and end-of-life care. A survey of British respiratory physicians also identified that the main reasons for seeking specialist palliative care for people with chronic lung diseases were for end-of-life care (63%) and psychological support (70%) [21]. Likewise, Australian junior doctors reported referring people with COPD to specialist palliative care to access community palliative care input (54%) and end-of-life care (45%) [34]. However, in the current study, respiratory doctors less commonly recommended referral for symptom management (42%), compared to 63% of British respiratory physicians and 62% of Australian junior doctors who referred for this reason [21, 34]. This would suggest that the ANZ respiratory doctors surveyed in this study not only feel comfortable providing a palliative approach, but also have greater confidence in managing difficult symptoms such as chronic breathlessness. However, there remains a significant need for specialist palliative care for people with COPD, particularly for psychosocial and existential support, addressing communication needs and for bereavement support of carers [11].

Advance care planning

The significant need for good communication and ACP in people with COPD and their carers is well-described [35, 36], and in this study was almost universally recognised. The responsibility for ACP rests with respiratory doctors as suggested by the majority of respondents in this study. Notably, while both specialties suggested similar topics should be covered within ACP and that it may involve several discussions, palliative medicine doctors were more likely to address challenging topics such as death and dying, prognosis, treatment limitations and place of future care as part of these discussions. Similarly, palliative medicine doctors recommended patient-led ACP discussions. Both specialties therefore report being engaged with ACP and their different approaches and skills appear to be complementary over the series of ACP conversations a patient may require. Therefore ideally respiratory doctors should initiate these discussions, and palliative medicine doctors can then develop and expand the conversation as the illness progresses and according to each person's needs and wishes.

Models of care

Confidence providing a palliative approach, managing difficult symptoms such as chronic breathlessness and awareness regarding the importance of ACP in people with advanced COPD does not necessarily translate into practice. A number of authors have documented the significant unmet palliative care needs reported by COPD patients [35] and the infrequent engagement in ACP discussions [21, 22, 25, 35, 37], suggesting a mismatch between our participants' responses and actual day-to-day clinical practice. Therefore it is not lack of awareness or confidence that is preventing clinicians from addressing the significant needs of people with advanced COPD. While lack of time may be a barrier, participants in this study raised concerns regarding the educational needs of doctors in each specialty and highlighted that current models of care are fragmented, with little collaboration between respiratory medicine, palliative medicine or primary care. Accessible, integrated, multi-disciplinary services, which embrace collaboration, trust and bi-directional education and support between both respiratory medicine and palliative care may overcome some of these issues [38]. Such integrated services include the Melbourne Advanced Lung Disease Service [39], and the London Breathlessness Support Service [40], both of which have demonstrated improved outcomes for people with COPD. However, larger, multi-site trials are required to fully assess these new models of care.

This study has some limitations. We had intended to survey British respiratory physicians, however, the British Thoracic Society declines to disseminate research surveys to its members. The response rate in this study, whilst similar to other online surveys of physicians [41–43], was low, thus limiting the generalisability of our findings. However, the gender and age characteristics of participants in this study were representative of the workforce demographics in all three countries [14, 17, 44–46]. Additionally, surveys require respondents to make black and white decisions to hypothetical scenarios, whereas in clinical practice these issues are not absolutely clear, instead requiring careful consideration.

Conclusions

Both respiratory and palliative medicine doctors recognised the significant palliative care and ACP needs of people with advanced COPD. Respiratory doctors reported being comfortable providing a palliative approach and acknowledged the role of both specialist palliative care and ACP, yet in reality people with advanced COPD rarely access these elements of care. Additionally, current models of care for people with COPD were considered inadequate and fragmented. Collaboration, trust, and bi-directional education between respiratory and palliative medicine, perhaps through integrated, multi-disciplinary services, are urgently required to address the unmet needs of people with advanced COPD.

Abbreviations

ACP: Advance care planning; ANZ: Australia and New Zealand; COPD: Chronic obstructive pulmonary disease

Acknowledgements

The authors would like to thank: Prof Danny Liew for initial suggestions regarding the questionnaire design; A/Prof Brian Le, A/Prof Lutz Beckert and Dr. Amanda Landers for providing local workforce data. We also thank the Thoracic Society of Australia and New Zealand, the Australian and New Zealand Society of Palliative Medicine, and the Association for Palliative Medicine of Great Britain and Ireland for supporting and distributing the survey to their members. We gratefully acknowledge the organisers of the following meetings who allowed us to distribute paper copies of the survey to attendees: the 13th Australian Palliative Care Conference (2015), the 3rd Australian Palliative Care Research Colloquium (2015), the Victorian Palliative

Medicine Advanced Trainees meeting (2015) and the Thoracic Society of Australia and New Zealand Victorian Branch Annual Scientific Meeting (2015).

Funding
Palliative Care Research Network provided research funding as a PhD scholarship for Dr. Natasha Smallwood. The funding body was not involved in any part of the study design, data collection, analysis or interpretation, or in writing the manuscript.

Authors' contributions
NS conceived the idea for the study, designed all aspects of the study, conducted the research survey, and analysed the data. DC, SB, AS, LI, and JP all contributed to the study design and set up. NS wrote the first draft of the manuscript, with all authors commenting on and contributing to successive drafts of the manuscript. NS oversaw the entire research study and JP is the guarantor. All authors had full access to all of the study data and take responsibility for the integrity of the data, data analysis and presentation of the data in this manuscript. All authors have approved this manuscript for publication.

Competing interests
Dr. Sara Booth is a member of the editorial board (Associate Editor) for BMC Palliative Care. The other authors declare that they have no competing interests.

Author details
[1]Department of Respiratory and Sleep Medicine, The Royal Melbourne Hospital, Melbourne, VIC 3050, Australia. [2]Department of Medicine (Royal Melbourne Hospital), University of Melbourne, Melbourne, VIC 3050, Australia. [3]IMPACCT - Improving Palliative, Aged and Chronic Care through Clinical Research and Translation, Faculty of Health, University of Technology Sydney, Ultimo, NSW, Australia. [4]University of Cambridge, Cambridge, UK. [5]Cambridge University Hospitals NHS Foundation Trust, Cambridge, UK. [6]Palliative Medicine, St Vincent's Hospital and Victorian Comprehensive Cancer Centre, University of Melbourne, Melbourne, Australia. [7]St Vincent's Hospital, Victoria Parade, Melbourne, VIC 3065, Australia.

References

1. GOLD, Global initiative for chronic obstructive lung disease (GOLD*). Global strategy for the diagnosis, management and prevention of COPD (2018 report). Available from:* http://www.goldcopd.org. Accessed June 2018. 2018.
2. Collaborators, G.B.D.C.R.D. Global, regional, and national deaths, prevalence, disability-adjusted life years, and years lived with disability for chronic obstructive pulmonary disease and asthma, 1990-2015: a systematic analysis for the global burden of disease study 2015. Lancet Respir Med. 2017;5(9): 691–706.
3. National End of Life Care Programme/National End of Life Care Intelligence Network. *Deaths from respiratory diseases: implications for end of life care in England. June* 2011. http://www.endoflifecare-intelligence.org.uk. Accessed April 2017.
4. Australian Institute of Health and Welfare (AIHW): *Poulos LM, Cooper SJ, Ampon R, Redell HK and Marks GB 2014. Mortality from asthma and COPD in Australia. Cat. no. ACM 30. Canberra: AIHW.*
5. Abernethy AP, Currow DC, Frith P, Fazekas BS, McHugh A, Bui C. Randomised, double blind, placebo controlled crossover trial of sustained release morphine for the management of refractory dyspnoea. BMJ. 2003; 327(7414):523–8.
6. Blinderman CD, Homel P, Billings JA, Tennstedt S, Portenoy RK. Symptom distress and quality of life in patients with advanced chronic obstructive pulmonary disease. J Pain Symptom Manag. 2009;38(1):115–23.
7. Johnson MJ, Yorke J, Hansen-Flaschen J, Lansing R, Ekstrom M, Similowski T, Currow DC. Towards an expert consensus to delineate a clinical syndrome of chronic breathlessness. Eur Respir J. 2017;49(5).
8. Johnson MJ, Bowden JA, Abernethy AP, Currow DC. To what causes do people attribute their chronic breathlessness? A population survey. J Palliat Med. 2012;15(7):744–50.
9. Hanania NA, Mullerova H, Locantore NW, Vestbo J, Watkins ML, Wouters EF, Rennard SI, Sharafkhaneh A. And C.L.t.I.P.S.E.s.i. evaluation of, *Determinants of depression in the ECLIPSE chronic obstructive pulmonary disease cohort.* Am J Respir Crit Care Med. 2011;183(5):604–11.
10. Kunik ME, Roundy K, Veazey C, Souchek J, Richardson P, Wray NP, Stanley MA. Surprisingly high prevalence of anxiety and depression in chronic breathing disorders. Chest. 2005;127(4):1205–11.
11. Disler RT, Green A, Luckett T, Newton PJ, Inglis S, Currow DC, Davidson PM. Experience of advanced chronic obstructive pulmonary disease: metasynthesis of qualitative research. J Pain Symptom Manag. 2014;48(6): 1182–99.
12. Lanken PN, Terry PB, Delisser HM, Fahy BF, Hansen-Flaschen J, Heffner JE, Levy M, Mularski RA, Osborne ML, Prendergast TJ, Rocker G, Sibbald WJ, Wilfond B, Yankaskas JR, Force ATSE-o-LCT. An official American Thoracic Society clinical policy statement: palliative care for patients with respiratory diseases and critical illnesses. Am J Respir Crit Care Med. 2008;177(8):912–27.
13. Palliative Care Australia. *Service provision in Australia: a planning guide. 2003. 2nd edition.* http://palliativecare.org.au/wp-content/uploads/2015/07/Palliative-Care-Service-Provision-in-Australia-a-planning-guide.pdf. Accessed 18/03/18.
14. Australian Institue of Health and Welfare. *2017. Medical practitioners workforce 2015.* http://www.aihw.gov.au/reports/workforce/medical-practitioners-workforce-2015/contents/what-types-of-medical-practitioners-are-there. Accessed 10/11/17.
15. Rosenwax L, Spilsbury K, McNamara BA, Semmens JB. A retrospective population based cohort study of access to specialist palliative care in the last year of life: who is still missing out a decade on? BMC Palliat Care. 2016;15:46.
16. Rush B, Hertz P, Bond A, McDermid RC, Celi LA. Use of palliative Care in Patients with end-Stage COPD and receiving home oxygen: National Trends and barriers to Care in the United States. Chest. 2017;151(1):41–6.
17. Australian Institute of Health and Welfare (AIHW). *2017.* Palliative care services in Australia. http://www.aihw.gov.au/reports/palliative-care-services/palliative-care-services-in-australia/contents/palliative-care-workforce. Accessed 10/11/17. 2017.
18. Bloom CI, Slaich B, Morales DR, Smeeth L, Stone P, Quint JK. Low uptake of palliative care for COPD patients within primary care in the UK. Eur Respir J. 2018;51(2).
19. Luddington L, Cox S, Higginson I, Livesley B. The need for palliative care for patients with non-cancer diseases: a review of the evidence. Int J Palliat Nurs. 2001;7(5):221–6.
20. Heffner JE, Fahy B, Hilling L, Barbieri C. Attitudes regarding advance directives among patients in pulmonary rehabilitation. Am J Respir Crit Care Med. 1996;154(6 Pt 1):1735–40.
21. Partridge MR, Khatri A, Sutton L, Welham S, Ahmedzai SH. Palliative care services for those with chronic lung disease. Chron Respir Dis. 2009;6(1):13–7.
22. Smallwood N, Taverner J, Bartlett C, Ross L, Irving L, Philip J. *Palliation of patients with Chronic Obstructive Pulmonary Disease (COPD).* Eur Respir J. 2016;48(Suppl. 60):3767.
23. Lunney JR, Lynn J, Foley DJ, Lipson S, Guralnik JM. Patterns of functional decline at the end of life. JAMA. 2003;289(18):2387–92.
24. Murray SA, Kendall M, Boyd K, Sheikh A. Illness trajectories and palliative care. BMJ. 2005;330(7498):1007–11.
25. Knauft E, Nielsen EL, Engelberg RA, Patrick DL, Curtis JR. Barriers and facilitators to end-of-life care communication for patients with COPD. Chest. 2005;127(6):2188–96.

26. Palliative Care Australia. 2010. Workforce for quality care at the end of life position statement. *Available at:* http://palliativecare.org.au/position-statements. Accessed May 2017.
27. Quill TE, Abernethy AP. Generalist plus specialist palliative care--creating a more sustainable model. N Engl J Med. 2013;368(13):1173–5.
28. Smallwood N, Currow D, Booth S, Spathis A, Irving L, Philip J. Differing approaches to managing the chronic breathlessness syndrome in advanced COPD: a multi-National Survey of specialists. COPD. 2018:1–9. https://doi.org/10.1080/15412555.2018.1502264.
29. NHS Health Research Authority & National Research Ethics Service. Does my project require review by a Research Ethics Committee? 2013. https://www.hra.nhs.uk/approvals-amendments/what-approvals-do-i-need/research-ethics-committee-review/. Accessed 1/6/2015.
30. Duenk RG, Verhagen C, Dekhuijzen P, Vissers K, Engels Y, Heijdra Y. The view of pulmonologists on palliative care for patients with COPD: a survey study. Int J Chron Obstruct Pulmon Dis. 2017;12:299–311.
31. Strang S, Ekberg-Jansson A, Strang P, Larsson L. Palliative care in COPD - web survey in Sweden highlights the current situation for a vulnerable group of patients. Ups J Med Sci. 2017;118(3):181–6.
32. Duenk RG, Verhagen C, Bronkhorst EM, Djamin RS, Bosman GJ, Lammers E, Dekhuijzen P, Vissers K, Engels Y, Heijdra Y. Development of the ProPal-COPD tool to identify patients with COPD for proactive palliative care. Int J Chron Obstruct Pulmon Dis. 2017;12:2121–8.
33. Fadul N, Elsayem A, Palmer JL, Del Fabbro E, Swint K, Li Z, Poulter V, Bruera E. Supportive versus palliative care: what's in a name?: a survey of medical oncologists and midlevel providers at a comprehensive cancer center. Cancer. 2009;115(9):2013–21.
34. Smallwood N, Gaffney N, Gorelik A, Irving L, Le B, Philip J. Doctors' attitudes to palliation and palliative Care in Patients with Advanced Chronic Obstructive Pulmonary Disease. J Pain Symptom Manag. 2017.
35. Maddocks M, Lovell N, Booth S, Man WD, Higginson IJ. Palliative care and management of troublesome symptoms for people with chronic obstructive pulmonary disease. Lancet. 2017;390(10098):988–1002.
36. Patel K, Janssen DJ, Curtis JR. Advance care planning in COPD. Respirology. 2012;17(1):72–8.
37. Philip J, Gold M, Brand C, Miller B, Douglass J, Sundararajan V. Facilitating change and adaptation: the experiences of current and bereaved carers of patients with severe chronic obstructive pulmonary disease. J Palliat Med. 2014;17(4):421–7.
38. Philip J, Crawford G, Brand C, Gold M, Miller B, Hudson P, Smallwood N, Lau R, Sundararajan V. A conceptual model: redesigning how we provide palliative care for patients with chronic obstructive pulmonary disease. Palliat Support Care. 2017:1–9.
39. Smallwood N, Thompson M, Warrender-Sparkes M, Eastman P, Le B, Irving L, Phillip J. Integrated respiratory and palliative care may improve outcomes in advanced lung disease. ERJ Open Res. 2018;4:00102-2017.
40. Higginson IJ, Bausewein C, Reilly CC, Gao W, Gysels M, Dzingina M, McCrone P, Booth S, Jolley CJ, Moxham J. An integrated palliative and respiratory care service for patients with advanced disease and refractory breathlessness: a randomised controlled trial. Lancet Respir Med. 2014;2(12): 979–87.
41. Ecenarro PS, Iguiniz MI, Tejada SP, Malanda NM, Imizcoz MA, Marlasca LA, Navarrete BA. Management of COPD in end-of-life care by Spanish pulmonologists. COPD. 2018:1–6.
42. Janssen DJ, de Hosson SM, bij de Vaate E, Mooren KJ, Baas AA. Attitudes toward opioids for refractory dyspnea in COPD among Dutch chest physicians. Chron Respir Dis. 2015;12(2):85–92.
43. Smallwood N, Gaffney N, Gorelik A, Irving L, Le B, Philip J. Junior doctors' attitudes to opioids for refractory breathlessness in patients with advanced chronic obstructive pulmonary disease. Intern Med J. 2017;47(9):1050–6.
44. Royal College of Physicians 2015. *Census of consultant physicians and specialty traines in the UK: Palliative Medicine 2013–2014.* https://www.jrcptb.org.uk. Accessed 10/8/16.
45. Royal College of Physicians 2016. *Census of consultant physicians and higher specialty trainees in the UK 2014–2015.* https://www.jrcptb.org.uk. Accessed 10/11/17.
46. Cullen, A., *The Medical Council of New Zealand: The New Zealand Medical Workforce in 2013 and 2014.* https://www.mcnz.org.nz/assets/News-and-Publications/Workforce-Surveys/2013-2014.pdf. Accessed 10/8/16.

Benchmarking time to initiation of end-of-life homecare nursing: a population-based cancer cohort study in regions across Canada

Hsien Seow[1,2,6*], Danial Qureshi[1,2], Lisa Barbera[2,3], Kim McGrail[4], Beverley Lawson[5], Fred Burge[5] and Rinku Sutradhar[2,3]

Abstract

Background: Several studies have demonstrated the benefits of early initiation of end-of-life care, particularly homecare nursing services. However, there is little research on variations in the timing of when end-of-life homecare nursing is initiated and no established benchmarks.

Methods: This is a retrospective cohort study of patients with a cancer-confirmed cause of death between 2004 and 2009, from three Canadian provinces (British Columbia, Nova Scotia, and Ontario). We linked multiple administrative health databases within each province to examine homecare use in the last 6 months of life. Our primary outcome was mean time (in days) to first end-of-life homecare nursing visit, starting from 6 months before death, by region. We developed an empiric benchmark for this outcome using a funnel plot, controlling for region size.

Results: Of the 28 regions, large variations in the outcome were observed, with the longest mean time (97 days) being two-fold longer than the shortest (55 days). On average, British Columbia and Nova Scotia had the first and second shortest mean times, respectively. The province of Ontario consistently had longer mean times. The empiric benchmark mean based on best-performing regions was 57 mean days.

Conclusions: Significant variation exists for the time to initiation of end-of-life homecare nursing across regions. Understanding regional variation and developing an empiric benchmark for homecare nursing can support health system planners to set achievable targets for earlier initiation of end-of-life care.

Keywords: Cancer, Palliative care, Benchmarking, End-of-life homecare nursing

Background

Providing end-of-life care in the home is an important policy issue because it can support many patients' preferences to die at home [1, 2], and has the potential for cost-savings by avoided hospitalizations [3–5]. In particular, homecare nursing is critical at end-of-life since it provides complex symptom management, education, and support, which can then help to avoid often unnecessary and expensive hospitalizations. Yet policymakers have little information or quality benchmarks about the delivery of end-of-life homecare nursing.

Research has shown that the use and intensity of end-of-life homecare nursing is strongly associated with a home death [6], and reduced hospitalizations near death [7]. Moreover, several studies have demonstrated that early initiation of palliative and end-of-life care in cancer patients has benefits, such as reduced symptoms, improved quality of life, and even longer survival [8–10]. Earlier initiation and more intensity of end-of-life homecare nursing specifically, has also been associated with reduced hospitalizations and hospital deaths [7, 11, 12]. Yet despite the growing evidence of the benefits of early initiation of end-of-life care by homecare nurses, little

* Correspondence:
[1]Department of Health Research Methods, Evidence, and Impact, McMaster University, Hamilton, ON, Canada
[2]Institute for Clinical Evaluative Sciences, Toronto, ON, Canada
Full list of author information is available at the end of the article

research describes the timing in when such care is initiated. This hinders health system planners from understanding regional variation in end-of-life home care access. Furthermore, there are no established benchmarks to compare or target against.

The purpose of this study is three-fold: i) to describe the regional variation in the mean time to first end-of-life homecare visit starting from 6 months before death among health regions across British Columbia (BC), Nova Scotia (NS), and Ontario (ON); ii) establish the three-province average with confidence limits for this outcome; and iii) determine a national empiric benchmark based on the best regional performers. Ultimately these data can be used by Canadian policy makers to set achievable targets and improve end-of-life home care access. The methods can be applied by other countries to determine their own benchmarks.

Methods

Study design

We conducted a retrospective cohort study of cancer decedents who received homecare nursing in the Canadian provinces of ON, NS and BC, which contain a total of 28 health regions. Our inclusion criteria were adult decedents (19 years or older) with a valid provincial health insurance number, who had at least one record of homecare nursing following their cancer diagnosis and within 6 months of their date of death during the study period between April 1, 2004 and March 31, 2009. Due to a time lag in capturing cancer-confirmed cause of death in cancer registries, these were the most recent data available at the time of study inception.

Data sources

To derive our cohort, we used a unique encrypted patient identifier within each province to link with multiple administrative databases. Starting with a provincial cancer registry for cancer type, cancer diagnosis, and confirmed cause of death from cancer, we then linked with the: provincial homecare database for homecare nursing use with standard or end-of-life intent; Canadian Institute for Health Information's Discharge Abstract Database for Charlson-Deyo score for comorbidity; and the provincial health insurance databases for demographics of age at death, sex, and postal code for both region and income quintile [13–16]. Individual level data were not merged across provinces.

Outcome

Our main outcome was mean number of days to first end-of-life homecare nursing visit, starting from 6 months (182 days) before death. Homecare nursing intent is recorded in each provincial homecare database. Standard intent nursing is provided to patients with service goals ranging from providing "short-term care" with a predictable recovery (e.g., wound care) to "preserving the client's level of function and autonomy" with a prognosis of very gradual decline (e.g., early onset of frailty) [17]. Whereas end-of-life nursing intent is provided to patients classified as "not responsive to curative treatment and are dying," with service goals being "to alleviate distressing symptoms to achieve the best quality of life by providing complex support in the last stages of their illness," and a typical prognosis of an "expected death within six months" [17]. Given this standardized homecare eligibility criteria, we aligned our outcome definition to start from 6 months from death; thus, a shorter mean time would represent earlier initiation, and the outcome has a maximum of 182 days representing death date. At each week, the number of patients receiving standard or end-of-life homecare nursing was identified. After first end-of-life homecare nursing visit, all subsequent nursing visits were considered end-of-life. Nursing visits were measured as time (hours/day) in ON, as nursing visits received in BC, and as authorized in NS over a month.

Statistical analyses

Through the use of descriptive statistics, baseline characteristics of each population under study were compared by province. The outcome was compared across health regions through the use of a bar chart graph and a X^2 test with $P < .05$ considered as statistically significant. The benchmark mean for the outcome of interest was determined using the pared-mean method, which derives benchmarks from the top decile of performers [18]. Five criteria are included for this method of benchmark development: 1) the level of the benchmark signifies excellence, that is, it is always better than the mean; 2) the benchmark is achievable and realistic; 3) high performers should be selected from all performers in a pre-defined way; 4) all high performers should contribute to the benchmark; and 5) high performers with a low number of cases should not excessively impact the benchmark level (but should contribute).

In order to construct benchmark levels, health regions were first ranked according to descending order of performance. Starting with the best performing health region (i.e. shortest mean time), the eligible population sizes in each region were summed sequentially until the combined population size of this subset of regions was at least 10% of the combined size of all health regions. Combining the number of patients from these best-performing regions, the benchmark mean was calculated as the weighted average of the mean time to initiation of end-of-life nursing among the best performing regions.

A funnel plot was created for the outcome, controlling for age and sex. The funnel plot displays the number that received end-of-life homecare in each region on the horizontal axis and the corresponding mean days to initiation of end-of-life homecare nursing on the vertical axis (as seen by the dots). This funnel plot also illustrates the overall mean of the outcome across all regions (as seen by the thick black line) and the expected 95% and 99.8% CIs (as seen by the curved black lines) calculated based on normal distribution control limits [19]. The benchmark mean calculated above was overlaid on the funnel plot, as indicated by the red line. Statistical analyses were performed using SAS 9.3 (SAS Institute, Cary, North Carolina, USA), R 3.0.1, and Microsoft Excel 2010.

Results

The study identified 85,339 cancer decedents who used any homecare nursing in the last 6 months of life, of which 61,903 of those used end-of-life care nursing (73%) to form our final cohort: 28% were from BC, 65% from ON, and 7% from NS. Table 1 shows the size and demographic information for the 28 regions examined in the three provinces. The average age was 71 years old, 48% were female, and approximately 20% had a comorbidity other than cancer.

Figure 1 displays the unadjusted mean number of days to initial end-of-life homecare visit (starting from 6 months before death) by the 28 regions, color-coded by province (shorter number of days to initiation equates to earlier access to end-of-life care). Large regional variations were observed. The longest mean time, 97 days, (ON- Mississauga Halton) is nearly twice as long as the shortest, 55 days (BC- Vancouver Coastal, and NS-South West). The majority of ON regions have the longest mean time to initial visit. BC and NS had the first and second shortest times, respectively.

Table 1 Cohort demographics

Province - Region #	Any Homecare Nursing Cohort, n	End-of-Life Homecare Nursing Sub-cohort, n (% of any nursing)	Median Age (IQR)	Female (%)	Wealthiest Income Quintile (%)	Deyo-Charlson Index of 1 or greater (%)
BC - 2	7104	6447 (91%)	71 (61–79)	48%	17%	14%
BC - 4	5902	5328 (90%)	73 (63–81)	47%	21%	13%
BC - 3	4225	3663 (87%)	72 (62–80)	49%	24%	14%
BC - 5	1242	1061 (85%)	68 (59–76)	44%	20%	20%
BC - 1	1021	878 (86%)	72 (64–80)	44%	12%	16%
NS - 9	1891	1633 (86%)	71 (61–80)	45%	20%	14%
NS - 8	824	701 (85%)	71 (62–80)	48%	14%	28%
NS - 3	478	406 (85%)	73 (64–81)	47%	15%	16%
NS - 4	450	375 (83%)	72 (62–80)	48%	18%	16%
NS - 2	412	372 (90%)	71 (62–81)	43%	12%	19%
NS - 1	377	315 (84%)	73 (62-(81)	47%	29%	11%
NS - 6	337	321 (95%)	73 (63–81)	42%	17%	22%
NS - 7	246	193 (78%)	76 (62–84)	45%	19%	23%
NS - 5	238	179 (75%)	71 (62–79)	48%	13%	21%
ON - 4	8256	5742 (70%)	71 (60–79)	48%	17%	18%
ON -9	6883	4696 (68%)	70 (60–80)	49%	15%	18%
ON - 11	6048	4487 (74%)	70 (62–78)	49%	22%	16%
ON - 8	5811	3885 (67%)	71 (60–80)	48%	21%	18%
ON - 7	4557	3307 (73%)	71 (59–79)	51%	30%	18%
ON - 2	5382	2710 (50%)	70 (60–78)	48%	18%	16%
ON - 3	3227	2565 (79%)	71 (60–78)	48%	21%	16%
ON - 1	3969	2552 (64%)	70 (64–79)	48%	18%	19%
ON - 6	3762	2459 (65%)	70 (59–77)	49%	29%	16%
ON - 13	3534	2121 (60%)	70 (62–79)	46%	13%	22%
ON - 10	3184	1846 (58%)	71 (60–78)	45%	15%	16%
ON - 12	2692	1752 (65%)	72 (60–78)	46%	24%	19%
ON - 5	2287	1302 (57%)	69 (61–79)	48%	12%	17%
ON - 14	1000	607 (61%)	70 (61–77)	46%	17%	23%

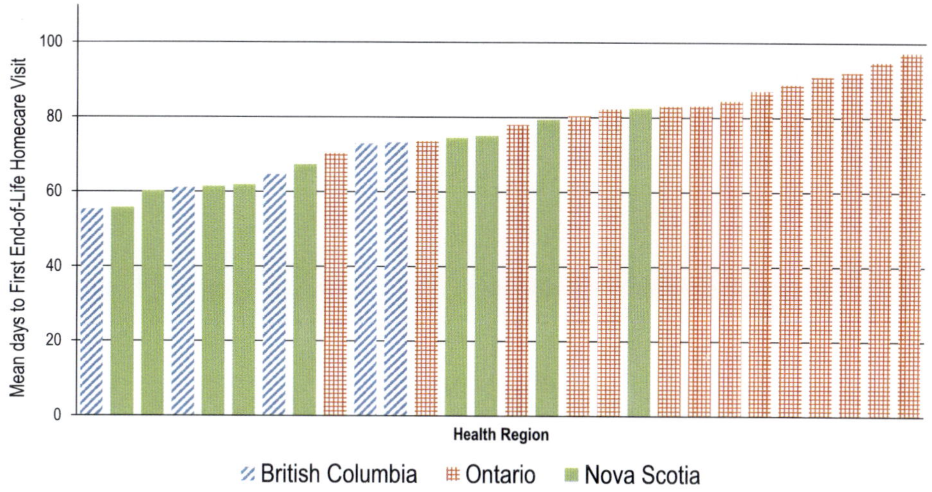

Fig. 1 Regional variation of mean days from 6 months prior to death to first end-of-life homecare visit

Figure 2 displays a funnel plot for the mean days to initial end-of-life homecare nursing visit, from 6 months before death, across the 28 regions controlling for age, sex, and region size. The funnel plot includes the following information: 1) the overall mean (straight black line), 2) the expected 95% Confidence Intervals (narrows as the number that received end-of-life care in each region increases), 3) the benchmark mean (straight red line), and 4) the mean of each region (dots, color-coded according to province). The overall three-province outcome average was 76 days after the six-month point (i.e. 106 days or 3.5 months before death). The empiric benchmark value based on best-performing regions was 57 days after the six-month point (i.e. 125 days or 4. 2 months before death). The best-performing regions belong to BC and NS. Most regions of ON are worse than the benchmark and overall mean. This contrasts with most regions of NS and BC, which are better than the overall mean. Regions with both small and large population sizes performed worse than the benchmark and worse than the overall indicator mean. Similarly, there were large and small regions at or near the benchmark.

Discussion

This population-based, end-of-life cancer study displays variations in timing of end-of-life homecare nursing among 28 regions across three Canadian provinces (BC, NS, ON). While past research has demonstrated the important benefits of early end-of-life homecare, this is the first study that compares the time to initiation of end-

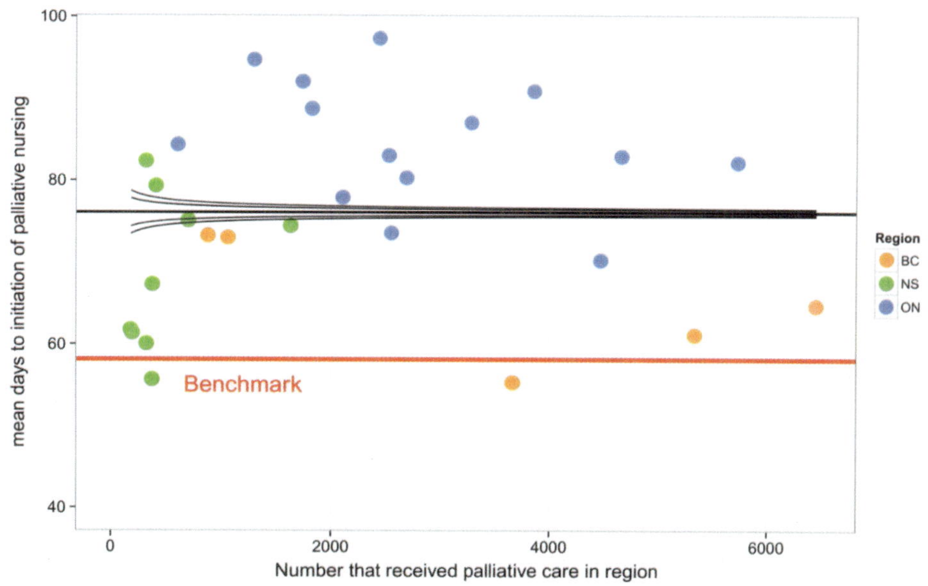

Fig. 2 Funnel plot of mean days to initial end-of-life homecare nursing visit by region

of-life homecare visits and establishes an empiric benchmark: 57 days after the six-month point (i.e. 125 days or 4.2 months before death). We found a nearly two-fold difference in the timing of when end-of-life homecare nursing was initiated among select regions. Starting from 6 months before death, BC generally has regions with the shortest times to initiation and ON has regions with the longest times to initiation (i.e. initiated closest to death) of end-of-life homecare. Ultimately this information is useful for health system planners aiming to monitor health system performance and improve policies related to end-of-life homecare access.

Prior cancer-based randomized controlled trials demonstrating the benefits of early palliative care (i.e. at late-stage diagnosis [9] or 8–12 weeks from diagnosis [8]) were conducted in hospital-based programs: Intervention patients received early palliative care and survived for a median of 11.6 months [9] and 14 months [8], respectively. In comparison, our patients received home-based end-of-life care for a far shorter period, ranging from 125 to 83 days before death. The variation in timing may reflect the differences between palliative approach to care versus end-of-life care and/or the differences between implementing a resource-intensive home-nursing program versus a hospital program.

Past research has also used similar benchmark methods to establish quality indicators for end-of-life cancer care, such as Emergency Department visits, physician visits, Intensive Care Unit admissions, and deaths in hospital [20]. This study extends those indicators by establishing "time to initiation of end-of-life homecare nursing" as an additional quality indicator, and is related to early initiation of supportive care rather than over-aggressive acute care. In prior research, BC was identified as having the lowest hospital death rate; our study corroborates this trend as the BC regions had among the shortest mean times to first end-of-life homecare nursing. Further research is required to understand differences in provincial policies that may explain variation. Other countries could apply these methods to determine their own regional variation and benchmarks and compare against Canadian rates.

The presentation of benchmark data using a funnel plot allows health system planners to observe their performance among regions of similar, smaller, or larger sizes. It is worth noting that the two regions better than the benchmark mean are very different in size ($n = 372$ and $n = 3663$), suggesting that region size is not necessarily the most important factor in early initiation of end-of-life homecare nursing. In fact, several small, medium, and large sized regions are near the benchmark. Another advantage of this approach is that often times, benchmark values are set by larger regions or based on crude unadjusted rates. As such smaller regions find it difficult to compare themselves to larger regions. Using this approach, other regions near to or worse than the overall mean can identify a realistic comparator mean, such as a region of similar size. As a result, this supports quality improvement by setting realistic targets that regions and/or provinces can aim to achieve and may help to reduce overall variation, particularly when using recent data and monitoring over time. Moreover, health system planners can compare against better performing regions and identify what policies they have that facilitate improved access.

This study is limited by including only cancer decedents in the analysis. Using a population-based decedent cohort prevents us from examining if and when individual patients ought to have received end-of-life home care nursing [21]. However, using retrospective decedent cohorts have been shown to be an efficient way to monitor performance at a population level [22], particularly as palliative care continues to be advocated earlier in the disease trajectory [9]. The quality of end-of-life homecare nursing is not described in administrative data. Additionally, we are unable to take other factors into account that may play a role in our results. For instance, patient preferences, level of need, refusal of services, or level of caregiver support or burnout are not available in our databases. As a result, we are not able to determine appropriateness of timing at an individual-level (more clinically relevant at a patient level), but rather we can only look at variation in timing at regional population level (more relevant for health system policy planner level). Further research should explore timing of homecare services based on comprehensive patient-level factors. Strengths of the study include using a population-based cohort from three provinces, comprising approximately 54% of the population in Canada. Hence, the results possess high external validity, which likely can be generalized to the entire Canadian population. Computing benchmark values through the use of real-world data gives insight into what is required for a practical and realistic target goal. Furthermore, the methods to explore regional variation and determine benchmarks would be relevant to other countries, particularly those with publicly-funded home care systems, though the actual benchmark values might differ.

Conclusions

In conclusion, we identified regional variation and empiric benchmarks for time to initiation of end-of-life homecare nursing using administrative health care data from three provinces. Identifying a benchmark using the best-performing regions is a beginning step. Understanding the reasons for variation, particularly provincial variation, could enable more equitable care. Exploring health system processes within best-performing regions could provide insights for other regions trying to initiate homecare services earlier. Ongoing surveillance efforts are essential to enable timely and realistic targets. National-level data sharing arrangements will allow more rapid access to regional and provincial comparisons and system performance measures.

Abbreviations

BC: British Columbia; NS: Nova Scotia; ON: Ontario

Acknowledgements

The authors would like to acknowledge the following people for their feedback during the preparation of this manuscript: Reka Pataky, Erin O'Leary, Ying Liu, and Konrad Fassbender.

Funding

This study was funded by the Canadian Cancer Society Research Institute (grant number 700689) and also supported by the Canadian Partnership Against Cancer's Applied Research in Cancer Control (grant number 019789). This study used databases maintained by the Institute for Clinical Evaluative Sciences, which receives funding from the ON Ministry of Health and Long Term Care. The British Columbia Cancer Agency and the BC Ministry of Health approved access to and use of the data facilitated by Population Data BC for this study. Portions of the data used in this report were made available by the NS Department of Health and Wellness and the Population Health Research Unit (now known as Health Data NS) of Dalhousie University. The opinions, results, and conclusions reported in this paper are those of the authors and are independent from the funding and data providing sources.

Authors' contributions

HS and LB designed the study and were responsible for the acquisition of data. HS, LB, and RS conducted the statistical analysis of the data, with all authors making important contributions to its interpretation. HS and DQ drafted the initial manuscript. LB, KM, BL, FB, and RS critically revised each draft of the manuscript and made significant contributions to its intellectual content. HS and DQ reviewed and approved the final draft of the manuscript. All authors read and approved the final manuscript.

Competing interests

The authors declare that they have no competing interests.

Author details

[1]Department of Health Research Methods, Evidence, and Impact, McMaster University, Hamilton, ON, Canada. [2]Institute for Clinical Evaluative Sciences, Toronto, ON, Canada. [3]University of Toronto, Toronto, ON, Canada. [4]University of British Columbia, Vancouver, BC, Canada. [5]Department of Family Medicine, Dalhousie University, Halifax, NS, Canada. [6]Department of Oncology, McMaster University, Hamilton, ON, Canada.

References

1. Brazil K, Howell D, Bedard M, Krueger P, Heidebrecht C. Preferences for place of care and place of death among informal caregivers of the terminally ill. Palliat Med. 2005;19(6):492–9.
2. Quality End-of-Life Care Coalition of Canada. Hospice Palliative Home Care in Canada: A Progress Report. Ottawa: Quality End-of-Life Care Coalition of Canada; 2008.
3. Kelley AS, Deb P, Du Q, Carlson MDA, Morrison RS. Hospice enrollment saves money for Medicare and improves care quality across a number of different lengths-of-stay. Health Aff. 2013;32(3):552–61.
4. Kerr CW, Donohue KA, Tangeman JC, Serehali AM, Knodel SM, Grant PC, Luczkiewicz DL, Mylotte K, Marien MJ. Cost savings and enhanced hospice enrollment with a home-based palliative care program implemented as a hospice–private payer partnership. J Palliat Med. 2014;17(12):1328–35.
5. Taylor DH, Ostermann J, Van Houtven CH, Tulsky JA, Steinhauser K. What length of hospice use maximizes reduction in medical expenditures near death in the US Medicare program? Soc Sci Med. 2007;65(7):1466–78.
6. Gomes B, Higginson IJ. Factors influencing death at home in terminally ill patients with cancer: systematic review. BMJ. 2006;332(7540):515–21.
7. Seow H, Barbera L, Howell D, Dy SM. Using more end-of-life homecare services is associated with using fewer acute care services: a population-based cohort study. Med Care. 2010;48(2):118–24.
8. Bakitas MA, Tosteson TD, Li Z, Lyons KD, Hull JG, Li Z, Dionne-Odom JN, Frost J, Dragnev KH, Hegel MT. Early versus delayed initiation of concurrent palliative oncology care: patient outcomes in the ENABLE III randomized controlled trial. J Clin Oncol. 2015;33(13):1438–45.
9. Temel JS, Greer JA, Muzikansky A, Gallagher ER, Admane S, Jackson VA, Dahlin CM, Blinderman CD, Jacobsen J, Pirl WF. Early palliative care for patients with metastatic non–small-cell lung cancer. N Engl J Med. 2010; 363(8):733–42.
10. Zimmermann C, Swami N, Krzyzanowska M, Hannon B, Leighl N, Oza A, Moore M, Rydall A, Rodin G, Tannock I. Early palliative care for patients with advanced cancer: a cluster-randomised controlled trial. Lancet. 2014; 383(9930):1721–30.
11. Chitnis X, Georghiou T, Steventon A, Bardsley M. Effect of a home-based end-of-life nursing service on hospital use at the end of life and place of death: a study using administrative data and matched controls. BMJ Support Palliat Care. 2013;3(4):422–30.
12. Seow H, Sutradhar R, McGrail K, Fassbender K, Pataky R, Lawson B, Sussman J, Burge F, Barbera L. End-of-life cancer care: temporal association between homecare nursing and hospitalizations. J Palliat Med. 2016;19(3):263–70.
13. Statistics Canada. Annual demographic estimates: Subprovincial areas 2005 to 2010. Ottawa: Statistics Canada; 2011. pp. 91–214.
14. British Columbia Ministry of Health. Home and Community Care (Continuing Care). Victoria: Ministry of Health; 2012.
15. Deyo RA, Cherkin DC, Ciol MA. Adapting a clinical comorbidity index for use with ICD-9-CM administrative databases. J Clin Epidemiol. 1992;45(6):613–9.
16. Wilkins R. PCCF+ version 3J User's guide (Geocodes/PCCF). Automated geographic coding based on the statistics Canada postal code conversion files, including postal codes to May 2002. Ottawa: Health Analysis and Measurement Group, Statistics Canada; 2002.
17. Canadian Institute for Health Information (CIHI). Development of National Indicators and Reports for Home Care: Phase 2 Indicator Descriptions. Ottawa: CIHI; 2002.
18. Kiefe CI, Weissman NW, Allison JJ, Farmer R, Weaver M, Williams OD. Methodology matters-XII. Identifying achievable benchmarks of care: concepts and methodology. Int J Qual Health Care. 1998;10(5):443–7.
19. Dover DC, Schopflocher DP. Using funnel plots in public health surveillance. Popul Health Metrics. 2011;9(1):58.
20. Barbera L, Seow H, Sutradhar R, Chu A, Burge F, Fassbender K, McGrail K, Lawson B, Liu Y, Pataky R. Quality indicators of end-of-life care in patients with cancer: what rate is right? J Oncol Pract. 2015;11(3):e279-e287.
21. Bach PB, Schrag D, Begg CB. Resurrecting treatment histories of dead patients: a study design that should be laid to rest. JAMA. 2004;292(22): 2765–70.
22. Earle CC, Ayanian JZ. Looking back from death: the value of retrospective studies of end-of-life care. J Clin Oncol. 2006;24(6):838–40.

Permissions

All chapters in this book were first published in PC, by BioMed Central; hereby published with permission under the Creative Commons Attribution License or equivalent. Every chapter published in this book has been scrutinized by our experts. Their significance has been extensively debated. The topics covered herein carry significant findings which will fuel the growth of the discipline. They may even be implemented as practical applications or may be referred to as a beginning point for another development.

The contributors of this book come from diverse backgrounds, making this book a truly international effort. This book will bring forth new frontiers with its revolutionizing research information and detailed analysis of the nascent developments around the world.

We would like to thank all the contributing authors for lending their expertise to make the book truly unique. They have played a crucial role in the development of this book. Without their invaluable contributions this book wouldn't have been possible. They have made vital efforts to compile up to date information on the varied aspects of this subject to make this book a valuable addition to the collection of many professionals and students.

This book was conceptualized with the vision of imparting up-to-date information and advanced data in this field. To ensure the same, a matchless editorial board was set up. Every individual on the board went through rigorous rounds of assessment to prove their worth. After which they invested a large part of their time researching and compiling the most relevant data for our readers.

The editorial board has been involved in producing this book since its inception. They have spent rigorous hours researching and exploring the diverse topics which have resulted in the successful publishing of this book. They have passed on their knowledge of decades through this book. To expedite this challenging task, the publisher supported the team at every step. A small team of assistant editors was also appointed to further simplify the editing procedure and attain best results for the readers.

Apart from the editorial board, the designing team has also invested a significant amount of their time in understanding the subject and creating the most relevant covers. They scrutinized every image to scout for the most suitable representation of the subject and create an appropriate cover for the book.

The publishing team has been an ardent support to the editorial, designing and production team. Their endless efforts to recruit the best for this project, has resulted in the accomplishment of this book. They are a veteran in the field of academics and their pool of knowledge is as vast as their experience in printing. Their expertise and guidance has proved useful at every step. Their uncompromising quality standards have made this book an exceptional effort. Their encouragement from time to time has been an inspiration for everyone.

The publisher and the editorial board hope that this book will prove to be a valuable piece of knowledge for researchers, students, practitioners and scholars across the globe.

List of Contributors

Ashleigh E. Butler and Helen Hall
The Louis Dundas Centre for Children's Palliative Care, University College London Great Ormond Street Institute of Child Health, London, UK
School of Nursing and Midwifery, Monash University, Melbourne, Australia

Beverley Copnell
School of Nursing and Midwifery, La Trobe University, Melbourne, Australia

Lisa Hjelmfors, Maria Friedrichsen and Tiny Jaarsma
Department of Social and Welfare Studies (ISV), Faculty of Health Sciences, Linköping University, 581 83 Linköping, Sweden

Anna Strömberg
Department of Medical and Health Sciences, Division of nursing, Faculty of Health Sciences, Linköping University, Linköping, Sweden
Department of Cardiology, Linköping University, Linköping, Sweden

Anna Sandgren
Department of Health and Caring Sciences, Center for Collaborative Palliative Care, Linnaeus University, Växjö, Sweden

Jan Mårtensson
Department of Nursing, School of Health Sciences, Jönköping University, Jönköping, Sweden

Camilla Kjellstadli and Steinar Hunskaar
Research Group for General Practice, Department of Global Public Health and Primary Care, University of Bergen, PO box 7804, N-5018 Bergen, Norway

Camilla Kjellstadli and Bettina Sandgathe Husebø
Centre for Elderly and Nursing Home Medicine, Department of Global Public Health and Primary Care, University of Bergen, N-5018 Bergen, Norway

Bettina Sandgathe Husebø
Bergen Municipality, Bergen, Norway

Hogne Sandvik and Steinar Hunskaar
National Centre for Emergency Primary Health Care, Uni Research Health, Kalfarveien 31, N-5018 Bergen, Norway

Elisabeth Flo
Department of Clinical Psychology, University of Bergen, N-5018 Bergen, Norway

Claire Poulalhon, Anne Fagot-Campagna and Philippe Tuppin
National sickness insurance fund, 26-50, avenue du Professeur André Lemierre, 75986 Paris cedex 20, France

Laureen Rotelli-Bihet
National Palliative care and end of life center, 75020 Paris, France

Sébastien Moine
Health Education and Practices Laboratory, Paris XIII University EA 3412, 93017 Bobigny cedex, France

Régis Aubry
Pain and palliative Care Department, Teaching Hospital, 25030, Besançon, France

Takashi Takeuchi
Section of Psychiatry and Behavioral Sciences, Graduate School of Medical and Dental Sciences, Tokyo Medical and Dental University, 1-5-45 Yushima, Bunkyo-ku, Tokyo 113-8519, Japan

Kanako Ichikura, Kanako Amano and Wakana Takeshita
Section of Liaison Psychiatry and Palliative Medicine, Graduate School of Medical and Dental Sciences, Tokyo Medical and Dental University, Tokyo, Japan

Wakana Takeshita
Graduate School of Human Sciences, Waseda University, Saitama, Japan

Kazuho Hisamura
Department of Medical Oncology, Kanazawa Medical University, Ishikawa, Japan

Kanako Ichikura
Department of Health Science, School of Allied Health Sciences, Kitasato University, Kanagawa, Japan

F. Weijers, C. Veldhoven, C. Verhagen, K. Vissers and Y. Engels
Department of Anesthesiology, Pain and Palliative Medicine, Radboud university medical center, Postbox 9101, internal code 549, 6500, HB, Nijmegen, the Netherlands

Emma Kirby, Katherine Kenny, Alex Broom and Holi Birman
Practical Justice Initiative, Faculty of Arts and Social Sciences, University of New South Wales, Level 3 Goodsell Building, University of New South Wales, Sydney, NSW 2052, Australia

Zarnie Lwin
Royal Brisbane and Women's Hospital, Brisbane, QLD, Australia

Zarnie Lwin and Phillip Good
University of Queensland, Brisbane, QLD, Australia

Phillip Good
St Vincent's Private Hospital Brisbane, Brisbane, QLD, Australia
Mater Health Services Brisbane, Brisbane, QLD, Australia

Inge Spronk, François G. Schellevis, Liesbeth M. van Vliet and Joke C. Korevaar
NIVEL (Netherlands Institute for Health Services Research), 3500BN Utrecht, The Netherlands

Jako S. Burgers
Dutch College of General Practitioners, Utrecht, The Netherlands. School CAPHRI, Department Family Medicine, Maastricht University, Maastricht, The Netherlands

François G. Schellevis
Department of General Practice & Elderly Care Medicine/ Amsterdam Public Health Research Institute, VU University Medical Center, Amsterdam, The Netherlands

Reetta P. Piili, Juho T. Lehto, Pirkko-Liisa I. Kellokumpu-Lehtinen
Faculty of Medicine and Life Sciences, University of Tampere, Tampere, Finland

Reetta P. Piili, Juho T. Lehto and Kellokumpu-Lehtinen Department of Oncology, Tampere University Hospital, Tampere, Finland

Reetta P. Piili
Department of Oncology, Tampere University Hospital, Palliative Care Unit, Teiskontie 35, R-building, 33520 Tampere, Finland

Tiina Luukkaala
Research and Innovation Center, Tampere University Hospital, Tampere, Finland
Health Sciences, Faculty of Social Sciences, University of Tampere, Tampere, Finland

Heikki Hinkka
Rehabilitation Center Apila, Kangasala, Finland

Marie Friedel, Jean-Marie Degryse and Isabelle Aujoulat
Institute of Health and Society- Institut de recherche Santé et Société (IRSS), Université catholique de Louvain, 30, Clos Chapelle-aux-Champs, Boite 1.30.13, B-1200 Brussels, Belgium

Marie Friedel
Haute Ecole Vinci, Institut Parnasse-ISEI, 41, Clos Chapelle-aux-Champs, 1200 Brussels, Belgium

Bénédicte Brichard
Cliniques universitaires St-Luc, 10, av Hippocrate, 1200 Brussels, Belgium

Christine Fonteyne
Hôpital universitaire des enfants Reine Fabiola, Equipe de liaison pédiatrique, 15, av. JJ Crocq, 1020 Brussels, Belgium

Marleen Renard
5Universitair Ziekenhuis Leuven, Department of Paediatric Hemato-Oncology, Kites-Team (Kinderen In Thuis En Supportieve zorgteam), Herestraat, 49, 3000 Leuven, Belgium

Jean-Paul Misson
Centre hospitalier régional de la Citadelle, 1, Bd du 12ème de Ligne, 4000 Liège, Belgium

Els Vandecruys
Universitair Ziekenhuis Gent, KOESTER - liaisonequipe Kinderziekenhuis Prinses Elisabeth, C. Heymanslaan, 9000 Ghent, Belgium

Els Vandecruys
Cliniques universitaires st Luc, Interface pédiatrique, 10, av Hippocrate, 1200 Brussels, Belgium

Katrien Moens
Scientific Institute of Public Health (ISP-WIV), 14, rue J. Wytsman, 1050 Brussels, Belgium

Jean-Marie Degryse
Katholieke Universiteit Leuven, Oude Markt 13, 3000 Leuven, Belgium

Anke J E de Veer, Renate Verkaik and Anneke L Francke
Netherlands Institute for Health Services Research (Nivel), 3500, BN, Utrecht, The Netherlands

Barbara Stringer
Center for Consultation and Expertise, Gouda, The Netherlands

Berno van Meijel
Inholland University of Applied Sciences, Amsterdam, The Netherlands
University Medical Center, VU, Department of Psychiatry, Amsterdam Public Health Research Institute, Amsterdam, The Netherlands
Parnassia Psychiatric Institute, The Hague, The Netherlands
GGZ-VS, Academy for Masters in Advanced Nursing Practice, Amsterdam, The Netherlands

Anneke L Francke
University Medical Center, VU, Department of Public and Occupational Health, Amsterdam Public Health Research Institute, Amsterdam, The Netherlands
Expertise Center for Palliative care, Amsterdam, The Netherlands

Britt Viola Danielsen and Anne Marit Sand
Department of Health and Caring Sciences, Faculty of Health and Social Sciences, Western Norway University of Applied Sciences, N-5020 Bergen, Norway

Jan Henrik Rosland
Department of Clinical Medicine, University of Bergen, Bergen, Norway
Sunniva Centre for Palliative Care, Haraldsplass Deaconess Hospital Bergen, Bergen, Norway

Oddvar Førland
Centre for Care Research - Western Norway, Western Norway University of Applied Sciences, Bergen, Norway
Faculty of Health Studies, VID Specialized University, Bergen, Norway

Sandra Stephanie Mai, Swantje Goebel and Martin Weber
Interdisciplinary Palliative Care Unit, III. Department of Medicine, University Medical Center of the Johannes Gutenberg University of Mainz, Mainz, Germany

Elisabeth Jentschke and Birgitt van Oorschot
Interdisciplinary Center for Palliative Medicine, University Hospital Würzburg, Würzburg, Germany

Karl-Heinz Renner
Department of Psychology, Bundeswehr University Munich, Neubiberg, Germany

Marianne Heins, Jolien Hofstede, Mieke Rijken, Joke Korevaar, Gé Donker and Anneke Francke
Netherlands Institute for Health Services Research (NIVEL), 3500 BN Utrecht, The Netherlands

Anneke Francke
Amsterdam Public Health research institute, VU University Medical Center, Amsterdam, the Netherlands
Expertise center palliative care, VU University Medical Center, Amsterdam, the Netherlands

Ilaria Massa, Oriana Nanni and Flavia Foca
Unit of Biostatistics and Clinical Trials, Istituto Scientifico Romagnolo per lo Studio e la Cura dei Tumori (IRST) IRCCS, Meldola, Italy

Marco Maltoni and Elisabetta Sansoni
Palliative Care Unit, Istituto Scientifico Romagnolo per lo Studio e la Cura dei Tumori (IRST) IRCCS, Meldola, Italy

Stefania Derni
Palliative Care Unit, AUSL Romagna, Forlì, Italy

Nicola Gentili
IT Unit, Istituto Scientifico Romagnolo per lo Studio e la Cura dei Tumori (IRST) IRCCS, Meldola, Italy

Giovanni Luca Frassineti, Andrea Casadei Gardini, Martina Valgiusti and Dino Amadori
Department of Medical Oncology, Istituto Scientifico Romagnolo per lo Studio e la Cura dei Tumori (IRST) IRCCS, Meldola, Italy

Elena Prati and Mattia Altini
Healthcare Administration, Istituto Scientifico Romagnolo per lo Studio e la Cura dei Tumori (IRST) IRCCS, Meldola, Italy

Davide Gallegati
Planning and Control, Istituto Scientifico Romagnolo per lo Studio e la Cura dei Tumori (IRST) IRCCS, Meldola, Italy

Jason Mills
Institute of Health and Biomedical Innovation, Queensland University of Technology, Kelvin Grove, QLD, Australia

Jason Mills, Timothy Wand and Jennifer A. Fraser
Susan Wakil School of Nursing and Midwifery, The University of Sydney, Camperdown, NSW, Australia

Jason Mills
School of Nursing, Faculty of Health, Queensland University of Technology, Kelvin Grove, QLD 4061, Australia

Naoki Sakakibara and Takahiro Higashi
Division of Health Services Research, Center for Cancer Control and Information Services, National Cancer Center, 5-1-1 Tsukiji, Chuo-ku, Tokyo 104-0045, Japan

Naoki Sakakibara
Department of Palliative Care, St. Luke's International Hospital, 9-1 Akashicho, Chuo-ku, Tokyo 104-8560, Japan

Itsuku Yamashita
Department of Palliative Care, Aomori Prefectural Central Hospital, 2-1-1 Higashitsukurimichi, Aomori City, Aomori 030-8553, Japan

Tetsusuke Yoshimoto
Department of Palliative and Supportive Care, Chukyo Hospital, 1-1-10 Sanjo, Minami-ku, Nagoya City, Aichi 457-8510, Japan

Motohiro Matoba
Department of Palliative Care, Japan Red Cross Medical Center, 4-1-22 Hiroo, Shibuya-ku, Tokyo 150-0012, Japan

Joseph M. Sawyer and Florence N. Todd Fordham
Marie Curie Palliative Care Research Department, UCL, 6th Floor, Wing B, Maple House, 149 Tottenham Court Road, London W1T 7NF, UK

Rahul Asgr
Society for Community Health Awareness Research and Action, Public Health, Bengaluru, Karnataka, India

John D. H. Porter
Departments of Clinical Research and Global Health and Development, London School of Hygiene and Tropical Medicine, Keppel Street, London WC1E 7HT, UK

Sheng-Yu Fan
Institute of Gerontology, College of Medicine, National Cheng Kung University, Tainan, Taiwan

Ying-Wei Wang
Department of Family Medicine, Buddhist Tzu Chi General Hospital, Hualien, Taiwan

I-Mei Lin
Department of Psychology, College of Humanities and Social Sciences, Kaohsiung Medical University, Kaohsiung, Taiwan

Dorthe Gaby
Emergency Department, Copenhagen University Hospital, Nordsjælland, Dyrehavevej 29, 3400 Hillerød, Denmark

Dorthe Gaby Bove, Marie Lavesen and Maria Omel Jellington
Department of Pulmonary & Infectious Diseases, Copenhagen University Hospital, Nordsjælland, Dyrehavevej 29, 3400 Hillerød, Denmark

Kristoffer Bastrup-Madsen Marsaa
Department of Palliative Medicine, Copenhagen University Hospital, Herlev and Gentofte Hospital, Herlev Ringvej 75, 2730 Herlev, Denmark

Suzanne Forsyth Herling
Neuroscience Centre, Copenhagen University Hospital, Rigshospitalet, Section 2091, Inge Lehmanns Vej 7, 2100 Copenhagen Ø, Denmark

Xiao Bin Lai
School of Nursing, Fudan University, Shanghai, China

Frances Kam Yuet Wong and Shirley Siu Yin Ching
School of Nursing, The Hong Kong Polytechnic University, Hung Hom, Hong Kong

Lucas Pieper, Julia Wager and Boris Zernikow
Department of Children's Pain Therapy and Paediatric Palliative Care, Witten/Herdecke University, Faculty of Health - School of Medicine, Witten, Germany

Julia Wager and Boris Zernikow
Paediatric Palliative Care Centre, Children's and Adolescents' Hospital Datteln, Dr.-Friedrich-Steiner-Str.5, 45711 Datteln, Germany

S. Aebischer Perone and F. Chappuis
Division of Tropical and Humanitarian Medicine, Geneva University Hospitals, Rue Gabrielle-Perret-Gentil 6, 1205 Geneva, Switzerland

R. Nikolic and R. Lazic
Primary Health Care Center, Dom zdravja Doboj, Nemanjina 18, 74000 Doboj, Bosnia and Herzegovina

E. Dropic
Fondacija fami, Kralja Aleksandra 52, 74000 Doboj, Bosnia and Herzegovina

T. Vogel, B. Lab and S. Lachat
Division of Tropical and Humanitarian Medicine, Geneva University Hospitals, Avenue de Beau-Séjour 22, Geneva, Switzerland

P. Hudelson
Transcultural consultation and interpretation, Geneva University Hospitals, Rue Gabrielle-Perret-Gentil 4, 1211 Geneva 14, Switzerland

C. Matis and S. Pautex
Geriatrics and community palliative care unit, Geneva University Hospitals, Avenue Cardinal-Mermillod 36, 1227 Carouge, Switzerland

Natasha Smallwood and Louis Irving
Department of Respiratory and Sleep Medicine, The Royal Melbourne Hospital, Melbourne, VIC 3050, Australia

Natasha Smallwood
Department of Medicine (Royal Melbourne Hospital), University of Melbourne, Melbourne, VIC 3050, Australia

David Currow
IMPACCT - Improving Palliative, Aged and Chronic Care through Clinical Research and Translation, Faculty of Health, University of Technology Sydney,Ultimo, NSW, Australia

Sara Booth
University of Cambridge, Cambridge, UK

Anna Spathis
Cambridge University Hospitals NHS Foundation Trust, Cambridge, UK

Jennifer Philip
Palliative Medicine, St Vincent's Hospital and Victorian Comprehensive Cancer Centre, University of Melbourne, Melbourne, Australia
St Vincent's Hospital, Victoria Parade, Melbourne, VIC 3065, Australia

Hsien Seow and Danial Qureshi
Department of Health Research Methods, Evidence, and Impact, McMaster University, Hamilton, ON, Canada

Hsien Seow, Danial Qureshi, Lisa Barbera and Rinku Sutradhar
Institute for Clinical Evaluative Sciences, Toronto, ON, Canada

Lisa Barbera and Rinku Sutradhar
University of Toronto, Toronto, ON, Canada

Kim McGrail
University of British Columbia, Vancouver, BC, Canada

Beverley Lawson and Fred Burge
Department of Family Medicine, Dalhousie University, Halifax, NS, Canada

Hsien Seow
Department of Oncology, McMaster University, Hamilton, ON, Canada

Index

A

Acceptability, 10-12, 15-16, 72, 74, 95, 123-124, 130-131

Administrative Health Data, 31

Algorithm-based Method, 20

B

Bereavement Support, 6, 9, 89, 199

Brainstorming, 13-14

Breast Cancer, 46, 69-72, 74-76

C

Capricious Trajectory, 99, 102-103

Cardiac Resynchronisation Therapy, 12, 17-18

Cardiology, 13-14, 16-19, 197-200

Cardiopulmonary Resuscitation, 177, 181-183, 202, 224, 226

Chronic Pulmonary Disease, 21

Circulatory Disease, 23, 28-29

Colorectal Cancer, 46, 49, 135, 140-141, 144

Communication Strategies, 11, 67

Communication Tool, 13-15

Communication Training, 14

Confidence Intervals, 135, 142, 233

D

Decision Aids (DAS), 70

Decision Support, 70-71, 75-76

Decompensation, 10, 31

Diagnostic Tests, 77

Dignity Therapy, 123-124, 128-132

Dnr, 177-183

Doctor-patient Interaction, 59

E

Emotional Distress, 5, 7, 49

End-of-life Care, 1-2, 8, 10-19, 25, 29-30, 32, 40, 53, 60, 77, 83, 86-87, 91, 94-95, 97, 99, 108-109, 111, 121, 123, 131, 139, 167, 175, 183, 194-196, 200-203, 213, 219-220, 222, 224-230, 232-235

Epidemiology, 20, 29, 108, 144-145

Epilepsy, 34, 36-37

F

Feasibility, 10-12, 16-19, 76, 93, 96, 123-125, 131-132, 155

G

General Practitioner, 21, 39, 50, 56-57, 80-81, 83, 91, 110, 120, 138-139, 153, 185

Grade, 69-70, 72-76

H

Heart Failure (HF), 10

Hf Trajectory, 10-18

Home Deaths, 20-23, 25-29, 91, 94, 110-112, 118, 122

Hospital Palliative Care (HPC), 31

I

Illness Trajectory, 10, 99, 106, 206

Implantable Cardioverter Defibrillator, 13, 17, 19

Improve Communication, 10-11

Internal Consistency, 42, 44

Interpretive Description, 184-185, 192-193

K

Kawakita Method, 43-44

L

Life Support Care, 77

Life-threatening Diseases, 194-195, 201

Limited Efficacy, 10-12, 15-16

Logistic Regressions Models, 20

Long-term Diseases (LTD), 32

M

Mdr-tb, 166-167, 170-171, 173, 175

Multiple Sclerosis, 31, 34, 36-38, 197

Myopathy, 34, 36-37

N

Nasogastric Tube, 77, 79, 81-82, 93

Ncodr, 21, 29

Neoplasms, 70, 75, 133

O

Occupational Stressors, 147, 154

P

Paediatric Liaison Teams (PLTS), 88

Paediatric Palliative Care (PPC), 88

Pain Interference, 159-160, 162-164

Pain Management Index (PMI), 159

Palliative Care Units (PCU), 123-124

Palliative Chemotherapy, 72-73, 76, 140

Palliative Home Care, 57, 110, 118, 176, 206, 220, 235
Palliative Medicine, 43, 49-50, 57, 77-78, 80-81, 83, 85, 87, 108, 121, 131, 157-158, 192, 211, 222-225, 227, 229
Paraplegia, 34, 36-37
Parental Bereavement, 6
Parenteral Fluids, 77, 87
Parkinson's Disease, 34, 36-37, 197, 202
Picu, 2-3, 5, 7-8
Pleural Effusion, 78, 207-208
Psychiatric Care, 99
Psychiatric Disorders, 34-37, 106
Psychological Problems, 41, 189

Q
Qpl, 10, 12-18

R
Radiant, 50, 52-56
Regression Analysis, 23, 77, 82
Rehabilitation, 32, 34-35, 38-39, 85, 228
Respiratory Disease, 23, 35, 38, 170, 193, 211
Retrospective Analysis, 30, 40, 140-141

S
Shared Decision Making (SDM), 69
Short Life Expectancy, 100, 110-112, 114, 118

T
Teaching Methods, 13, 15
Terminal Diagnosis, 59, 62, 64-65
Therapeutic Benefits, 7
Transferability, 7, 157, 197
Tuberculosis (TB), 166

U
User Perspective, 10